MEDICAL ETHICS:
Sources of Catholic Teachings
THIRD EDITION

MEDICAL ETHICS:
Sources of Catholic Teachings
THIRD EDITION

Kevin D. O'Rourke, O.P., J.C.D., S.T.M.
Philip Boyle, Ph.D.

GEORGETOWN UNIVERSITY PRESS / WASHINGTON, D.C.

Imprimatur:

+Michael Sheridan
Auxiliary Bishop
Saint Louis
January 1999

Georgetown University Press, Washington, D.C. 20057-1079
© 1999 by Georgetown University Press. All rights reserved.
Printed in the United States of America
10 9 8 7 6 5 4 3 2 1   1999
THIS VOLUME IS PRINTED ON ACID-FREE OFFSET BOOK PAPER.

Library of Congress Cataloging-in-Publication Data

Medical ethics : sources of Catholic teaching / edited by Kevin D.
    O'Rourke, Philip Boyle.—3rd ed.
        p.   cm.
    Includes bibliographical references and index.
    ISBN 0-87840-722-7 (pbk.)
    1. Medical ethics. 2. Medicine—Religious aspects—Catholic
Church. 3. Christian ethics—Catholic authors. 4. Pastoral
medicine—Catholic Church. I. O'Rouke, Kevin D. II. Boyle,
Philip.
R725.56.075   1999
241'.642—dc21   98-44647
                                                   CIP

Contents

Contents

Contents _____

Preface

Catholic health care professionals frequently encounter serious ethical problems. These problems arise whether the professionals in question are working in Catholic health care facilities or in health care facilities sponsored by the state, community, or private corporations. When faced with a serious ethical problem, the sincere Catholic seeks to make a judgment of conscience enlightened by faith. When making such a judgment, many of the facts necessary for a valid decision will be drawn from the medical situation. For example, when faced with a decision whether or not to withdraw life-support equipment, the medical condition of the patient will be the most important factor. After discerning the medical facts, the key element of the decision of conscience concerning removal of life support will be the values of Catholic tradition which are expressed in the principles of medical ethics offered in the teachings of the Church. These principles of medical ethics are not preconceived solutions to the problems, but rather they are general statements drawn from faith and experience which must be applied to particular cases. They are a source of Christian wisdom drawn from the application of the teaching of Christ to human problems.

This book seeks to help Catholic health care professionals understand, internalize, and apply the principles of Catholic teaching to the many ethical issues they encounter in their research and practice. Insofar as possible, this collection of teachings will help Catholic health care professionals "give a reason to the faith that is in them" (1 Pt 4:15). The third edition of this book answers the request of many students and scholars but also is prompted by statements from recent encyclicals and magisterial statements such as *The Splendor of Truth*,[1] *The Gospel of Life*,[2] and the *Catechism of the Catholic Church*[3] promulgated by Pope John Paul II since the last edition.

The Catholic Church presents the substance of its moral teaching in the context of theological reasoning. While faith calls forth an assent of intellect and will on the part of Catholics to the substance of the teaching of the Church, theological reasoning helps one penetrate the meaning of the teaching and apply it more effectively. The Church, then, seeks to present more than a set of rules as it presents moral teachings. The depth and beauty offered by documents of the Church in opposition to a set of rules may be perceived if one reads the Encyclicals *On Human Life* of Pope Paul VI or *The Gospel of Life* of Pope John Paul II and compares it with Directive 19 of the *Ethical and Religious Directives* of 1971. While the encyclicals prohibit contraception, this teaching is presented in the context of the meaning of self-giving which occurs under grace in matrimony. Directive 19, on the other hand, simply expresses a rule prohibiting the use of any action "which as an end or as a means, (serves) to render procreation impossible" and does not offer reasons. Our experience leads us to believe that many health care professionals are acquainted with the

xiv *Ethical and Religious Directives* of the Church (p. 128) but only in regard to particular negative prohibitions. For example, most health care professionals, whether Catholic or not, are aware that Catholic teaching prohibits contraceptive sterilization and direct abortion. Some are even aware that the Church declares artificial reproduction to be morally flawed. However, only a few health care professionals are acquainted with the theological reasons which support the teachings of the Church. As a result, many health care professionals have a well-developed knowledge of science or medicine, but have an underdeveloped understanding of the teachings of the Church. Our hope is that this collection of teachings will help health care professionals increase their understanding of Catholic ethical principles so that it parallels their professional knowledge and acumen.

In order to put this collection of Church teachings in proper perspective, there are two introductory chapters. The first chapter presents the general teachings of the Church about the human person and explains how the concept of the human person and human action relates to the various issues of medical ethics. While the references to Sacred Scripture in this section are not intended to be conclusive proof texts, they do provide some indication of faith commitment for the statements of the Church Magisterium.

The second chapter concerns formation of conscience. In contemporary society, there are many erroneous thoughts about the source of ethical norms and the methods of conscience formation. Moreover, many Catholics believe that the teachings of the Church are to be apprehended as "over and against" their own consciences. Thus, they believe they are to form their own consciences before consulting the teachings of the Church. Briefly, we try to describe the erroneous systems of forming ethical decisions, state why these systems are inadequate, and describe the role that the teachings of the Church play in the formation of conscience for sincere Catholics. Finally, in this second chapter we seek to emphasize the fact that decisions of conscience are always about particular actions which involve particular facts and judgments. Thus, the teachings of the Church are never to be considered as preconceived solutions to serious problems. Rather, they are general statements, reflecting the teaching of Christ and the wisdom of Christian experience, but they must be applied to difficult situations by compassionate individuals.

In many cases, we have cited only those parts of the document which present the theological reasons for a particular teaching. When parts of the document have been omitted we follow *The Chicago Manual of Style* (14th Edition), which states: ". . . in a quotation of several paragraphs, the omission of an intervening paragraph or paragraphs is adequately indicated by a period and three ellipsis points at the end of the paragraph preceding the omitted part. And if a paragraph in the quotation, other than the first paragraph, begins with a sentence that does not open a paragraph in the original, it should be preceded by three dots following the usual paragraph indention. It is thus possible on occasion to use ellipsis points at the end of one paragraph *and* at the beginning of the next in a block quotation." For example, when presenting the matter on contraception, we have selected only those sections of the Encycli-

cal *On Human Life* that contain the theological reasoning, not those that contain
exhortations or pastoral applications. The reference to the complete text is cited,
however, for those who wish to study the entire document.

The particular teachings in this collection are drawn from statements of
the Second Vatican Council, encyclicals and allocutions emanating from Papal
Magisterium, and a few statements from bishops' conferences such as the *Ethical
and Religious Directives for Catholic Health Care Services* of 1994, and pontifical
commissions. Within each section, we sought to arrange the teachings by reason
of importance, that is, by reason of perceived authority. Some may question
why we have not stated which teachings of the Church are infallible or irreformable and which are reformable, that is, which merit an assent of faith and which
merit "assent of intellect and will" (*Dogmatic Constitution on the Church*, no. 25).
This division of Church teaching does not reflect our approach to truth and
morality. In this regard we echo the words of Dominican Yves Congar: "Infallibility affects truth in the same way legalism affects morality"; that is, just as
in moral matters one misses the meaning and motivation of Christian behavior
if one concentrates only on the written law, so also where proper moral decision
making is concerned, one misses the fullness of Christ's teaching if one accepts
only those statements of the Church which are certainly infallible and questions
those that are not proposed as revealed truth. As indicated in Chapter 2, all
statements which reflect the tradition of the Church and the effort of the Church
to lead people to holiness should be accepted by Catholics at least with respect
and often with "assent of intellect and will" (cf. Chapter 2, p. 23).

The teachings in the collection drawn from the statements of Pope Pius
XII are numerous. He seemed to enjoy studying and commenting upon the
ethical issues arising from medicine. While his statements are not as contemporary as some others cited in this volume, they offer a credible expression of
Church teaching because the reasoning contained in them reflects the perennial
truths of Catholic theology which have not been disproved or mitigated by
later statements of the Vatican Council, papacy, or bishops.

NOTES AND REFERENCES

1. Pope John Paul II. "The Splendor of Truth" (*Veritatis Splendor*), *Origins* 23: no.
18 (Oct. 14, 1993).

2. Pope John Paul II. "The Gospel of Life" (*Evangelium Vitae*), *Origins* 24: no. 42
(Apr. 6, 1995).

3. *Catechism of the Catholic Church*, Liguori, MO: Ligouri Publications, 1994.

Sources

The statements in the book, for the most part, are contained *in toto* in the following books and periodicals:

Flannery, Austin, OP, ed., *Vatican Council II: The Conciliar and Post Conciliar Documents*, Vol. 1. Northport, N.Y.: Costello Publishing Co., 1975.

Flannery, Austin, OP, ed., *Vatican Council II: More Post Conciliar Documents*, Vol. 2. Northport, N.Y.: Costello Publishing Company, 1982.

The Monks of Solesmes, ed., *The Human Body: Papal Teachings*. Boston, MA: St. Paul Editions, Daughters of St. Paul, 1960 and 1979.

National Catholic News Service. *Origins: NC Documentary Service*. Washington, D.C., United States Catholic Conference, 1981–1998.

Nolan, Hugh J., ed., *Pastoral Letters of the United States Catholic Bishops 1962–1974*, Vol. III. Washington, D.C.: United States Catholic Conference, 1983.

Nolan, Hugh J., ed., *Pastoral Letters of the United States Catholic Bishops 1975–1983*, Vol. IV. Washington, D.C.: United States Catholic Conference, 1984.

The Catholic Health Association. *Health Progress* (originally *Hospital Progress*). St. Louis, MO: The Catholic Health Association, 1985–1987.

The Pope Speaks: The Church Documents Quarterly. Huntington, IN: Our Sunday Visitor, Inc., 1958–1986.

The Vatican Commission for Health Care Workers. *Dolentium Hominum*. Vatican City: Vatican Press, 1992.

Pontifical Council for Pastoral Assistance to Health Care Workers. *Charter for Health Care Workers*. Vatican City: Vatican Press, 1995.

Verspieren, Patrick, ed., *Biologie Medicine et Ethique* (a valuable collection containing the complete text of papal teachings in regard to medical ethics). Paris: LeCenturion, 1987.

Part I: Understanding Church Teaching

1: The Values Underlying the Teachings of the Catholic Church in Regard to Medical Ethics

INTRODUCTION

The Christian life consists of human fulfillment in Christ Jesus, not in following rules. While good Christians observe the laws of God and the Church, these laws have a much deeper meaning than their prescriptive statements. They present the teaching of Jesus, the Word, and the grace-prompted experience of the Christian faithful as applied to specific human life situations. Hence, Christian life is a loving response to the word and grace of God, especially as the word and grace of God are manifested to us through the person of Jesus Christ. This loving response leads to personal human fulfillment as well as to fulfillment as a friend of God.

Catholics believe that the word and grace of God in the person of Jesus Christ are revealed to us through Sacred Scripture and tradition and that the Church authentically interprets both Scripture and tradition.[1] "Sacred Scripture is the speech of God as it is put down in writing under the breath of the Holy Spirit. And tradition transmits in its entirety the word of God which has been entrusted to the apostles by Christ the Lord and the Holy Spirit. It transmits it to the successors of the apostles so that, enlightened by the spirit of truth, they may faithfully preserve, expound, and spread it abroad by their preaching."[2] Tradition has been expressed through the centuries in Patristic writings, in theological writings, and in the official statements of the Church. In order to present a meaningful handbook of medical ethics for Catholic health care professionals, we must be concerned with the specific teachings of the Catholic Church concerning medical ethics. But in order to understand the full meaning of these teachings in regard to the practice of medicine and the pursuit of health, we must probe the teachings of Scripture, tradition, and theology which are the basis for Church statements on these subjects. The most important teachings concern the nature of the human person and his or her relationship to God and others.

In order to understand the human person in his or her fullness, we need to consider some important facets of human life. Thus, in this chapter we shall consider briefly what it means to be human as well as the meanings of health, sickness, death, and human sexuality. These general considerations will offer the framework for understanding the Church's teaching in regard to specific issues in medical ethics. Indeed, in one sense the specific normative teachings presented in Church documents are only applications of the general ideas about person, sickness, health, death, and sexuality. Our aim, then, in compiling this handbook is not to list rules of the Catholic Church that health care professionals

4   must obey if they are to be faithful Catholics. Rather, we are more interested in presenting the statements of the Church in regard to medical ethics in the context of the Christian vision of the human person. As a result of this perspective, Catholic health care professionals will be able to understand and internalize the pertinent Christian teachings, thus enabling them to make informed decisions of conscience concerning health care situations.

THE CHRISTIAN VIEW OF PERSON

All the teaching of the Church in regard to medical ethics results from the Christian understanding of the worth and activity of the human person.[3] The Christian view of the human person is based on the biblical teaching that each human being is created by God in his own image and likeness, differing from the animals by possessing a spiritual intelligence and free will (cf. Gn 1:26–31). Although the human body is brought into being through the cooperation of human parents, the creation of the human soul is a direct act of God (cf. Gn 2:7; 2 Mt 7:22–23), who calls each person into existence in relation to God himself (cf. Ps 22:10–11). Each person is unique and irreplaceable (cf. Mt 10:29–31), and all are called not only to personal maturity but also to eternal life (cf. 1 Tm 2:4). In order to attain fulfillment and eternal life, human beings have freedom of choice which is "an exceptional sign of the image of God in man."[4] Through free choice, each person shapes his or her own character and destiny. If there were no human freedom, there would be no morality because good and evil result from human choice. In making choices, Christians believe that God's grace helps all to overcome the weakness of human nature. The differences of sex, race, or individual talents in no way detract from this basic equality of all human beings (cf. Rom 2:11; Gal 4:38; Eph 6:9). Because of each person's relationship to God, human life is sacred. From this overriding value follows the specific teaching of the Church that it is a heinous crime to directly intend the death of an innocent person.

The worth of human persons was confirmed when God sent his Divine Son to assume human nature (cf. Heb 4:14–16). In recalling us to our dignity and restoring to us the hope of perfect happiness, which God intended when he created us, Jesus Christ worked miracles of healing (cf. Mk 1:32–39) and was concerned with even the most neglected and powerless members of society (cf. Mt 26:31–46).

MORAL NORMS

Theology seeks to study the explicit and implicit teachings of Sacred Scripture in regard to the human person in order to formulate moral norms expressing the actions which help or hinder the human person. In their writings, theologians utilize human learning as well as Scripture and tradition. Hence, in order to understand the Word of God more clearly in regard to the human person, theologians utilize the psychology and sociology of human behavior. In order to know more precisely about the human person, the Catholic view of person taught in Sacred Scripture and tradition is often expressed in theology by considering the needs of the human person and the powers or functions human beings possess in order to fulfill these needs. Briefly, the powers or functions which enable people to fulfill their needs are divided into four general categories: the physiological (biological), the psychological (emotional), the social, and the spiritual (creative).[5] Being precise about human needs and functions enables theologians to formulate more clearly moral norms for helpful human behavior. Theologians use the findings of human arts and sciences as well as Sacred Scripture to express their interpretations of the faith. Thus, human reason is a vital part of theological science and hence a vital factor in Church teaching. Faith and human reason work together to enable us to express the truth about human destiny and fulfillment in Christ. Over the years the Church sometimes accepted the teachings of theologians and included them in conciliar documents or official statements. Thus, teachings which the theologians formulate on the basis of Sacred Scripture, traditions, and human disciplines sometimes become the teachings of the Church.

NEEDS AND GOODS

Moral norms seek to direct us toward fulfillment of our human needs. Hence, a knowledge of human needs is necessary in order to formulate moral norms for the Christian life. St. Thomas Aquinas, one of the great theologians of the Church, described the fundamental needs of the human person as follows: to preserve life, to procreate children, to know the truth, and to live in society.[6] In numerous statements, Church teaching speaks about the human person and his or her spiritual, social, psychological, and physiological needs and functions as the "measure and criteria of good and evil in human affairs."[7] Some modern theologians suggest that human needs direct persons to fundamental "goods" which fulfill humans, thus emphasizing that fulfilling a true human need is of moral worth.[8] If we understand the human person and his or her needs and the goods which fulfill these needs, then we understand what is necessary for human fulfillment.

NATURAL AND CULTURAL NEEDS

In order to understand the needs and functions of the human person from a Christian perspective, we must realize that each level of human need comprises a complex of natural and cultural needs—the cultural needs being rooted in the natural needs but greatly expanding them. It cannot be emphasized too strongly that the four levels of human needs—physiological, psychological, social, and spiritual—and the corresponding functions directed to fulfilling them are not related as stories in a building, but are related as dimensions of a cube. Thus, the powers or activities of the human person can no more be separated from one another than can the length, breadth, and height of a cube. Every human act or event has all four dimensions. A human spiritual activity, whether it be a creative, scientific, artistic, or graced act of faith, hope, or love, also involves biological, psychological, and social activity.

6   Moreover, the relationship between these levels of need and the function of the human personality are ordered hierarchically so that spiritual activities are the deepest, most central, and the most integrating; biological activities are the least unified and the most peripheral; and psychological and social activities have intermediate positions. At the same time, the higher activities in this hierarchy are rooted in and depend on the lower in a network of interrelations. Nevertheless, each level has a certain genuine autonomy and differentiation in its structure and modes of functioning. St. Thomas makes it clear that there is an order among these needs, the lower being subordinate to the higher. Though needs are fulfilled through human functions, there must be an integration of functions, lest the person lead an unbalanced life. For example, a person may so emphasize fulfilling intellectual needs to the extent that he forgoes physiological or social needs and thus never develops as an integral human person. The good of the whole person requires that all the basic aspects of human personality be simultaneously respected, even when it is necessary to subordinate or even sacrifice in some measure a lower to a higher function.[9] This general teaching of Catholic theology concerning the integration of human functions is expressed in the "principle of totality" and is extremely important in medical ethics, being the principle by which surgery is justified and contraceptive sterilization rejected. A specific statement of the integration of human functions may be expressed as follows: "Except to save life itself, the fundamental functional capacities which constitute the human person should not be destroyed, but preserved, developed, and used for the good of the whole person and of the community."[10]

PERSON IN COMMUNITY

Human beings do not respond to the word and grace of God and reach fulfillment in isolation from other persons.[11] They have a social need which must be considered in order to understand the teaching of the Church concerning the human person. Because we realize that effective social relationships are an essential element in human fulfillment, we must consider the Christian vision of person in community. The provision of health care by Catholic institutions and Catholic health care professionals should be shaped by the Catholic notion of community. Do human beings have a responsibility to provide health care for others in the community? Can we speak about a right to health care? In order to speak intelligently about these questions as Catholics and Christians, we need an accurate notion of community.

Jesus indicated our need for community and the key to successful community living when he said: "Treat others the way you would have them treat you" (Mt 7:12); and "You shall love your neighbor as yourself" (Mt 22:39). According to this teaching, we are not asked to love our neighbor and not love ourselves, but to love our neighbor *as* we love ourselves. In other words, if we really love ourselves, not selfishly, but intelligently, we will realize that we cannot be happy in isolation, because we are created as social beings. We can attain integral human fulfillment only in a community of people, and that

means that we each must not only respect the rights of others, but must be   7
actively concerned to promote each other's welfare: the needs that the person
could not attain by himself or herself.

In our twentieth-century world, two extreme views about the relation of
person to community are in constant competition. One is collectivism. Generally,
collectivism favors a system in which the state closely regulates all human
activity in that the welfare of individual persons is strictly subordinated to the
welfare of the total community (the rights of persons can be sacrificed to the
interests of the nation).

The other extreme, individualism, favors individual freedom and considers responsibility to the community as a burden or interference. Though individualism does not eliminate all community responsibility, it seeks to keep it at a
minimum.[12] The ideal for individualism is the detached and self-sufficient
person. We often hear individualism called "the democratic way of life." In
defense of individualism, many argue that the goal of government should be
to protect and foster the maximum of individual freedom, because any restriction on freedom is believed to be an attack on the well-being of the individual.

Both of the aforementioned views of community—collectivism and individualism—are inconsistent with Christian teaching insofar as health care is
concerned. The subordination of persons to collectivism in the name of equality
will lead persons to a life of drudgery and oppression. Individualism, on
the other hand, produces individuals who never experience fulfilling social
relationships and victimizes the poor and less talented in society who are never
allowed to participate fully in the good and prosperity of the community.[13]

In macroeconomic affairs, collectivism is epitomized in the term "communism," or liberal socialism, and individualism is epitomized in the term "free
market capitalism." Many Catholics are under the impression that the Catholic
Church favors capitalism because it opposes socialism and communism. They
are unacquainted with the fully developed, recent social teaching of the Church
which must be considered in any Catholic approach to today's ethical problems,
including those in the medical field. The popes and bishops who apply the
Catholic tradition in regard to the human community urge us to work for a
world community based on spiritual goods or values and economic cooperation. They link human health and world poverty as the most fundamental
ethical problems of our time, problems which are often ignored in the United
States by ethicists and health care professionals alike while attention is devoted
to more esoteric problems such as genetic engineering and heart transplants.[14]

The social teaching of the Catholic Church, derived from the teaching of
Jesus, insists therefore that the human community, including its government,
must be actively concerned in promoting the health and welfare of every one
of its members so that each member can contribute to the common good of
all. This concern cannot be a matter of a mere trickle-down, by which the weak
live on the leavings of the powerful, but must be aimed directly at enabling
the weak to share in the goods of life. The Christian view of person in community, then, should influence the manner in which we plan health care and the

8 way we seek to care for the poor. This teaching of the Church in regard to the individual and community is summed up in the "principle of common good and subsidiarity."

The principle of common good and subsidiarity may be expressed as follows: Human communities exist only to promote and share the common good among all their members ("from each according to ability, to each according to need") in such a way that:

1. decision making rests vertically first with the person, then with the lower social levels, and horizontally with functional social units; and
2. the higher social units intervene only to supply the lower units with the goods they cannot achieve by themselves, while at the same time working to make it easier in the future for lower units and individuals to satisfy these needs by their own efforts.

This principle is the basis for many teachings of the Church in regard to allocation of resources and responsibility of the community to offer health care to the indigent. The practical implications for specific moral norms can be seen when the Church speaks about the right to health care and how it is to be implemented or concern for the aging.[15]

THE CHRISTIAN NOTION OF HEALTH

The Christian notion of health also serves as the basis for specific normative statements of the Church. Generally speaking, *health* is optimal human functioning, but the term may be used in a narrower sense or in a wider, more holistic sense. In the narrower sense, health refers only to the physiological and psychological functions of the person; therefore, a healthy person is one who meets all the requirements for "normal" psychological and physiological functioning. He or she has a "normal" pulse rate, "normal" stamina, "normal" blood count, and so on. In a wider sense, health includes social and spiritual functions as well as physiological and psychological functions. In Sacred Scripture, health is used in the wider sense of the term. Jesus was the Divine Healer who came to the world to help us become fully human, to help us realize our human dignity as creatures made in the image of God (cf. Lk 11:33). From a Christian perspective, then, health envisions optimal functioning of the human person to meet physiological, psychological, social, and spiritual needs in an integrated manner.[16]

While Christian teaching encourages a balanced development of all human power, it is clear from faith and experience that this is something very difficult to accomplish (cf. Rom 7:14). We all live with handicaps, ranging from minor to severe; though everyone seeks health, we are all wounded. But the tribulations we suffer, though we do not welcome them, are not meaningless. As we shall see, the ultimate reason for tribulation and suffering is spiritual growth in Jesus Christ (cf. Jn 16:33). As Christians, then, our health goals must always be realistic and we must realize that living with infirmities and deprivations in an integrated manner is necessary for pursuing human health.

Fulfilling all our natural and acquired needs will never be a possibility. For   9
many people life will not be "normal" in the limited sense of health, but it will
be fulfilling in the holistic notion of health if people use the powers they do
possess to love God and neighbor.

Many health care professionals are concerned almost exclusively with
health in the narrower sense, confining their major interest to the physiological
and psychological functions. While a certain concentration on health in this
narrower sense is required on the part of health care professionals if they are
to be good scientists,[17] they must also become cognizant of the social and
spiritual functions of their patients if they are to be truly concerned about their
patients as persons and help them to a better life.[18] Thus, the physician may
be better informed concerning the needs of a person at the physiological or
psychological levels because of his or her greater scientific knowledge. But if
one is to use the Christian view of the person as a norm of action, fulfilling
these physiological and psychological needs should be subordinated to the
social and spiritual needs of the patient. This realization of the hierarchy of
needs influences the teaching of the Church in regard to informed consent and
proxy consent.

THE CHRISTIAN NOTION OF SICKNESS AND DEATH

When discussing the Christian view of health, whether expressing meanings or delineating responsibilities, there is always a sense of loss lurking in
the background. We know that health is a great human value and that by
striving for health and enabling others to have access to health care we are
returning the love God has shown us by wisely using the gifts he has bestowed
upon us. Indeed, we remember that Jesus often used healing in the physiological
sense to remind us of his power to heal spiritually (cf. Lk 5:10). He demonstrated
that illness could be an occasion to prove God's love for his people and not a
sign of punishment. Yet, a sense of loss is present because it is obvious from
human experience that all efforts to promote and increase health will not
prevent the inevitability of death. How are Christians to think about this
paradox?

"Death was not God's doing; he takes no pleasure in the extinction of the
living. For this he created all" (Wis 1:13–14). "God had not wished to include
in man's destiny suffering and death."[19] Whence, then, came suffering and
death? St. Paul says, "Through one man sin entered the world and with sin
death, death thus coming to all men inasmuch as all sinned" (Rom 5:12). Even
if man had not sinned (original sin), life in this world would have ended; yet
with original sin, fear of death distorts human vision and choices.[20] This original
sin was essentially a sin of pride, the will to be like God; the sin of not using
God's gifts to come closer to God in community, but of using these gifts to set
up the human individual in self-centered domination of the world apart from
God. It is this misuse of God's gifts, from the beginning of the human race to
this day, that has prevented humankind from overcoming the natural causes
of death and has transformed what might have been a joyful completion of
this life and a serene passage into a greater life, into a blind, terrifying mystery.[21]

10 Although people have turned their backs on God, he has not turned from them but has offered them forgiveness and restoration. Yet in his mercy, he cannot deny their human freedom but has called them to return to him, not simply by restoring them to grace, but by a long history of struggle and learning from experience, an experience in which sickness and suffering are inevitable. For the Christian and for all who travel the same road in less clear ways, God has revealed in Christ the direction of their journey and the power of grace by which it can be traveled. In baptism, according to St. Paul (cf. Rom 6:1–11), through the cross of Christ man has died and been reborn in a new creation that will be completed in the resurrection of the body in eternal life. Men and women live now in such unity with Christ that all the events of their lives take on meaning from his life and death Consequently, both the joy and the suffering of this life have a Christian meaning: its joys are signs of the hope for everlasting life in his kingdom, which is already present here on earth in promise; and its sorrows are a sharing in his cross through which a victorious resurrection is to be achieved (cf. Rom 8:11–25).

Jesus came to conquer suffering and death. In what sense has he succeeded? People still get sick and continue to suffer, and death is inevitable. Jesus conquered sickness, suffering, and death in the sense that he gave them a new meaning, a new power (cf. Jn 4:25). By believing in Jesus as Savior, by joining suffering and death to his, humankind overcomes the evil aspect of suffering and death through hope in the resurrection. Through Jesus' sacrifice, man is able to conquer the evil that is associated with sickness and death. Though the results of original and actual sin are still present in life, they neither dominate it nor serve as punishment. Rather, suffering and death are transformed into the very actions that help humankind fulfill its destiny.

The Catholic teaching on death and the responsibility of health care professionals for the dying is summarized in the following statement from a Church document on this subject:

> . . . Life is a gift of God, and on the other hand, death is unavoidable; it is necessary therefore that we, without in any way hastening the hour of death, should be able to accept it with full responsibility and dignity. It is true that death marks the end of our earthly existence, but at the same time it opens the door to immortal life. Therefore all must prepare themselves for this event in the light of human values, and Christians even more so in the light of faith.
>
> As for those who work in the medical profession, they ought to neglect no means of making all their skill available to the sick and the dying; but they should also remember how much more necessary it is to provide them with the comfort of boundless kindness and heartfelt charity. Such service to people is also service to Christ the Lord, who said: "As you did it to one of the least of these my brethren, you did it to me" (Mt 25:40).[22]

This general outlook on death as an inevitable experience and the door to eternal life underlies the distinction that the Church makes between euthanasia and allowing a person to die. Moreover, this attitude underlies the various specific statements of Church teaching when offering guidance in regard to prolonging life-support systems for patients with serious illnesses. **11**

At one time human death was described as the separation of body and soul. This is still an adequate notion of death if we realize that the human soul is the unifying force in the composite of body and soul. Thus, when the unification of the human composite is no longer evident, it may be discerned that the human soul no longer informs the human body. This teaching of the Church has practical implications in regard to the declaration of human death through criteria which assess human brain activity. It also influences the teaching regarding organ transplants, which often follow a declaration of brain death.

In their attempts to specify more clearly what it means to die, modern theologians have concentrated on death as a personal human act, an act that terminates earthly existence but also fulfills it. Since the person is not merely passive in the face of death, death is different for the just than for the sinner. In the view of many theologians, death is an active consummation, a maturing self-realization that embodies what each person has made of himself or herself during life.[23] Death becomes a ratification of life, not merely an inevitable process. It is an active event in which the freedom of the person is intimately involved and in which the person is united to Christ. Dying with Christ is a deep, personal experience, a consequence of, but not a penalty for, sin. This is a new approach to death, yet it is thoroughly in keeping with the Christian tradition. Indeed, this view of death seems to describe more clearly the experience of Christ, who offered his life, rather than have it taken from him, who fulfilled his love and generosity in the final act of obedience to the Father. This concept of death has pastoral implications for Catholic health care professionals and Catholic health care facilities.

THE CHRISTIAN NOTION OF SEXUALITY

Sound, healthy sexuality is central to the human person and human community. The Christian notion of sexuality, especially as it relates to the goodness of marriage, to sexual activity within marriage, and to sexual activity that is not authentically marital, has normative ramifications for health care. While there is no systematic teaching about Christian sexuality in either Sacred Scripture or tradition, certain themes concerning sexuality are identifiable.[24]

First, Christian teaching is unequivocal: sexuality is good; in other words, its proper use is necessary for human fulfillment. The Old Testament presents human sexuality as a gift from God. Genesis 1–3 teaches that God created persons as male and female and blessed their sexuality as a great and good gift. Furthermore, the Church has always taught that the union of man and woman in marriage is good. It is good because as Scripture makes clear, God himself instituted marriage and gave it its defining characteristics. It is holy because the Lord Jesus made marriage a sacrament of his relation with the Church and a source of grace (cf. Mk 10:2–21; 1 Cor 7:10). In marriage, and especially in the act of conjugal love between husband and wife, there exists the symbol that shows us the irreplaceable, irrevocable, and fruitful love of Christ for his people (cf. Eph 5:22–23).

12   Second, sexuality is at the heart of the human person and fundamental to basic human relations. The recent teaching of the Church identifies the effect of sexuality on the person and community:

> The human person . . . is so profoundly affected by sexuality that it must be considered one of the principal formative influences in the life of a man or woman. In fact, sex is the source of the biological, physiological, and spiritual characteristics which make a person male or female and which thus considerably influence each individual's progress toward maturity and membership of society.[25]

Through their sexuality men and women are called by God to either marriage or the single state. John Paul II writes:

> God inscribed in the humanity of man and woman the vocation, and thus the capacity and responsibility, of love and communion. Love (community) is therefore the fundamental and innate vocation of every human being. . . . Christian revelation recognizes two specific ways of realizing the vocation of the human person, in its entirety, to love: marriage and virginity or celibacy.[26]

These statements point to both a general and a specific perspective on sexuality, each with normative consequences. Generally considered, sexuality affects the core of every person by bestowing identity and necessary responsibilities. The Church teaches that sexuality, in the general sense of the term, was given to us to help us love and serve one another whether we freely choose to marry or to live the single life of service to society. In this sense all persons, even celibates, are sexual people.

Used in a more specific sense, however, the term sexuality refers to the act of marital intercourse and the genital acts which lead to sexual intercourse. When speaking about sexuality in the specific sense, the Church maintains:

> The only "place" in which this self-giving in its whole truth is made possible is marriage, the covenant of conjugal love freely and consciously chosen, whereby man and woman accept the intimate community of life and love willed by God himself.[27]

This statement and the previous one indicate that sexuality is at the heart of the basic relationships which form the human community. The community formed in marriage is unlike any other institution inasmuch as it is created by God and signifies uniquely God's irrevocable, irreplaceable, and fruitful love for his people. Normatively, any action which would promote either the quality of marriage, the divine institution, or sacramental sign value, would be encouraged; any action which would jeopardize these elements of marriage would be proscribed.

Disagreement about the fundamental characteristics of sexuality and marriage creates tension in our world where there are various analyses of the conjugal act as it fulfills human needs. Contemporary thought maintains that conjugal acts fulfill one or more of the following needs:

1. Conjugal acts are a search for sensual pleasure and satisfaction, releasing physical and psychic tensions.
2. Conjugal acts are a search for the profound completion of the human person through an intimate, personal love expressed by bodily union. Ordinarily, conjugal love is also conceived as the complementing of male and female by one another so that each achieves a more complete humanity.
3. Conjugal acts are a social necessity for the procreation of children and creation of the family so as to expand the human community and guarantee its future beyond the death of individual members.
4. Conjugal acts are a symbolic (sacramental) mystery, indicating the relationship of persons to God.

Each of these characteristics of conjugal love is commonly recognized in all great religions and philosophies of life and is protected and developed in every viable culture. Today, however, the interrelationship and priority of sexuality and marriage is the subject of severe disagreement. In our modern culture, these values of sexual activity are generally thought to be combined in conjugal acts by sheer accident through the purposeless process of biological evolution. Consequently, many argue that we are free to combine or separate these different values according to our own purposes and preferences. Thus, some maintain that it seems entirely reasonable to use sex purely for the sake of pleasure apart from any relation to love or family; or to use it to reproduce (e.g., in vitro fertilization) apart from the marital act; or to use it as an expression of love, without any relation to marriage or family.

The teaching of the Church in regard to sexuality agrees with contemporary thought in recognizing these same four values of conjugal acts. But the teaching of the Church differs in its conviction that sexuality is a gift of the Creator, who in his wisdom and love for humanity created in his image has so intertwined these values that we cannot separate them without injury to that same image. Thus, when the Church expresses positive or negative norms in regard to sexuality and its expression, the Church seeks to delineate the actions which will be personally fulfilling or debilitating for individuals.

Clearly, there is a social aspect to procreation, because through responsible procreation the human community is built and perfected. Implicit in sexual activity therefore is the important and difficult responsibility to procreate children and educate them about the values of Christian life. Because it is often difficult to accomplish this important task, the Church teachings on the procreative value of human sexuality are quite extensive. The basis for Church teaching is not a negative view of human nature but rather a positive effort to help people respond to the teaching of Christ in regard to sexual activity. Human culture and customs have undergone many revolutions, but such changes cannot alter the basic structure of human sexuality and marital love without destroying humanity itself. This understanding of the Church in regard to human sexuality is the basis for the teaching in regard to contraception, artificial insemination, co-creation of children, family life, and in vitro fertilization.

14   Sexuality is only one element of Christian life; Christians must also be concerned about many other issues, such as social justice and the quest for peace. But sexuality exercises a deep and pervasive influence in the life of each person, hence, there are many Church statements on the subject. These statements about sexual activity must be considered seriously by Christian health care professionals.

CONCLUSION

Clearly, there is more to Catholic teaching than the bold statement of a precept. One needs to understand the principles and values underlying the Church's teachings in order to apply those teachings accurately to daily life.

In this chapter, we have presented briefly the principles and values of the Catholic faith which are the basis for statements of the Church in regard to medical ethics. In the next chapter we shall consider the particular act through which the teaching of the Church can be applied: namely, the formation of conscience.

NOTES AND REFERENCES

1. Cf. Vatican Council II, "Dogmatic Constitution on Divine Revelation," nos. 9 and 10, in *Vatican Council II: The Conciliar and Post Conciliar Documents*, Vol. 1, Austin Flannery, OP, ed., (Northport, NY: Costello Publishing Co., 1975), p. 755.

2. *Vatican Council II*, "Dogmatic Constitution on Divine Revelation," no. 9, p. 755.

3. Cf. Vatican Council II, "Pastoral Constitution on the Church in the Modern World," no. 12, in *Vatican Council II: The Conciliar and Post Conciliar Documents*, Vol. 1, Austin Flannery, OP, ed., (Northport, NY: Costello Publishing Co., 1975), p. 913.

4. *Vatican Council II*, "Pastoral Constitution on the Church in the Modern World," no. 17, p. 917.

5. Cf. Benedict M. Ashley, OP, and Kevin D. O'Rourke, OP, *Health Care Ethics*, 2nd ed., (St. Louis, MO: Catholic Health Association, 1982), p. 18.

6. Cf. St. Thomas Aquinas, *Summa Theologicae* I–II, q.94, a.2.

7. Pope John Paul II, "A Patient Is a Person" (Oct. 27, 1980), *The Pope Speaks* 26: no. 1 (1981), pp. 1–5.

8. Cf. Germain Grisez, *The Way of the Lord Jesus*, Vol. 1, (Chicago, IL: Franciscan Herald Press, 1983), p. 115.

9. Cf. Benedict M. Ashley, OP, *Theologies of the Body*, (St. Louis, MO: Pope John XXIII Medical-Moral Research and Education Center, 1986), p. 925.

10. Ashley and O'Rourke, *Health Care Ethics*, p. 44.

11. Cf. *Vatican Council II*, "Pastoral Constitution on the Church in the Modern World," no. 24, p. 925.

12. Cf. Robert Bellah et. al., *Habits of the Heart*, (New York: Harper & Row, 1985).

13. Cf. National Conference of Catholic Bishops, "Catholic Social Teaching and the U.S. Economy" (Oct. 7, 1985), *Origins*, 16: no. 24, Nov. 27, 1986, p. 409.

14. Cf. Pope John Paul II, "Health Care: Ministry in Transition" (Sept. 14, 1987), *Origins* 17: no. 17, Oct. 8, 1987, p. 291; National Conference of Catholic Bishops, "Pastoral Letter on Health and Health Care" (Nov. 16–19, 1981), *Origins* 11: no. 25, Dec. 3, 1981, pp. 396–402.

15. Cf. National Conference of Catholic Bishops, "Catholic Social Teaching and the U.S. Economy," p. 259.

16. Cf. Pope John Paul II, "The Ethics of Genetic Manipulation" (Oct. 29, 1983),
Origins 13: no. 23, Nov. 17, 1983, p. 385.

17. Cf. Edmund D. Pellegrino and David C. Thomasma, *A Philosophical Basis of Medical Practice*, (New York: Oxford Press, 1981), pp. 51–80.

18. Cf. Pellegrino and Thomasma, *A Philosophical Basis of Medical Practice*, pp. 51–80.

19. Pope Pius XII, "Christian Principles and the Medical Profession," in *The Human Body: Papal Teachings*, The Monks of Solesmes, eds., (Boston, MA: St. Paul Editions, Daughters of St. Paul, 1960), p. 57.

20. Cf. Karl Rahner, SJ, *On the Theology of Death*, (New York: Herder & Herder, 1965), pp. 42–43.

21. Cf. Rahner, *On the Theology of Death*, pp. 42–52.

22. Sacred Congregation for the Doctrine of the Faith, "Declaration on Euthanasia" (May 5, 1980), in *Vatican Council II: More Post Conciliar Documents*, Vol. 2, Austin Flannery, OP, ed., (Northport, NY: Costello Publishing Company, 1982), p. 516.

23. Cf. Rahner, *On the Theology of Death*, pp. 42–43.

24. Cf. Joseph Jensen, OSB, "Human Sexuality and the Scriptures," in *Human Sexuality and Personhood*, (St. Louis, MO: Pope John XXIII Medical-Moral Research and Education Center, 1981), pp. 15–36.

25. Sacred Congregation for the Doctrine of the Faith, "Declaration on Certain Questions of Sexual Ethics," no. 1 (Dec. 29, 1975), in *Vatican Council II: More Post Conciliar Documents*, Vol. 2, Austin Flannery, OP, ed., (Northport, NY: Costello Publishing Company, 1982), p. 486.

26. John Paul II, "The Christian Family in the Modern World," no.11 (Nov. 22, 1981), in *Vatican Council II: More Post Conciliar Documents*, Vol. 2, Austin Flannery, OP, ed., (Northport, NY: Costello Publishing Company, 1982), p. 822.

27. *ibid*

2: Formation of Conscience

INTRODUCTION

Nurses, physicians, and other health care workers constantly confront the moral dimensions of their profession. Critical issues, ranging from ethical care for the newborn to determining the proper care for the terminally ill, demand that people think through the ethical or moral issues of health care and make judgments of conscience. In making any decision of conscience concerning proper health care, clinicians look to medical judgments such as diagnosis and prognosis; they consider the desires of the patient or of the appropriate proxy decision maker concerning possible treatment alternatives; and they reflect on the fundamental ethical norms of the medical profession, such as "do no harm." Sometimes judgments of conscience are easily reached because there is no dispute over treatment; the medical condition of the patient is clear and his or her choices of treatment simply ratify the medical decision. Often, however, insufficient evidence exists to make a clear decision of conscience. In some cases uncertainty may arise because there are insufficient objective medical criteria to indicate the best way to treat the patient. At other times the legitimate subjective preferences of the patient can add ambiguity to the situation. Finally, ethical principles utilized in the past sometimes do not seem to apply because technology has advanced so rapidly. In such situations, Catholic health care professionals, responding to grace and faith, realize the impasse and look to the teaching of the Church for help in making their decisions. Catholic health care professionals believe that the teaching of the Church is founded upon Sacred Scripture and tradition. Thus, they rely upon Church documents for insights to apply Sacred Scripture and tradition to contemporary health care issues. In so doing, Catholic health care professionals broaden their perspective for decision making and root their decisions of conscience more firmly in the eternal values preached by Jesus.

When reflecting upon the teaching of the Church, Catholic health care professionals do not surrender their rights of conscience.[1] But in order to help health care professionals to understand more accurately the relationship between formation of conscience and the authority of the documents contained in this book, several issues must be considered. First, the various mistaken notions of conscience which diminish the human capacity to arrive at objective moral truth or which eliminate the possibility of objective moral discourse must be identified. Second, after exploration of the various erroneous methods of forming conscience, an accurate understanding of conscience formation will be presented. Finally, the role that faith plays in the formation of a Christian conscience will be thoroughly examined. Once this is done, it will become more clear how each of the documents in this book should be utilized in decision making.

"To follow my conscience" has many different meanings. Each meaning presupposes a different theory of ethical decision making and results in a different method of forming conscience. Briefly, we shall explain some of the more popular methods of forming conscience and indicate the insufficiency of the ethical theories from which they proceed.

For some people "to follow my conscience" means to follow feelings or emotions. Thus, according to this theory, the norm for moral good or evil is always subjective and cannot be communicated rationally to others. In the United States, this method of moral decision making is followed by many and often approved because the public is usually willing to forgive even serious injuries if the perpetrators of the action "feel deeply about it." So, for example, popular opinion sometimes favors those who commit "mercy killings" because of their subjective anguish. The ultimate purpose of their actions may be understandable; to eliminate suffering. But they choose an evil action to accomplish their goal; namely, killing an innocent person.

Another popular meaning of "to follow my conscience" is to follow the law or to follow custom. Thus, some will maintain that the action of the Supreme Court in the Roe vs. Wade case, which made abortion legal in the United States, also made abortion morally good. Some will maintain that greater permissiveness in society allows one to engage in extramarital or premarital sexual relations in good conscience, hence giving custom the force of ethical sanction. Law and custom overall are not sufficient norms in themselves for forming conscience.

"To follow my conscience" for others implies a blind obedience to direct inspiration from God. Some might defend an instance of stealing by saying that God ordered them to act in this manner. The implication of this ethical theory is that God bypasses human reason when instructing a person's conscience.

For others, "to follow my conscience" implies that the simple choice of an action makes it right or wrong. In this theory the ultimate recourse of conscience becomes personal freedom and autonomy; a decision of conscience is a good decision as long as the individual makes a personal decision. Thus, some people choose to destroy public property in order to protest a public policy; simply on the basis that they have reached the decision of conscience autonomously, they believe they are morally justified.

These views of conscience are in conflict and often disregard consideration of the goods or needs which are preeminent in human life, such as life, health, procreation, knowledge, community, friendship, and integrity. Formation of conscience should prompt people to fulfill these basic needs and achieve the good of the human person in a balanced manner, thus enabling people to become integrated and fulfilled human beings. Formation of conscience which is based totally upon feelings is inadequate because it leads to subjective ethical assessments which cannot be defended in moral dialogue and which often neglect fundamental human goods. Formation of conscience founded totally upon custom and law rather than upon fundamental human needs or goods

18   is extrinsic and minimalistic, and does not lead to total personal fulfillment. While some existing social norms are conducive of human fulfillment others, such as abortion and sexual promiscuity, lead to actions which are destructive of what is truly human. Overemphasizing personal freedom often leads to disregard for the needs and rights of others, thus destroying community as well as personal integrity. Experience demonstrates that people who use freedom as the sole warrant for formation of conscience are usually acting in ways that cannot be justified by faith or reason; hence, personal freedom alone is also an insufficient basis for ethical decision making. Finally, maintaining that formation of conscience is the direct inspiration of God eliminates the need for human reason. While it is valid to maintain that God speaks to our hearts and inspires us, this does not imply that God bypasses our reasoning process when he speaks to us, nor does it allow us to forsake evaluating our judgment of conscience by means of the principles of reason and faith.

Though formation of conscience is faulty if it is founded only upon emotion, divine command, law, custom, or personal autonomy, a sound and accurate theory of ethics and decisions of conscience nonetheless involves an appreciation of feelings, law, custom, divine instruction, and personal freedom. All these elements must be taken into account when making decisions of conscience, *but in addition* something more fundamental is needed for valid ethical theory and ethical decisions of conscience. Ethics, understood as a systematic reflection on moral living, primarily directs people to human happiness and fulfillment and integration of self with others and God. As stated in the previous chapter, ethics enables people to fulfill the fundamental goods of human living in a reasonable or balanced manner. Hence, the resource which is fundamental for accurate decisions of conscience is human reason, by which we consider whether our actions are directed toward achieving human goods. While emotions are present in reasonable decisions of conscience, they should accompany the reasonable judgment, not overpower it. Thus, we know that righteous anger may help one make a better judgment of conscience concerning what is morally good or evil. For example, righteous anger aroused by degradation of the homeless may give one the courage to work for better public housing. But we also know from experience that anger may be so strong that it overrides reason and makes impossible a balanced moral judgment. For example, when one is angry because of some slight given by another, one has a difficult time being kind and compassionate to the person who caused the slight. Laws and customs are considered when one makes a reasonable judgment of conscience, but they are not the "last word." Rather, reason evaluates laws and customs to make sure they contribute to the true good of human persons in community. Not even divine faith should be considered apart from reason when a judgment of conscience is made. When Christians make decisions of conscience, divine faith influences reason, but does not supplant it. As we shall see, faith "sheds a new light on all human activity,"[2] but does not eliminate the light of reason.

In sum, a sound account of "following conscience" shows it to be grounded in a reasoned assessment of needs or goods that fulfill human persons; it directs

people to be interrelated with self, others, and God. "Following conscience"   **19**
must be more than following feelings; it must be a judgment of reason. "Following conscience" must involve more than an intuition or a divine command; it
must proceed from principles of reason and faith to practical conclusions.
"Following conscience" involves more than a subjective personal decision; it
involves an analysis of objective reality. Finally, "following conscience" should
not be confused with following societal customs; rather, it requires following
sound patterns of moral thinking which consider the goods that fulfill the
human person. Hence, "following conscience" directs persons to choose, to
promote, and to protect goods that fulfill fundamental human needs; "following
conscience" never destroys, impedes, or sets aside goods or actions that fulfill
the human person.

FORMING A CHRISTIAN CONSCIENCE

Conscience, in a Christian sense, is awareness of moral truth.[3] More specifically, conscience is the final practical judgment determining which actions
are morally right or wrong; that is, which actions will fulfill a person and meet
human needs in a balanced manner. This act of moral judgment includes several
components: awareness of principles and norms, understanding the particular
facts of the issue in question, and forming a practical judgment that an action
fulfills human need, or is good, and which dictates that the will should choose
this action. The first component, awareness of principles and norms, traditionally has been referred to in Sacred Scripture as the law of the heart. People,
enlightened by the gift of wisdom, receive and retain God's law in their hearts.
It is also referred to as the habit of *synderesis*.[4] Nonbelievers also admit an
awareness of certain moral principles and norms written in their hearts which
they do not need to learn in a school. The general desire "to do good and avoid
evil" is such a norm (*synderesis*). The first step in the formation of conscience
involves using basic principles or norms. Some of these principles are general,
such as "love God and neighbor," and must be transposed into more particular
principles before one can act; for example, "tell the truth," which expresses a
way to show love for God and neighbor. The general and particular principles
utilized in forming decisions of conscience are action principles rather than
speculative principles; they indicate which actions are morally good, because
those actions fulfill our needs as human beings. Many fundamental principles
which inform conscience formation are the result of God's teaching us through
Sacred Scripture or the Church. But principles of conscience also are deduced
by our natural ability to reason practically. Thus, each person has the ability
and inclination to form decisions of conscience utilizing general principles and
particular norms which indicate moral good or evil. Those who "listen to God
in their heart" have their natural capacity to form principles improved and
strengthened by the Word of God.

The second component of conscience formation involves understanding
the special circumstances or facts of a situation and the practical possibilities
for action. For example, before telling the truth to another person, one must

20 know the truth. In medicine, knowing the truth in regard to the results of a particular procedure is difficult because of the variables which may influence the outcome. However, a physician may be able to convey either definite probabilities or possibilities to a patient based on medical research and experience. Thus, "telling the truth" to a patient in these circumstances will require specialized knowledge and experience about particular facts.

Finally, forming a decision of conscience is completed by means of a practical judgment dictating a particular action which will fulfill a particular human need; either do this or do not do that.

Making a particular practical judgment that is an accurate and valid judgment that an act is good requires knowledge of actions which fulfill human needs and also requires balanced or well-disposed human affections. Probably, well-disposed human affections, or virtues, are the most overlooked component of moral decision making. If a person's emotions or affections are not disposed toward morally good actions, then one will have a difficult time choosing actions which truly fulfill human needs and thus are morally good. For example, making accurate ethical judgments which involve the rights of other persons will be very difficult for a selfish or greedy person, who may think, "Should I pay back the money I owe a friend, or use the money to satisfy my desire for some luxury?" The emotional inclination of a selfish person would be to favor himself or herself; hence, his or her emotions will often override an accurate judgment of conscience and lead one to reject the good and choose evil. Thus, a person strongly attracted to sexual pleasure may determine that a particular liaison leads to acts of adultery and therefore should be avoided. But after making this accurate moral analysis, the person's strong desire for sexual pleasure may override the initial decision of conscience. Instead of following the valid and accurate decision of conscience, the person with misguided affections starts the decision-making process over again and arrives at a judgment which is more compatible with his or her affections. Thus, forming and following a good conscience is more than an intellectual reasoning process. One's affective powers are intimately involved as well. For this reason, the process used to form one's affective powers is also important because it involves many decisions of conscience. Experiencing the value of good actions, prayer, liturgy, and association with good people are means to influence one's affective powers toward the morally good. The entire process of disposing one's affections and carrying out good decisions of conscience is known as the prudential process,[5] a topic which merits further study by concerned Catholics.

Since conscience is one's final practical judgment about right and wrong, an honest person has no alternative other than to follow conscience even if it involves suffering; not to follow one's judgment would be to act against conscience. One is always bound to follow one's conscience even if commanded by authority to do otherwise. In this context, the statement of the Second Vatican Council on conscience should be understood:

> Deep within his conscience man discovers a law which he has not laid upon himself but which he must obey. Its voice, ever calling him to love and to do what is good and to avoid evil, tells him inwardly at the right

moment: do this, shun that. For man has in his heart a law inscribed by
God. His dignity lies in observing this law, and by it he will be judged.[6]

This passage is unequivocal: conscience is the awareness of a law that is discovered within the human person. The term "law," used here in its broadest sense, does not describe an alien authority, but emphasizes each person's internal, natural impetus to do good and seek fulfillment as a human being. People sometimes conceive law to be an undue restraint, and they equate conscience with freedom; thus, they posit intrinsic opposition between law and conscience. However, an accurate view of conscience does not set in opposition to law; rather, it uses law as one of the integral components in arriving at the last best judgment about what action integrally fulfills the human person, and in an analogous sense a final decision of conscience becomes a "law."

CONSCIENCE IS NOT INFALLIBLE

Maintaining that one ought to follow one's conscience does not imply that conscience is infallible. To follow one's conscience presupposes that one has not chosen to remain ignorant of one's responsibility, but rather that one has struggled to make an honest effort to inform one's conscience accurately. At the same time, mistakes are possible in formulating the principles, in understanding the facts involved in the choice, or in reasoning from this information to a practical moral judgment whether to perform or avoid an action, and one's affections may not be well-disposed to the good. Thus, mistakes, which are or are not the responsibility of the individual person, may occur in the forming of conscience. The potential for human error underlies the need for caution and care. The Second Vatican Council teaches: "Yet it often happens that conscience goes astray through ignorance which it is unable to avoid, without thereby losing its dignity. This cannot be said of the man who takes little trouble to find out what is true and good, or when conscience is by degrees almost blinded through the habit of committing sin."[7]

From experience it is clear that our knowledge of facts is not always accurate, yet judgments of conscience depend upon particular facts. Still, at any given time, we must make decisions with the knowledge available. Even wise people can look back and realize that their judgments of conscience could have been better informed. Sometimes empirical evidence is not as accurate as first perceived. For instance, a physician might recommend a therapeutic regime based on a drug initially approved as safe by the FDA. Later, however, because of new evidence, it is indicated that the drug has harmful side effects. Even conscientious people, through no fault of their own, may make judgments of conscience resulting from mistakes of fact.

In other cases, people may misunderstand moral principles. For instance, a health care professional might interpret a specific norm such as "let the autonomous competent patient decide what treatment is best" to mean that *any* request a patient makes about his or her health care is acceptable. This is a misunderstanding of the norm of patient autonomy. Patient autonomy means the patient can request either morally licit treatments or what is considered good professional practice. Interpreting the norm of autonomy to mean that

22 the health care professional must do everything the patient requests absolutizes autonomy in an unwarranted fashion. When a judgment of conscience is based upon false information or moral misunderstandings, the person does not act in bad faith because the person would have acted otherwise had he or she understood the facts. In the proper formation of conscience, one must always gather and check facts as well as reconsider one's position through prayer, especially if one's judgment of conscience seems to conflict with those formed by other good people in similar circumstances.

The foregoing brief analysis of formation of conscience illustrates that the process of forming and following one's conscience is the touchstone of morality and human fulfillment. But it is a process that involves our reason and emotions, and it must be a careful process because error may result from many different factors, such as misunderstanding of principles or honest mistakes of factual knowledge or undisciplined emotions. Hence, in a certain sense, "Did I form my conscience prudently?" is as important a question as "Did I follow my conscience?"

FAITH AND ASSENT IN THE FORMATION OF CONSCIENCE

"Following conscience" for Catholics implies that the dimension of faith is introduced into the process of conscience formation through the teaching of the Church. "For faith throws a new light on all things and makes known the full ideal which God has set for man, thus guiding the mind toward solutions that are fully human."[8] Hence, when forming conscience, Catholics consider not only the basic moral principles and the particulars of the situation, but also the teachings of the Church. Tradition includes the teaching of the Church, the writings of the theologians, and the example offered by holy people of the past and present.[9] Do these sources of faith-related information come from outside the person? Do they interfere with freedom of conscience? In the act of faith one establishes a profound personal and internal relationship with God revealing himself through the teaching Church. Sacred Scripture and tradition, as presented by the Church, communicate to us at our deepest level of being; these sources of truth help us to broaden our perspectives and to organize our lives for total human fulfillment in Jesus Christ. Because faith is an internal act of the person, the wisdom communicated by reason of faith is internal to the person. Grace perfects nature; it does not replace the actions of nature. Rather than interfere with the free act of conscience, then, faith-related information strengthens the internal and personal aspects of a decision of conscience.

Catholics admit that Scripture and tradition inform their conscience and help them understand which actions fulfill them in Christ. Nonetheless, Catholics may find it difficult at times to understand the meaning or the precise authority of a particular document or statement which intends to communicate the teaching of faith. What authority is to be given to a specific document? Is it ever possible not to follow the teaching of bishops or the Holy Father? The Second Vatican Council addressed these concerns by discussing the essential characteristics of the relationship between the teaching of the Church and the conscience of the individual.

VARIOUS LEVELS OF TEACHING

When listening to the teaching of the Church, one must realize that the Church is a dynamic communion of people and that the Church grows in understanding of the truth. For example, applying traditional revealed principles to new circumstances will result in new teachings. Not until chemical contraceptions were invented did the Church develop an integral teaching in regard to artificial birth control, founded upon the unitive and procreative goals of the marital act. Because the Church is a living and dynamic society, all teachings of the Church do not have the same authority. The Second Vatican Council sought to distinguish the various levels of Church teaching;[10] but an even more well-developed explanation of Church teaching has been promulgated recently by the Congregation for Doctrine of the Faith. According to this document,[11] the Church teaches with three different levels of authority:

1. infallible or definitive teaching which requires an assent of faith;
2. authoritative teaching, or non-definitive teaching, which concerns teachings related to the truths of faith. The proper response to this teaching is religious assent of will and intellect; not the same as an act of faith but reverential respect for the power of the Holy Spirit in the teaching Church;
3. pastoral teaching, which combines principles with contingent facts resulting in "non-irreformable" teaching, calls for habitual "adherence of the faithful."

The varying levels of Church lead the Church to advise: "One must take into account the proper character of every exercise of the magisterium, considering the extent to which its authority is engaged. It is also to be kept in mind that all acts of the magisterium derive from the same source, that is, from Christ who desires that his people walk in truth. For this same reason, magisterial decisions in matters of discipline, even if they are not guaranteed by the charism of infallibility, are not without divine assistance and call for adherence of the faithful."[12]

The impact of the various levels of Church teaching is an important theological study, but beyond the purpose of this work. Interested persons will find a clear exposition in Francis Sullivan's *Magisterium: Teaching Authority in the Catholic Church*; John Boyle's *Church Teaching Authority*; and the document referred to above, "Instruction on the Ecclesial Vocation of the Theologian."[13]

Because there are different levels of authority in Church teaching, some interpret this to mean that one should form one's conscience separately and then compare it to the Church's teaching. According to this conception, the teaching of the Church becomes a set of laws or imposed social standards that are external to the person. But when one makes a fundamental option of faith one accepts the truth that the Spirit of God lives within the believing person and that the Holy Spirit informs and nurtures the person through the teaching Church. Therefore, "the assent of mind and will" to Church teachings prompted by faith is not an assent to *external authority* or to an external blueprint for

24   Christian behavior, but rather it is an internal acceptance at the deepest core of the person. Faith informs conscience; it does not usurp the right of conscience. Faith and reason are not in opposition or in conflict with one another. Pope John Paul II sought to emphasize this fact in a recent addition to the Code of Canon Law. This new statement in the Code, c. 750, #2, states that those teachings set forth definitively, as well as those set forth as divinely revealed, must be firmly accepted and held by Catholics.[14]

It is important to distinguish an act prompted by faith in the Church from an act of "following orders." "Assent of mind and will" is *not* blind obedience. To form a Christian conscience does not mean that one receives an exact blueprint which specifies how one ought to act in every situation. To define the formation of a Christian conscience as following orders or as replacing one's conscience with ecclesial statements of extrinsic authority is an inappropriate understanding of faith as well as an inappropriate understanding of the human person's ability to make decisions of conscience. No matter how certain and definite a moral teaching of the Church might be, it must still be applied to particular individual actions. Because each act of conscience is a practical, personal judgment, individuals must apply the teaching of the Church to decisions about specific singular actions in the process of forming their consciences.

For example, the Church teaches that killing an innocent human being (murder) is a serious moral evil. But when making decisions whether or not to prolong life, health care professionals often must determine the particular facts of the case and decide if withdrawing or withholding care is euthanasia or if it is allowing a patient to die because further care would be medically futile or impose a grave burden with little benefit. Difficulty concerning the application of Church teaching leads some Catholics to require artificial nutrition and hydration for all patients in irreversible comas, while other Catholics interpret the use of artificial nutrition and hydration in certain circumstances as an optional means to prolong life. Often the teaching of the Church is not specific, and the decision of conscience prudently formed in regard to particular decisions by one Christian may differ from that of another.[15] These differences of conscience frequently occur when the rights of management and the rights of labor are in conflict.

While there is no razor's edge to separate the levels of Church teaching, prudent believers seek to evaluate the character, frequency, and manner of teaching as they form their conscience. Statements issued by the Roman Congregations and Commissions of the Church which are not signed by the Holy Father do not in themselves have the same authority as statements issued by the Holy Father or bishops in their pastoral teachings, but their statements are to be heeded by Catholics as a guide to forming their consciences. Often they summarize papal teaching and apply the teaching to particular issues. In the texts collected in this book there are some statements from Roman Congregations and Pontifical Commissions (e.g., p. 44; pp. 431), and their authority should be evaluated according to the foregoing norms; in other words, these statements do not acquire any additional authority simply because they are included in a collection.

Can one ever withhold assent of will and intellect from a Church teaching because one thinks the teaching is in error? When one's moral evaluation of an action conflicts with Church teaching, one has a primary responsibility to reflect on the matter and to ask whether sufficient justification exists to withhold assent.[16] Occasionally, one might withhold assent for one of the following reasons:

1. A teaching has not been taught for very long and has not been proposed by many bishops. Some conflict of opinion is inevitable if certain people consider a teaching to be very serious but it is too new to command universal assent.

2. Sometimes the teaching requiring assent and the faith tradition it is based upon is not effectively presented. One might then withhold assent until one was certain what precisely was being taught.

3. Sometimes certain teachings are presented which are merely the opinions of an individual; for example, a bishop may speak as a civic leader or as a private theologian. In this case assent is not obligatory.[17]

4. Some Church teachings are presented as general principles with the practical application being uncertain while some authorities maintain the statement must be understood in a specific manner. For example, the Church teaches that we should "respect the life" of every person, but applying this norm to many of the "withholding life support" issues is difficult. Some bishops have maintained that, as a result of Church teaching, food and water must always be given to patients,[18] but this specific indication is not part of Church teaching.

5. The understanding of a teaching may deepen. For example, the Church teaching for centuries permitted *capital punishment* by the state. However, reflection on more fundamental principles within the faith tradition, such as the respect for and dignity of human life, suggests that capital punishment may be at odds with a basic doctrine, namely respect for human life.[19] Because there is a deeper understanding of a more fundamental principle of faith, believers may legitimately withhold assent from those in the Church who teach that capital punishment is permissible.

Thus, several grounds exist for withholding assent from a teaching of the Church. But before doing so legitimately, one must have serious reasons which are in accord with Church tradition. Otherwise, one may be rejecting the voice of the Holy Spirit within the Church. A person cannot withhold assent simply to replace the teaching of the Body of Christ with a personal view or with the norm of a permissive society. People often dissent from a teaching of the Church because it is difficult to follow, or counter culture, not because they are able to prove that it is inconsistent with basic Catholic teaching. When the recent statement on in vitro fertilization was issued by the Church, for example, many people declared it to be wrong, though they had not read the document and

26 did not understand the basis for the Church teaching. Some will hold that one ought always to prefer one's own personal conscience to the teaching of the Church. If this were a habitual practice, what role would faith have in informing one's conscience? Can a person consistently put aside the Church's teaching and still remain a Catholic? Furthermore, if one prefers one's own interpretation of faith to that of the Magisterium of the Church, one is preferring one's own opinions to the faith of the multitude of believers which has been handed down through the centuries and is found in the faith tradition of the living Body of Christ. To withhold assent from a Church teaching, one must have a more fundamental reason than "the teaching is difficult to follow."

SUMMARY

In this chapter, we have explained how the teaching of the Church informs the conscience of an individual Catholic. The following concepts are fundamental.

First, conscience is the final practical judgment about a particular course of action. Forming an accurate decision of conscience involves reasoning about moral principles, understanding the particulars of the case, and reaching a specific decision which declares something is to be done or avoided to fulfill the person's human needs. The affections and will, as well as reason, are involved in making balanced moral decisions. Following the decision of a rightly formed conscience is a moral imperative. If one reaches a decision which seems difficult, this in itself is not a sufficient reason to forgo following the decision of conscience.

Second, conscience can be in error concerning moral good because one can misunderstand the principles, misjudge the particular facts, or be indisposed to moral good by reason of misguided affections. The affections may also prevent one from following an accurate decision of conscience. One is culpable for an erroneous decision of conscience only if it is within one's capability to have prevented the error.

Third, faith adds new insights into what will integrally fulfill a person: it informs one's conscience with a broad understanding of the principles that affect certain choices.

Fourth, assent to the teaching of the Church does not imply that formation of conscience is a simple act of obedience. Assent does require, however, a prayerful consideration and integration of the Church's teaching.

Fifth, even in matters that are not proposed *ex cathedra*, Catholics give assent of will and intellect to propositions set forth by the Magisterium. This assent is influenced by the character, frequency, and manner in which the document is proposed.

Finally, withholding assent may be licit on some occasions, but not simply because a teaching is difficult to follow. If what is taught is in conflict with a more fundamental principle of belief, assent may be withheld.

The Church documents in this book are of varying importance and contain both moral principles and normative conclusions. Health care professionals reviewing the documents should evaluate them seriously because they are the

distillation of centuries of faith experience. While the importance of these
teachings may be less clear at times, they do provide us with an important
source of wisdom. We use this wisdom in forming our consciences and we
pray with the help of the Holy Spirit that the judgments we make about the
many ethical questions we face will be accurate and morally sound.

Notes and References

1. For a summary of the scriptural and patristic sources that underlie the teachings on conscience found in St. Thomas Aquinas's writings and in Vatican documents, see Phillippe Delhaye, *The Christian Conscience* (New York: Desclee, 1968), pp. 36–99.

2. Vatican Council II, in *Vatican Council II: The Pastoral Constitution on the "Church in the Modern World,"* no. 11, p. 912.

3. Cf. Vatican Council II, "Pastoral Constitution on the Church in the Modern World," no. 16, in *Vatican Council II: The Conciliar and Post Conciliar Documents*, Austin Flannery, OP, ed., p. 916.

4. Cf. *Summa Theologicae* I, q. 79, a. 12.

5. Benedict M. Ashley, OP, and Kevin D. O'Rourke, OP, *Health Care Ethics*, 4th ed. (Washington, D.C.: Georgetown University Press, 1997), p. 58.

6. *Vatican Council II*, "Pastoral Constitution on the Church in the Modern World," no. 16, p. 916.

7. *Ibid.*, p. 917.

8. Vatican Council II, "Pastoral Constitution on the Church in the Modern World," no. 11, p. 912.

9. *Vatican Council II*, "Dogmatic Constitution on Divine Revelation," no. 8, pp. 754–55.

10. Cf. *Vatican Council II*, "Dogmatic Constitution on the Church," no. 25, pp. 379–81.

11. Congregation for the Doctrine of the Faith, "Instruction on the Ecclesial Vocation of the Theologian," *Origins* 20:8 (July 5, 1990).

12. *op. cit.*

13. Cf. Francis A. Sullivan, *Magisterium: Teaching Authority in the Catholic Church*, (Mahwah, NJ: Paulist Press, 1983); John Boyle, *Church Teaching Authority*, (Notre Dame, IN: University of Notre Dame Press, 1995).

14. Cf. John Paul II, Apostolic Letter *Ad Tuendam Fidem Origins* 28: no. 8 (July 16, 1998).

15. *Vatican II*, "Pastoral Constitution on the Church in the Modern World," no. 43, p. 944.

16. Congregation for the Doctrine of the Faith, "Instruction on the Ecclesial Vocation of the Theologian," *Origins* 20: no. 8 (July 5, 1990), pp. 117–126.

17.

18. Cf. National Conference of Catholic Bishops Committee for Pro-Life Activities, "Nutrition and Hydration: Moral and Pastoral Reflections," *Origins* 21: no. 44 (Apr. 9, 1992), pp. 705–12.

19. Pope John Paul II, "The Gospel of Life," no. 55, *Origins* 24: no. 42 (Apr. 6, 1995), pp. 708–09.

Part II: Specific Teachings of the Church

3: Abortion

DOCUMENT 1:

SOURCE: Pope John Paul II, "The Gospel of Life" (Mar. 25, 1995), *Origins* 24: no. 42, Apr. 6, 1995, pp. 696, 710, 711, 723.

18. . . . Decisions that go against life sometimes arise from difficult or even tragic situations of profound suffering, loneliness, a total lack of economic prospects, depression, and anxiety about the future. Such circumstances can mitigate even to a notable degree subjective responsibility and the consequent culpability of those who make these choices, which in themselves are evil. But today the problem goes far beyond the necessary recognition of these personal situations. It is a problem which exists at the cultural, social and political level, where it reveals its more sinister and disturbing aspect in the tendency, ever more widely shared, to interpret the above crimes against life as legitimate expressions of individual freedom, to be acknowledged and protected as actual rights. . . .

19. . . . We can find them in an overall assessment of a cultural and moral nature, beginning with the mentality which carries the concept of subjectivity to an extreme and even distorts it, and recognizes as a subject of rights only the person who enjoys full or at least incipient autonomy and who emerges from a state of total dependence on others. But how can we reconcile this approach with the exaltation of man as a being who is "not to be used"? The theory of human rights is based precisely on the affirmation that the human person, unlike animals and things, cannot be subjected to domination by others. We must also mention the mentality which tends to equate personal dignity with the capacity for verbal and explicit, or at least perceptible, communication. It is clear that on the basis of these presuppositions there is no place in the world for anyone who, like the unborn or the dying, is a weak element in the social structure, or for anyone who appears completely at the mercy of others and radically dependent on them, and can only communicate through the silent language of a profound sharing of affection. In this case it is force which becomes the criterion for choice and action in interpersonal relations and in social life. But this is the exact opposite of what a state ruled by law, as a community in which the "reasons of force" are replaced by the "force of reason," historically intended to affirm.

At another level, the roots of the contradiction between the solemn affirmation of human rights and their tragic denial in practice lie in a notion of freedom which exalts the isolated individual in an absolute way and gives no place to solidarity, to openness to others and service of them. While it is true

32 that the taking of life not yet born or in its final stages is sometimes marked by a mistaken sense of altruism and human compassion, it cannot be denied that such a culture of death, taken as a whole, betrays a completely individualistic concept of freedom, which ends up by becoming the freedom of "the strong" against the weak who have no choice but to submit. . . .

58. . . . The moral gravity of procured abortion is apparent in all its truth if we recognize that we are dealing with murder and, in particular, when we consider the specific elements involved. The one eliminated is a human being at the very beginning of life. No one more absolutely innocent could be imagined. In no way could this human being ever be considered an aggressor, much less an unjust aggressor! He or she is weak, defenseless, even to the point of lacking that minimal form of defense consisting in the poignant power of a newborn baby's cries and tears. The unborn child is totally entrusted to the protection and care of the woman carrying him or her in the womb. And yet sometimes it is precisely the mother herself who makes the decision and asks for the child to be eliminated, and who then goes about having it done.

It is true that the decision to have an abortion is often tragic and painful for the mother insofar as the decision to rid herself of the fruit of conception is not made for purely selfish reasons or out of convenience, but out of a desire to protect certain important values such as her own health or a decent standard of living for the other members of the family. Sometimes it is feared that the child to be born would live in such conditions that it would be better if the birth did not take place. Nevertheless, these reasons and others like them, however serious and tragic, can never justify the deliberate killing of an innocent human being.

61. . . . Even scientific and philosophical discussions about the precise moment of the infusion of the spiritual soul have never given rise to any hesitation about the moral condemnation of abortion.

62. . . . The revised canonical legislation continues this tradition when it decrees that "a person who actually procures an abortion incurs automatic (*latae sententiae*) excommunication. . . ." In the Church the purpose of the penalty of excommunication is to make an individual fully aware of the gravity of a certain sin and then to foster genuine conversion and repentance.

. . . Therefore, by the authority which Christ conferred upon Peter and his successors, in communion with the bishops—who on various occasions have condemned abortion and who in the aforementioned consultation, albeit dispersed throughout the world, have shown unanimous agreement concerning this doctrine—I declare that direct abortion, that is, abortion willed as an end or as a means, always constitutes a grave moral disorder, since it is the deliberate killing of an innocent human being. This doctrine is based upon the natural law and upon the written word of God, is transmitted by the Church's tradition and taught by the ordinary and universal magisterium. . . .

99. . . . I would now like to say a special word to women who have had an abortion. The Church is aware of the many factors which may have influenced your decision, and she does not doubt that in many cases it was a painful and even shattering decision. The wound in your heart may not yet have

healed. Certainly what happened was and remains terribly wrong. But do not give in to discouragement and do not lose hope. Try rather to understand what happened and face it honestly. If you have not already done so, give yourselves over with humility and trust to repentance. The Father of mercies is ready to give you his forgiveness and his peace in the sacrament of reconciliation. You will come to understand that nothing is definitively lost, and you will also be able to ask forgiveness from your child, who is now living in the Lord. With the friendly and expert help and advice of other people and as a result of your own painful experience, you can be among the most eloquent defenders of everyone's right to life. Through your commitment to life, whether by accepting the birth of other children or by welcoming and caring for those most in need of someone to be close to them, you will become promoters of a new way of looking at human life.

DOCUMENT 2 / Abortion

Source: Pope Pius XI, *Encyclical Letter on Christian Marriage* (Dec. 31, 1930), *The Human Body: Papal Teachings*, pp. 31–34.

... Another very grave crime is to be noted ... which regards the taking of the life of the offspring hidden in the mother's womb. Some wish it to be allowed and left to the will of the father or the mother; others say it is unlawful unless there are weighty reasons which they call by the name of medical, social, or eugenic "indication." Because this matter falls under the penal laws of the state by which the destruction of the offspring begotten but unborn is forbidden, these people demand that the "indication," which in one form or another they defend, be recognized as such by the public law and in no way penalized. There are those, moreover, who ask that the public authorities provide aid for these death-dealing operations, a thing, which, sad to say, everyone knows is of very frequent occurrence in some places.

As to the "medical and therapeutic indication" to which, using their own words, we have made reference ... however much we may pity the mother whose health and even life is gravely imperiled in the performance of the duty allotted to her by nature, nevertheless what could ever be a sufficient reason for excusing in any way the direct murder of the innocent? This is precisely what we are dealing with here. Whether inflicted upon the mother or upon the child, it is against the precept of God and the law of nature: "Thou shalt not kill." The life of each is equally sacred, and no one has the power, not even the public authority, to destroy it. It is of no use to appeal to the right of taking away life for here it is a question of the innocent, whereas that right has regard only to the guilty; nor is there here question of defense of bloodshed against an unjust aggressor (for who would call an innocent child an unjust aggressor?); again there is no question here of what is called the "law of extreme necessity" which could even extend to the direct killing of the innocent. Upright and skillful doctors strive most praiseworthily to guard and preserve the lives of both mother and child; on the contrary, those show themselves most unworthy of the noble medical profession who encompass the death of one or the other, through a pretense at practicing medicine or through motives of misguided pity.

All of which agrees with the stern words of the Bishop of Hippo in denouncing those wicked parents who seek to remain childless, and failing in this, are not ashamed to put their offspring to death: "Sometimes this lustful cruelty or cruel lust goes so far as to seek to procure a baneful sterility, and if this fails the fetus conceived in the womb is in one way or another smothered or evacuated, in the desire to destroy the offspring before it has life, or if it already lives in the womb, to kill it before it is born. If both man and woman are party to such practices, they are not spouses at all; and if from the first they have carried on thus, they have come together not for honest wedlock,

but for impure gratification; if both are not party to these deeds, I make bold
to say that either the one makes herself a mistress of the husband, or the other
simply the paramour of his wife."

What is asserted in favor of the social and eugenic "indication" may and
must be accepted, provided lawful and upright methods are employed within
the proper limits; but to wish to put forward reasons based upon them for
the killing of the innocent is unthinkable and contrary to the divine precept
promulgated in the words of the apostle: Evil is not to be done that good may
come of it.

Those who hold the reins of government should not forget that it is the
duty of public authority by appropriate laws and sanctions to defend the lives
of the innocent, and this all the more so since those whose lives are endangered
and assailed cannot defend themselves. Among whom we must mention in
the first place infants hidden in the mother's womb. And if the public magis-
trates not only do not defend them, but by their laws and ordinances betray
them to death at the hands of doctors or of others, let them remember that God
is the judge and avenger of innocent blood which cries from earth to heaven.

DOCUMENT 3 / Abortion

SOURCE: Congregation for the Doctrine of the Faith, "Declaration on Procured Abortion" (Nov. 18, 1974), *Vatican Council II*, Vol. 2, 1982, pp. 441–43.

INTRODUCTION

1. The problem of procured abortion and of its possible legal liberalization has become almost everywhere the subject of impassioned discussions. These debates would be less important were it not a question of human life, a primordial value, which must be protected and promoted. . . .

. . . The Church is too conscious of the fact that it belongs to her vocation to defend man against everything that could destroy or diminish his dignity to remain silent on such a topic. . . .

IN THE LIGHT OF FAITH

5. "Death was not God's doing, he takes no pleasure in the extinction of the living" (Wis 1:13). Certainly God has created beings who have only one lifetime and physical death cannot be absent from the world of those with a bodily existence. But what is immediately willed is life, and in the visible universe everything has been made for man, who is the image of God and the world's crowning glory (cf. Gn 1:26–28). On the human level, "it was the devil's envy that brought death into the world" (Wis 2:24). Introduced by sin, death remains bound up with it: death is the sign and fruit of sin. But there is no final triumph for death. Confirming faith in the resurrection, the Lord proclaims in the Gospel: "God is God, not of the dead, but of the living" (Mt 22:32). And death like sin will be definitively defeated by resurrection in Christ (cf. 1 Cor 15:20–27). Thus we understand that human life, even on this earth, is precious. Infused by the creator, life is again taken back by him (cf. Gn 2:7; Wis 15:11). It remains under his protection: man's blood cries out to him (cf. Gn 4:10) and he will demand an account of it, "for in the image of God man was made" (Gn 9:5–6). The commandment of God is formal: "You shall not kill" (Ex 20:13). Life is at the same time a gift and a responsibility. It is received as a "talent" (cf. Mt 25:14–30); it must be put to proper use. In order that life may bring forth fruit, many tasks are offered to man in this world and he must not shirk them. More important still, the Christian knows that eternal life depends on what, with the grace of God, he does with his life on earth.

6. The tradition of the Church has always held that human life must be protected and cherished from the beginning, just as at the various stages of its development. . . .

. . . In the *Didache* it is clearly said: "You shall not kill by abortion the fruit of the womb and you shall not murder the infant already born. . . ."

7. In the course of history, the fathers of the Church, her pastors and her doctors have taught the same doctrine—the various opinions on the infusion

of the spiritual soul did not cast doubt on the illicitness of abortion. It is true 37
that in the Middle Ages, when the opinion was generally held that the spiritual
soul was not present until after the first few weeks, a distinction was made in
the evaluation of the sin and the gravity of penal sanctions. In resolving cases,
approved authors were more lenient with regard to that early stage than with
regard to later stages. But it was never denied at that time that procured
abortion, even during the first days, was objectively a grave sin. This condemnation was in fact unanimous . . . . Most recently, the Second Vatican Council,
presided over by Paul VI, has most severely condemned abortion: "Life must
be safeguarded with extreme care from conception; abortion and infanticide
are abominable crimes. . . ."

IN THE ADDITIONAL LIGHT OF REASON

8. Respect for human life is not just a Christian obligation. Human reason
is sufficient to impose it on the basis of the analysis of what a human person
is and should be. Constituted by a rational nature, man is a person, a subject
capable of reflecting on himself and of determining his acts and hence his own
destiny: he is free. . . .

11. The first right of the human person is his life. He has other goods and
some are more precious, but this one is fundamental—the condition of all the
others. It does not belong to society, nor does it belong to public authority in
any form to recognize this right for some and not for others: all discrimination
is evil, whether it be founded on race, sex, color or religion. It is not recognition
by another that constitutes this right. This right is antecedent to its recognition;
it demands recognition and it is strictly unjust to refuse it.

12. . . . The right to life is no less to be respected in the small infant just
born than in the mature person. In reality, respect for human life is called for
from the time that the process of generation begins. From the time that the
ovum is fertilized, a life is begun which is neither that of the father nor of the
mother; it is rather the life of a new human being with his own growth. It
would never be made human if it were not human already.

13. This has always been clear, and discussions about the moment of
animation have no bearing on it. . . .[19]

---

[19] This declaration expressly leaves aside the question of the moment when the
spiritual soul is infused. There is not a unanimous tradition on this point and authors
are as yet in disagreement. For some it dates from the first instant, for others it could
not at least precede nidation. It is not within the competence of science to decide between
these views, because the existence of an immortal soul is not a question in its field. It
is a philosophical problem from which our moral affirmation remains independent for
two reasons: (1) supposing a later animation, there is still nothing less than a *human*
life, preparing for and calling for a soul in which the nature received from parents is
completed; (2) on the other hand it suffices that this presence of the soul be probable
(and one can never prove the contrary) in order that the taking of life involve accepting
the risk of killing a man, not only waiting for, but already in possession of his soul.

38   **REPLY TO SOME OBJECTIONS**

14. Divine law and natural reason, therefore, exclude all right to the direct killing of an innocent man. However, if the reasons given to justify an abortion were always manifestly evil and valueless the problem would not be so dramatic. The gravity of the problem comes from the fact that in certain cases, perhaps in quite a considerable number of cases, by denying abortion one endangers important values which men normally hold in great esteem and which may sometimes even seem to have priority. We do not deny these very great difficulties. It may be a serious question of health, sometimes of life or death, for the mother; it may be the burden represented by an additional child, especially if there are good reasons to fear that the child will be abnormal or retarded; it may be the importance attributed in different classes of society to considerations of honor or dishonor, of loss of social standing, and so forth. We proclaim only that none of these reasons can ever objectively confer the right to dispose of another's life, even when that life is only beginning. . . .

DOCUMENT 4 / Abortion

SOURCE: Congregation for the Doctrine of the Faith, "Instruction on Respect for Human Life in Its Origin and on the Dignity of Procreation" (Feb. 22, 1987), *Origins* 16: no. 40, Mar. 19, 1987, pp. 701–02.

... This Congregation is aware of the current debates concerning the beginning of human life, concerning the individuality of the human being, and concerning the identity of the human person. The Congregation recalls the teachings found in the *Declaration on Procured Abortion*: "From the time that the ovum is fertilized, a new life is begun which is neither that of the father nor of the mother; it is rather the life of a new human being with his own growth. It would never be made human if it were not human already. To this perpetual evidence ... modern genetic science brings valuable confirmation. It has demonstrated that, from the first instant, the program is fixed as to what this living being will be: a man, this individual man with his characteristic aspects already well determined. Right from fertilization is begun the adventure of a human life, and each of its great capacities requires time ... to find its place and to be in a position to act."

This teaching remains valid and is further confirmed, if confirmation were needed, by recent findings of human biological science which recognize that in the zygote resulting from fertilization the biological identity of a new human individual is already constituted.

Certainly no experimental datum can be in itself sufficient to bring us to the recognition of a spiritual soul; nevertheless, the conclusions of science regarding the human embryo provide a valuable indication for discerning by the use of reason a personal presence at the moment of this first appearance of a human life: how could a human individual not be a human person? The Magisterium has not expressly committed itself to an affirmation of a philosophical nature, but it constantly reaffirms the moral condemnation of any kind of procured abortion. This teaching has not been changed and is unchangeable.

Thus the fruit of human generation, from the first moment of its existence, that is to say from the moment the zygote has formed, demands the unconditional respect that is morally due to the human being in his bodily and spiritual totality. The human being is to be respected and treated as a person from the moment of conception; and therefore from that same moment his rights as a person must be recognized, among which in the first place is the inviolable right of every innocent human being to life.

This doctrinal reminder provides the fundamental criterion for the solution of the various problems posed by the development of the biomedical sciences in this field: since the embryo must be treated as a person, it must also be defended in its integrity, tended and cared for, to the extent possible, in the same way as any other human being as far as assistance is concerned. **39**

DOCUMENT 5 / Abortion

Source: National Conference of Catholic Bishops Ad Hoc Committee on Pro-Life Activities, "Pastoral Guidelines for the Catholic Hospital and Catholic Health Care Personnel" (Apr. 11, 1973), *Pastoral Letters of the United States Catholic Bishops,* Vol. III, 1983, pp. 370–74.

1. The decision of the U.S. Supreme Court on Jan. 22, 1973, in regard to the abortion laws of Texas and Georgia radically changed the legal and political discussion of the past decade. For all practical purposes, the Court has given its approval to abortion on request, and the sweeping opinion of the Court has left many states in legal disarray regarding abortion.

2. Legally, the question of responsibility has been made ambiguous by the Court's opinion. The Supreme Court held that the right of privacy encompasses a woman's decision to obtain an abortion. The Court also stated that the abortion decision is "primarily a medical decision and basic responsibility for it must rest with the physician." In its opinion, during the first three months, once the woman has decided to abort and the physician has been consulted, anyone may perform the abortion procedure. Thus according the the Court, in such a case the physician is primarily and basically responsible, though he may have the least to do with the abortion itself.

3. In terms of moral teaching, the American bishops have declared that the "opinion of the Court is wrong and is entirely contrary to the fundamental principles of morality. . . . Whenever a conflict arises between the law of God and any human law we are held to follow God's law." Catholics, then, may not obey laws that require them to act in violation of their conscience.

4. Catholic hospitals cannot comply with laws requiring them to provide abortion services; and Catholic physicians, nurses, and health care workers who work in facilities that provide abortions and sterilizations may not take part in such procedures in good conscience. Thus, in light of the legal safeguards respecting the moral responsibilities of Catholic hospitals and health care personnel, there is reason for a specific application of moral principles.

5. In this analysis, the application of the moral principles on conscientious objection to abortion is approached in terms of the *responsibilities* of Catholic hospitals and health care personnel to give witness to their faith and moral convictions, and the *restrictions* imposed by moral convictions on policies and behavior. Sterilization is treated separately, and a special section is added on excommunication.

I. Principles of Responsibility for Catholic Hospitals

1. Catholic hospitals must witness to the sanctity of life, the integrity of the human person, and the value of human life at every stage of its existence.

2. Catholic hospitals should commit themselves to a special effort in   **41**
providing compassion and care for pregnant women and their unborn children.
This would include providing a full range of prenatal, obstetric, and postnatal
services. It would also involve spiritual assistance and sacramental administration. In this regard, the designation of sisters or nurses as special ministers of
the Eucharist in keeping with the latest norms of the Holy See might be especially helpful in making it possible for women to receive the Eucharist frequently
during their stay in the hospital (cf. *Immensae Caritatis*, Sacred Congregation
of the Sacraments, Jan. 29, 1973).

3. Catholic hospitals should show a willingness to extend privileges to
physicians and health care workers who share this commitment to serving
life, particularly in situations where such health care workers find that their
opposition to abortion or sterilization procedures places them at a disadvantage
in other hospitals or facilities.

4. Catholic hospitals must give public notice of their commitment to the
sanctity of life and their refusal to provide abortion or sterilization services.

5. The Catholic hospital has a responsibility to clearly enunciate its policies
for all physicians holding privileges and for all health care personnel employed
by the hospital.

II. Responsibilities of Physicians, Nurses, and Health Care Workers

1. Physicians, nurses, and health care workers should give public witness
to their belief in the sanctity of life, the integrity of every person, and the value
of human life at every stage of its existence by their compassion and care for
their patients.

2. Physicians, nurses, and health care workers should provide encouragement and support for women and their children. They should be especially
attentive to the tensions created for women by society's depreciation of the
value of life. When advisable, they should seek the assistance of the chaplain
in making available the Church's spiritual assistance and sacramental administration.

3. Physicians, nurses, and health care workers who work in hospitals that
provide abortion or sterilization services should notify the hospital in writing
of their conscientious refusal to participate in such actions. When efforts are
made to compel participation in these procedures, health care personnel should
protest this violation of conscience to their superiors and to the administrator.

4. In their professional associations and contacts, Catholic physicians,
nurses, and health care workers should candidly and charitably explain their
convictions to their colleagues when called upon to do so. Charity also requires
that they refrain from judging the motives of their colleagues or patients who
do not agree with or will not accept their conscientious convictions. Catholics
must expect that their faith and moral convictions on the sanctity of life may
result in their being misjudged, treated unfairly, or alienated. Such is the price
of Christian witness in today's world.

5. An aborted fetus showing signs of life, at any stage of pregnancy, is
entitled to Baptism.

42   III. Restrictions that Follow from Moral Convictions

1. No Catholic hospital may provide abortion services, nor may any Catholic hospital make its facilities or personnel available for abortions.

2. A Catholic hospital should make it clear to all staff and health care workers that abortions and sterilizations are prohibited, and that agreement to this policy is a condition for privileges.

3. Abortion, the deliberate expulsion of the fetus from the womb of its mother to terminate the pregnancy, is a serious and immoral action. Catholics who perform or obtain abortions, or persuade others to do so, commit a serious sin. Among those who assist the woman, primary responsibility for the abortion procedure rests with the doctor who advises and/or assists the woman to have an abortion.

4. All who willingly and deliberately assist in abortion procedures share the sinfulness of the abortive act. This is particularly true of the attending surgeon and the health care personnel who administer abortifacient drugs or other abortion procedures.

5. Nurses and health care personnel may not assist in abortion procedures. Particular questions of conscience should be taken up with a confessor.

6. Cooperation in the sinful act of abortion would not ordinarily extend to preparing patients for the procedure or providing after-care. However, because in many instances abortion is promoted as an alternate method of birth control and thus a denial of the value of the child, the cooperation of the Catholic health care worker may be interpreted as agreement that the unborn child is of subordinate value and has no right to life. Christian witness may well require Catholic nurses to avoid even those actions that—although not necessarily evil—may be interpreted as a compromise of Christian values.

EXCOMMUNICATION

1. Because abortion is a serious evil, both for those who take part in it and for society, the Church has sought to dissuade people from utilizing it by placing it in a special moral category. Under Church law, those who perform or obtain an abortion or deliberately persuade others to do so place themselves in a state of excommunication. Ordinarily this involves the woman who obtains an abortion, the doctor who performs the abortion, the person who persuades a woman to have an abortion, and any person who cooperates to the extent that the abortion would not otherwise take place without his or her cooperation.

2. Excommunication is a special penalty, and conditions under which it applies must be strictly interpreted. Generally it does not apply to nurses and other assistants, nor can it be extended to legislators. It does not apply in any way to sterilization procedures.

CONCLUSION

1. Human life exists in a person, who must be respected and cared for and, at times, reconciled to God and the community. Catholic hospitals and health care workers have distinguished themselves in the past in the provision of competent medical care motivated by respect for the person and Christian

charity. Along with the added responsibilities they will face in an increasingly 43
permissive abortion atmosphere there are also opportunities for Christian witness, for competent care based on charity, for encouraging women and health
care workers who refuse to take part in abortions, and for reconciling and
showing mercy to those who have failed. Now, more than in the past, Catholic
health care workers, and perhaps especially those in hospitals not under Catholic auspices, will be ministers of God's word and mediators of his grace. They
deserve the support and assistance of the entire Church.

2. Finally, though these guidelines have attempted to cover a wide range
of problems, there are many cases that do not fall within the specified categories.
In these cases, the standard principles of moral theology need to be applied.
Parish priests, hospital chaplains, and sisters involved in the ministry to the
sick should be available to explain and apply the principles and to encourage
and support doctors, nurses, and health care workers.

4: Addiction

DOCUMENT 1:

Source: Pontifical Council for the Family, "From Despair to Hope: Family and Drug Addiction," *Origins* 22: no. 12, Sept. 3, 1992, pp. 206–13.

. . . We do not intend to deal with the drug problem in an exhaustive manner. There are already many serious studies about this. We simply wish to highlight certain aspects of our educative and pastoral mission and make public the widespread concern and hope which motivates all of us.

. . . Here we mention only some aspects of this complex and distressing problem. Specifically, we refer to the following: the person, the family and society.

A. THE PERSON

Drugs are not the drug user's main problem. Drug consumption is merely a deceptive answer to the lack of a positive meaning of life. The human person, unique and unrepeatable, with his or her own interior life and specific personality, is really at the center of the problem of drug dependence. However, the person is the object of the love of God the Father, who in his redemptive plan calls each one to the sublime vocation of being a son in the Son. Yet, by drug use, the realization of this vocation is gravely compromised, together with happiness in this world. The reason is that drug addiction has deleterious effects upon mental receptivity and the correct use of the intellect and will of the human person who is the "image of God" (Gn 1:27).

. . . There are many personal motives which lead individuals to begin using drugs. However, in every user—whatever their age and frequency of drug use—there is one constant basic motive: a certain crisis of values and the person's lack of interior harmony. Different combinations of motives, according to personal weaknesses, in every drug user render him or her incapable of living a normal life. An "unmotivated" and "indifferent" state of mind is created in the drug user, unleashing an internal moral and spiritual imbalance. This produces an immature and weak character which causes the drug user to take on unstable attitudes toward his or her own responsibilities.

. . . Certain specialists have observed that drug users live in a mental state equivalent to an endless adolescence. This state of immaturity originates and develops within the context of defective upbringing. The immature person is one who often comes from families which, even in spite of the parents' will, did not succeed in transmitting values. These families failed either because they did not exercise adequate authority or because they found themselves living in a "passive" society, with a lifestyle which is consumerist and permissive, secularized and without ideals. Basically, the drug user is one who is sick because of a lack of love: He or she did not know love; he or she does not know how to love correctly because he or she was never loved correctly.

. . . The endless adolescence, characteristic of the drug user, is frequently manifested in a fear of the future or in the refusal of new responsibilities. The behavior of these young people often reveals the manifestation of a painful helplessness due to a lack of trust and expectation with regard to social structures to which they no longer feel they belong. Who can be blamed if many young people have no desire to grow up and become adults? Have these young people been given sufficient reason to hope in tomorrow, to invest in the present so as to gain in the future, to be stable, feeling solidly grounded in a past which they feel belongs to them? Nonetheless, hidden behind shocking attitudes, often deviant and unacceptable, one can perceive a spark of idealism and hope in these people.

B. THE FAMILY

Among the personal and environmental factors which contribute to drug use, the principal one is, without a doubt, the absolute or relative lack of family life. The family is the key element in the formation of a person's character and attitudes toward society. Let us consider some of these more important factors.

The drug user frequently comes from a family which does not know how to react to stress because it is unstable, incomplete or divided. Today the negative effects of matrimonial and family crises are increasing alarmingly: easy separation and divorce, living together, the inability to give a well-rounded upbringing to prepare one for facing ordinary problems, the lack of dialogue, etc. Factors that can predispose for the choice of drugs are periods of silence, fear to communicate, competitiveness, consumerism, stress resulting from excessive work, selfishness; in a word, the inability to raise children in an open and wholesome way. In many cases children do not feel understood and find themselves without family support. Furthermore, faith and the value of suffering and sacrifice, so important for maturation, are presented as negative values. Parents who are not up to their task constitute a real shortcoming with regard to the formation of their children's character. And what is to be said about the warped and deviant behavior of certain families in the area of sexuality.

. . . Besides the family of origin, special attention must also be given to the family established by the drug users themselves. In many instances these couples are composed of partners, both of whom are users. Many of these, although still young, are already separated or divorced or merely living together. In this context the problems of drug users' children take on particular importance, especially their upbringing. The problems of the orphan children of deceased drug users are also important.

Particular attention must be given to pregnant women who are drug users. Many of them are unwed or simply abandoned. Unfortunately, abortion is often proposed to them instead of coming to their aid with concrete solidarity and assistance so that they may accept the life of the child and respect it.

46 C. SOCIETY

Such widespread drug dependence is an indication of the current state of society. Today the person and the family find themselves living in a "passive" society, that is to say, a society without ideals, permissive, secularized, where the search for escape expresses itself in so many different ways, of which one is the flight to drug addiction.

The age we live in exalts a freedom which "is no longer seen positively as a striving for good . . . , but is rather defined as an emancipation from all conditions which prevent each one from following his own reason." Utilitarianism and hedonism, together with individualism and selfishness, are extolled. The quest for an illusory good under the banner of the greatest pleasure ends up by favoring the strongest and creates conditions of frustration and dependence among the majority of citizens. In this way, reference to moral values and to God himself is erased both in society and in human relations.

In today's society an artificial consumerism, which is contrary to the health and dignity of man and favors the spread of drugs, has taken root (cf. *Centesimus Annus*, N. 36). This consumerism creates false needs and urges man, especially the young, to seek satisfaction only in material goods, thus causing dependence on them. Furthermore, a certain economic exploitation of young people easily spreads in this materialistic and consumerist context. In many places, youth unemployment favors the spread of drug dependence.

No attentive observer fails to notice that today's society favors the promotion of unbridled hedonism and a confused meaning of sexuality. The exercise of sexuality has been separated from conjugal communion and from its intrinsic orientation to procreation, so that all that remains is a superficial enjoyment to which even the dignity of persons is often subordinated.

In a society in search of immediate gratification and personal convenience at all costs, a society which is more interested in "having" than in "being," it is not surprising that its culture of death considers abortion and euthanasia as goods and rights. The meaning of life has been lost, and the person is emptied of his dignity, which leads to frustration and a one-way street to self-destruction. In such a society, drugs are an easy and immediate but deceptive answer to the human need for satisfaction and true love.

. . . The mass media often exercise a negative influence favoring the spread of drug use, above all among young people. With direct and indirect messages, and through the industry of entertaining the young, the mass media create models, set up idols and define "normality" by means of a system of pseudo values. In this way the young absorb a bizarre and distorted concept of life and society. Moreover, we should not overlook the violence which is served up to the public every day in particular video cassettes.

Some of us participating in this meeting are convinced that there is danger, on the part of the mass media, of presenting an image of the drug user which only leads to criminalizing him or her as the one alone who is to blame. The talents, intelligence and other capabilities of so many young drug users cannot be denied; and these should be taken into consideration in any rehabilitation initiative.

. . . Given the religious implications of the problems connected with drugs, in speaking about responsibility one cannot fail to mention the silence, lack of action and inadequacies that still exist in the pastoral care of the Church in the area of drugs.

Under the aspects of person, family and society, the drug phenomenon highlights the urgent need for "wisdom" to regain an awareness of the primacy of the moral values concerning the person. The Holy Father, John Paul II, affirms: "The great task that has to be faced today for the renewal of society is that of recapturing the ultimate meaning of life and its fundamental values. . . . The education of the moral conscience, which makes every human being capable of judging and of discerning the proper ways to achieve self-realization according to his or her original truth, thus becomes a pressing requirement that cannot be renounced" (*Familiaris Consortio*, 8). With the help of this wisdom the new emerging culture "will not distract people from their relationship with God, but will lead them to it more fully" (ibid.). This is the authentic "new humanism," which can only be "an authentic family humanism," to which pertains a "new mentality . . . essentially positive, inspired by the great values of life and man" (ibid.).

5: Aging

DOCUMENT 1:

SOURCE: National Conference of Catholic Bishops, "Society and the Aged: Toward Reconciliation" (May 5, 1976), *Pastoral Letters of the United States Catholic Bishops*, Vol. IV, 1984, pp.138–42.

I. The Aged

1. America today faces a great paradox: It is an aging nation which worships the culture, values, and appearance of youth. Instead of viewing old age as an achievement and a natural stage of life with its own merits, wisdom, and beauty, American society all too often ignores, rejects, and isolates the elderly.

4. . . . The elderly are denied their God-given right to develop their potential to the fullest at every stage of life; at the same time, society is denied the fruits of that development.

II. Human Rights and the Elderly

10. The elderly do not forfeit their claim to basic human rights because they are old. . . .

> "Every man has the right to life, to bodily integrity, and to the means which are suitable for the proper development of life; these are primarily food, clothing, shelter, rest, medical care, and finally the necessary social services. Therefore, a human being also has the right to security in cases of sickness, inability to work, widowhood, old age, unemployment, or in any other case in which he is deprived of the means of subsistence through no fault of his own." (Pope John XXIII, *Peace on Earth*)

A. The Right to Life

12. On one level, the elderly, along with the sick and the handicapped, are the targets of a "mercy killing" mentality which would dispose of the unwanted. Even well-meaning legislative efforts to cope with complex questions about when and when not to use extraordinary technological and therapeutic means to preserve life pose genuine dangers, particularly since some would place fateful decisions solely in the hands of physicians or the state.

15. The elderly have a right to "new life": not just to material survival, but to education, recreation, companionship, honest human emotions, and spiritual care and comfort.

D. The Right to Health Care

21. Health care is a basic right, but it is often regarded as an expensive luxury. Despite passage a decade ago of Medicare, millions of elderly people still lack adequate medical care.

24. Nursing home care is a serious problem. Well-publicized scandals 49 have arisen concerning the operations of some nursing homes, where patient care is sacrificed while operators amass huge profits. Large numbers of elderly people are institutionalized needlessly for want of simple services, such as visiting nurses or homemakers, which would help them remain in their homes.

25. Mental health care for the elderly is even more inadequate than physical health care. An estimated one-third of the elderly in mental hospitals are there because they have nowhere else to go. Physical illnesses such as diabetes, anemia, or simply over-medication may produce behavior patterns in the elderly which are mistaken for senility.

E. The Right to Eat

26. A 1971 Administration Task Force on Aging declared that the elderly are the most severely malnourished group in society. Poor nutrition is a major factor in the incidence of poor health among them.

27. The food stamp program, hot meals program, and other efforts are a help to the elderly, but they still do not reach all those in need. The elderly are also threatened by new food stamp proposals. Some would increase the amount the elderly must pay for food stamps or create unreasonable assets limitations which would force them either to forfeit food stamps or sell their valuables, possibly their homes; other proposed regulations determining food stamp benefit levels could result in a decrease in benefits for many of the elderly.

28. Inadequate income is not the only reason why many of the elderly have poor diets. Lack of proper kitchen facilities, nutrition education, or simple lack of companionship and incentive to eat are also factors.

III. The Role of the Church
D. As Public Policy Advocates

51. Many of the needs of the elderly will only be met adequately when the needs of others are met through a national policy guaranteeing full employment, a decent income for those unable to work, equitable tax legislation, and comprehensive health care for all. . . .

6: AIDS

DOCUMENT 1:

Source: John Paul II, "Africa's AIDS Crisis," *Origins* 22: no. 36 (Feb. 18, 1993), pp. 613–14.

... Dear brothers and sisters, because of our incorporation into Christ through baptism Christians are given a share in the mystery of Christ's cross, the mystery by which he chose to redeem the world. Because it was by suffering that Jesus brought grace and mercy to us all, each of us "is also called to share in that suffering through which the redemption was accomplished" (*Salvifici Doloris*, 19). Through the cross a transcendent dimension and salvific meaning has been brought to human suffering, giving it a purpose and value never before imagined. "Thus, each man, in his suffering, can also become a sharer in the redemptive suffering of Christ" (ibid.).

Christians are therefore invited to look not merely at themselves, but to see with the eyes of faith the great good that can be accomplished if they offer their sufferings in union with the cross of Christ as a pleasing sacrifice to God our Father. How many people there are in Uganda who can be helped by our prayers! I am thinking of the orphans, the young men seeking employment, the families struggling to survive, the people addicted to alcohol or drugs, the men and women who have never heard the Gospel of Christ, the elderly, the lonely and especially those whose illness may be even greater than our own. "I appeal to you, therefore, brethren, by the mercies of God, to present your bodies as a living sacrifice, holy and acceptable to God, which is your spiritual worship" (Rom 12: 1).

Those who generously embrace the cross of Jesus Christ and offer their sufferings in union with the saving power of his eternal sacrifice can help bring new life to the people of Uganda and to men and women throughout the world. St. Paul saw clearly how much the Church was enriched by the sufferings of Christians when they are borne with patience and love: "Now I rejoice in my sufferings for your sake, and in my flesh I complete what is lacking in Christ's afflictions for the sake of his body, that is, the church" (Col 1:24). The Church needs the spiritual gift which only the sick are able to offer. Bear your sufferings in union with the Lord, confident that one day you will be glorified with him. For "the sufferings of the present time are not worth comparing with the glory that is to be revealed to us" (Rom 8:18).

And now I would like to address in particular those among you who are suffering from AIDS. I know well that within one decade this dreaded disease

has already affected so many of your people and left thousands of children without parental care. Many of you are already bedridden, many others diag- **51** nosed as seropositive, others living in constant fear of contracting the disease. There is only one who can give you hope and confidence in the midst of such pain, fear and even death itself. He is Christ, who said: "Come to me, all you who labor and are heavy laden, and I will give you rest. Take my yoke upon you, and learn from me; for I am gentle and lowly in heart, and you will find rest for your souls. For my yoke is easy and my burden light" (Mt 11:28-30).

Never lose heart! At times the yoke may not seem easy or the burden light, but the Lord assures you, as he did St. Paul: "My grace is sufficient for you, for my power is made perfect in weakness" (2 Cor 12:9). Christ is at your side; do not doubt his presence or the strength of his grace!

The scourge of AIDS challenges everyone. As the bishops of Uganda have rightly observed, "This situation, which is affecting everyone, needs to be confronted in solidarity, with much love and care for the victims, with much generosity to the orphans and with much commitment to a renewed way of Christian moral living" (Pastoral letter "Let Your Light Shine," 28). Indeed all people of good will are called to reflect on the deeper social and moral issues associated with this disease. Parallel to the spread of AIDS, there is a dangerous crisis of values in some societies, as many people grow crippled in spirit, indifferent to the virtues and spiritual values which alone can guarantee true happiness and the authentic progress of society. This spiritual crisis especially affects the young, on whom the future of your country depends.

You who suffer from AIDS have an important role to play in this vital struggle for the well-being of your country! Offer your sufferings in union with Christ for your brothers and sisters who are especially at risk! Your suffering can be a grace-filled opportunity to bring about the moral rebirth of Ugandan society. I invoke the comforting and strengthening gifts of God's unfailing love upon those who suffer from AIDS and upon all those who are generously engaged in caring for them. At the same time I appeal to those who are working to find an effective scientific response to this illness not to delay and above all not to allow commercial considerations to detract from their committed efforts.

The cross and resurrection of Jesus Christ shed light on the true meaning and value of human suffering. The Lord invites everyone to join him on the road to Calvary and to share in the joy of Easter. On that journey we are never alone; the Blessed Virgin Mary, who stood at the foot of her Son's cross, is ever at our side. Invoking her intercession and that of St. Charles Lwanga and all the Uganda martyrs, I impart my apostolic blessing to you, your loved ones and all who care for you, as a pledge of God's grace and comfort.

DOCUMENT 2 / AIDS

SOURCE: United States Catholic Conference Administrative Board, "The Many Faces of AIDS: A Gospel Response" (Dec. 11, 1987), *Origins* 17: no. 28, Dec. 24, 1987, pp. 483–87.

. . . What does the Gospel tell us about these representative faces of AIDS?

First, Jesus has revealed to us that God is compassionate, not vengeful. Made in God's image and likeness, every human person is of inestimable worth. All human life is sacred, and its dignity must be respected and protected. The teaching of Jesus about human sexuality and the moral norms taught by the Church are not arbitrary impositions on human life, but disclosures of its depth.

Second, the Gospel acknowledges that disease and suffering are not restricted to one group or social class. Rather, the mystery of the human condition is such that, in one way or another, all will face pain, reversal, and ultimately the mystery of death itself. Seen through the eyes of faith, however, this mystery is not closed in upon itself. Through sharing in the cross of Christ, human suffering and pain have a redemptive meaning and goal. They have the potential of opening a person to new life. They also present an opportunity and a challenge to all, calling us to respond to suffering just as Jesus did—with love and care.

Third, while preaching a Gospel of compassion and conversion, Jesus also proclaimed to those most in need the good news of forgiveness. The father in the parable of the prodigal son did not wait for his son to come to him. Rather, he took the initiative and ran out to his son with generosity, forgiveness, and compassion. This spirit of forgiveness Jesus handed on to his followers.

For Christians, then, stories of persons with AIDS must not become occasions for stereotyping or prejudice, for anger or recrimination, for rejection or isolation, for injustice or condemnation. They provide us with an opportunity to walk with those who are suffering, to be compassionate toward those whom we might otherwise fear, to bring strength and courage both to those who face the prospect of dying as well as to their loved ones. . . .

Our reflections are threefold. First, we present some facts about AIDS and comment on what they say to us. Then we address issues associated with the prevention of the disease. Finally we explore appropriate care for persons with AIDS. At various points throughout this statement, we indicate the responsibilities and obligations of all the members of the Church and society. In an appendix we address certain significant related questions. All that we say in this statement is not intended to be the last word on AIDS, but rather our contribution to the current dialogue. . . .

. . . First, while it is understandable that there is fear and uncertainty about a disease as new and deadly as AIDS, we encourage all members of our society to relate to its victims with compassion and understanding, as they 53 would to those suffering from any other fatal disease.

Second, we are alarmed by the increase of negative attitudes as well as acts of violence directed against gay and lesbian people since AIDS has become a national issue. We strongly condemn such violence. Those who are gay or lesbian or suffering from AIDS should not be the objects of discrimination, injustice, or violence. All of God's sons and daughters, all members of our society, are entitled to the recognition of their full human dignity.

Third, because there is presently no positive or sound medical justification for the indiscriminate quarantining of persons infected with the AIDS virus, we oppose the enactment of quarantine legislation or other laws that are not supported by medical data or informed by the expertise of those in the health care or public health professions. The best of our civic heritage of extreme caution and restraint in restricting human and civil rights should be the norm in this situation as in all others. We urge legislators to act judiciously rather than to react out of a sense of hysteria or latent prejudice. Especially acute is the problem of health insurance. We decry the exclusion of certain groups of persons from health insurance coverage. At the same time we recognize the problems faced by the insurance industry as well as those who pay premiums because of the cost of treatment. This exemplifies the weakness of our health care delivery system. This problem must be addressed in a way that will provide adequate and accessible health care for all.

Fourth, we oppose the use of the HIV-antibody test for strictly discriminatory purposes. However, if safeguards are provided to prevent such discrimination and to maintain the needed degree of confidentiality, such tests may play an important role in basing patient care on facts rather than fear or stereotypes. Testing for the AIDS virus, with appropriate counseling beforehand and afterward, should be readily available to all who request it. Those who undergo such testing and receive a negative report can be reassured and educated on risk factors for contracting the virus. Those who receive a positive test result can be promptly offered counseling and care. There may be sound public health reasons for recommending the use of the HIV-antibody test in certain situations, either because some persons have a heightened risk of becoming infected or because precautions may have to be taken by others (e.g., prospective spouses, hospital staffs) if the test results are positive. Nevertheless, we agree with many public health authorities who question the appropriateness and effectiveness of more sweeping proposals such as widespread mandatory testing.

Fifth, we are greatly concerned that some in the health care professions or working in health care institutions refuse to provide medical or dental care for persons exposed to the AIDS virus or presumed to be "at risk." We call upon all in the health care and support professions to be mindful of their general moral obligation, while following accepted medical standards and procedures, to provide care for all persons, including those exposed to the AIDS virus. Similarly, although funeral directors may find it necessary to take appropriate precautions, they are not justified in refusing to accept or prepare for burial the bodies of deceased persons with AIDS.

54   Sixth, to the extent possible, persons with AIDS should be encouraged to continue to lead productive lives in their community and place of work. They also have the right to decent housing, and landlords are not justified in denying them this right merely because of their illness.

Seventh, we support collaborative efforts by governmental bodies, health providers, and human service agencies to provide adequate funding and care for persons with AIDS. We also encourage the development of hospice like programs that will afford persons with AIDS dignified and effective care and treatment. We call for the development of programs to care for infants and children with AIDS, especially those facing life and death without parental care.

Eighth, because of the virtually epidemic proportions of AIDS, we acknowledge the need for cooperative efforts by private and public entities to discover ways to treat and cure this disease and to commit adequate funding for basic research, applied research, and general education.

Ninth, we call on the federal government to provide additional funding for the care of those infected with the HIV virus who do not have health insurance as well as expanded income support for those impoverished by illness related to the AIDS virus. We also ask the federal government to take the lead in funding the necessary research and educational efforts as well as ensuring protection for those exposed to the AIDS virus against discrimination in insurance, employment, health care, education, and housing. The federal government should also provide funding for voluntary testing and ensure the confidentiality of such testing.

Tenth, current programs and services need to be expanded to assist the families of those with AIDS while they are alive and also to support them in their bereavement. In addition, new programs, services, and support systems need to be developed to deal with unmet and poorly met needs. To accomplish this, parishes and Catholic health care providers and agencies are encouraged to collaborate with others to ensure that there is continuity of health care and pastoral services to families and persons with AIDS in response to the unique set of psychological, social, and spiritual issues that may arise during the illness.

Eleventh, hospitals, because of their responsibility to care for the sick, and Catholic hospitals, because of their special mission and philosophy, have a unique call and role in caring for persons with AIDS. Hospitals have the responsibility and obligation to ensure that persons with AIDS and their families are cared for compassionately. Hospital personnel and church personnel also ought to go beyond their institutions to become facilitators, advocates, educators, and conveners to ensure that currently unmet and poorly met needs will be addressed in their communities by collaboration and networking with others in developing programs, services, and funding.

Twelfth, as a society, we need effective educational media programs to help reduce fear, prejudice, and discrimination against persons with AIDS, ARC, antibody-positive persons and those perceived to be in high-risk groups. . . .

. . . These are sensitive issues. In a brief statement like this we cannot apply the Church's teaching to all possible human behavior. Instead, in accord with the Church's traditional wisdom and moral teaching, we will offer some general principles and concrete guidelines. We speak to an entire nation, whose pluralism we recognize and respect.

These observations come from our profound care for those who place themselves or might be placed in danger of contracting AIDS: intravenous drug users and their partners, children born and unborn, and persons involved in sexual contact which is physically dangerous or morally wrong. In other words, the primary concern of our observations is people's moral and physical well-being, not their condemnation, however much we might disagree with their actions.

Consistent with the insights and values found in the Scriptures, our religious tradition, and a philosophy of the human person that is consonant with both, we believe that the best source of prevention for individuals and society can only come from an authentic and fully integrated understanding of human personhood and sexuality, and from efforts to address and eliminate the causes of intravenous drug abuse. We are convinced that the only measures that will effectively prevent this disease at present are those designed to educate and to change behavior. . . .

If, then, we are to address the prevention of AIDS in an effective way, we must deal with those human and societal factors which reduce or limit the quality of human life. When people think their lives devoid of meaning or when they find themselves in oppressive and despair-inducing poverty, they may turn to drugs or reach out for short-term physical intimacy in a mindless effort to escape the harsh conditions in which they live.

The Church and society need to address these realities. We have a responsibility first of all to help people realize that, whatever their circumstances, God's gift of life is precious, and there is more to life than its sometimes depressing or superficial dimensions. . . .

. . . Second, in our society we must offer everyone a fully integrated understanding of human sexuality. Every person, made in God's image and likeness, has both the potential and the desire to experience interpersonal intimacy that reflects the intimacy of God's triune love. This reflection in human love of the divine love gives special meaning and purpose to human sexuality. Human sexuality is essentially related to permanent commitment in love and openness to new life. It is most fully realized when it is expressed in a manner that is as loving, faithful, and committed as is divine love itself. That is why we call upon all people to live in accord with the authentic meaning of love and sexuality. Human sexuality, as we understand this gift from God, is to be genitally expressed only in a monogamous heterosexual relationship of lasting fidelity in marriage.

In light of this understanding of the human person, we are convinced that unless, as a society, we live in accord with an authentic human sexuality, on which our Catholic moral teaching is based, we will not address a major source of the spread of AIDS. Any other solution will be merely short term, ultimately ineffective, and will contribute to the trivialization of human sexuality that is already so prevalent in our society.

56   That is why we oppose the approach to AIDS prevention often popularly called "safe sex." This avenue compromises human sexuality—making it "safe" to be promiscuous—and, in fact, is quite misleading. As the National Academy of Sciences has noted in its study of AIDS, "many have argued that it is more accurate to speak in terms of 'safer' sex because the unknowns are still such that it would be irresponsible to certify any particular activity as absolutely safe."

What kind of approach will we support?

As pastors of dioceses throughout the United States, we commit ourselves and our resources, within our moral restraints and prudent judgment, to provide education to limit the spread of AIDS and to offer support for persons with AIDS.

We will also support legislation and educational programs that seek to provide accurate information about AIDS. This is both legitimate and necessary. Pertinent biological data and basic information about the nature of the disease are essential for understanding the biological and pathological consequences of one's personal choices, both to oneself and to others.

Nonetheless, as we have intimated above, we also have a responsibility as religious leaders to bring analysis to bear upon the moral dimensions of public policy. In our view, any discussion of AIDS must be situated within a broader context that affirms the dignity and destiny of the human person, the morality of human actions, and considers the consequences of individual choices for the whole of society.

Since AIDS is transmitted through intravenous drug use, we support and urge increased public support for drug treatment programs, the elimination of the importation of illicit drugs and every effort to eliminate the causes of addiction in all communities, especially those of the poor.

Since AIDS is also transmitted through sexual practices, legislation and public guidelines should encourage private and public institutions to go beyond mere biological education. Such legislation or guidelines must respect, however, the inalienable right of parents to be the first educators of their children regarding the meaning and purpose of human sexuality. . . .

Because we live in a pluralistic society, we acknowledge that some will not agree with our understanding of human sexuality. We recognize that public educational programs addressed to a wide audience will reflect the fact that some people will not act as they can and should; that they will not refrain from the type of sexual or drug abuse behavior which can transmit AIDS. In such situations educational efforts, if grounded in the broader moral vision outlined above, could include accurate information about prophylactic devices and other practices proposed by some medical experts as potential means of preventing AIDS. We are not promoting the use of prophylactics, but merely providing information that is part of the factual picture. Such a factual presentation should indicate that abstinence outside of marriage and fidelity within marriage as well as the avoidance of intravenous drug abuse are the only morally correct and medically sure ways to prevent the spread of AIDS. So-called "safe sex" practices are at best only partially effective. They do not take into account

either the real values that are at stake or the fundamental good of the human person. . . .

In sum, it is our judgment that the best approach to the prevention of AIDS ought to be based on the communication of a value-centered understanding of the meaning of human personhood. Such a perspective provides a suitable context for the consideration of legislation or educational policy. . . .

We also wish to say a word about the responsibilities of those who find themselves "at risk" of having been exposed to the AIDS virus. Earlier we stated something of the meaning and purpose of human sexuality. If a person chooses not to live in accord with this meaning or has misused drugs, he or she still has the serious responsibility not to bring injury to another person. Consequently, anyone who is considered to be "at risk" of having been exposed to the AIDS virus has a grave moral responsibility to ensure that he or she does not expose anyone else to it. This means that such a person who is considering marriage, engaging in intimate sexual contact, planning to donate blood, organs, or donating semen has a moral responsibility to be tested for exposure to the AIDS virus and should act in such a way that it will not bring possible harm to another. . . .

CARE FOR PERSONS WITH AIDS AND ARC

. . . Persons with AIDS, their families, and their friends need solidarity, comfort, and support. As with others facing imminent death, they may experience anger toward and alienation from God and the Church as they face the inevitability of dying. It is important that someone stand with them in their pain and help them, in accord with their religious tradition, to discover meaning in what appears so meaningless. Offering or ensuring this human companionship is especially important lest those who would diminish respect for life by encouraging euthanasia or suicide determine how to "care" for persons with AIDS. . . .

In sum, by collaborating with other agencies and programs we hope that the Church will provide an appropriate example about the manner in which those suffering from AIDS, and their families and friends, are cared for as well as the nature of that care. Through this collaboration we will help provide the kind of care and services that place persons with AIDS in appropriate settings that best meet their needs. In addition, we encourage the use of church facilities as sites for providing various levels and kinds of care. . . .

DOCUMENT 3 / AIDS

Source: New York Bishops, "Statement on Public Schools' Condom Distribution," *Origins* 22: no. 32 (Jan. 21, 1993), pp. 553–56.

. . . We firmly believe, on both moral and practical grounds, that distributing condoms to young people is not the proper approach to the AIDS epidemic. It is just one more example of society's quick-fix, Band-Aid approach to problems. To help our youth understand issues of human sexuality, we must look deeper and work harder to send the right message. The right message is that human sexuality is beautiful, powerful, sacred, and good. It is a gift of God that must be used responsibly and morally.

. . . The message such programs send to young people is, "We have no faith in you." They tell adolescents that we've given up, sold out, and assume they will do wrong. It signals total disregard for the dignity of our young people by suggesting they are incapable of moral behavior consistent with their Judeo-Christian ethic. Have we deemed our youth hopelessly beneath our expectations and challenge?

At a time of adolescent uncertainty, sexual maturation, and unparalleled questioning, we should be offering young people clear guidance and strong direction. We should be giving them a message of hope, faith, self-worth, and self-respect. We believe in the dignity of our young. We believe that with proper guidance, with parental involvement, and with programs built upon the concept of deepening self-esteem, our youth will respond to the message to live their lives consistent with healthy sexual attitudes and the values that encourage sexual abstinence.

There is a better way.

. . . We should be teaching our children reverence and awe for such an act; it reflects the total commitment shared by a husband and wife. It is a totally selfless, unconditional love which is expressed in sexual intercourse, a sign of the fidelity, acceptance, commitment, and closeness shared by married lovers. We must give our children the understanding that the more powerful the gift, the more cautious and responsible we must be in using it.

The emotional bonding which occurs in physical genital activity between two persons may not be fully understood by those who promote condoms for teenagers. Teens who engage in premarital sexual activity feel this bonding, too, and are often deeply hurt when the casual, uncommitted relationship ends. Feelings of emptiness, loss, and guilt are not uncommon when one gives of oneself totally to another, only to be tossed aside for a new "steady". . . .

Practical Dimensions

Evidence reveals that condoms do not provide a reliable safeguard against pregnancy or against a deadly disease like AIDS, for a number of reasons. The

failure rate of condoms in preventing pregnancy has been estimated at anywhere from 10 percent to 52 percent, with failure calculated as the percentage of
women who experience an unintended pregnancy while using the contraceptive
method over one year's time. In 1981 the National Center for Health Statistics
found the rate to be 10.1 percent. Today, family-planning advocates cite a rate of
14.6 pregnancies during the first year of use. And a recent study in Manchester,
England, found that 52 percent of condom users had experienced breakage or
slippage during the first three months of use. . . .

. . . Passing out condoms to adolescents in school under the guise of "safe
sex" is much like encouraging them to play Russian Roulette—both games are
deadly. In addition to not being used correctly, condoms often break, tear,
slip, get damaged during shipping and handling, and are exposed to extreme
elements of heat and cold, which cause cracking, drying, loss of tension and
shrinkage. Periodically, defective condoms are widely distributed by manufacturers, only to be recalled within a short time. For some, the recall may come
too late.

Alternative to Condoms

As Church, we firmly believe that we must discuss sex openly and honestly with children, answering all of their questions. Several of our dioceses
have instituted human sexuality curricula in their Catholic schools and religious
education programs. These comprehensive programs reflect sound scientific
and psychological information, the teachings of the Church, and a clear understanding of the challenges facing adolescents today. They emphasize the value
of each individual person, the gift of sexuality, parental involvement, and the
importance of family.

There are other programs, not specifically Church affiliated, which teach
the value of chastity and the positive, healthy outcomes of refraining from
premarital sexual activity. Project Respect, based in Illinois, has recently demonstrated a 45 percent lower pregnancy rate among high school sophomores and
juniors using the "Sex Respect" curricula. Fertility Appreciation for Families,
a program which promotes abstinence, respect for life, moral values and discussion with parents, recently found pregnancy rates among the 15–19 year-old
participants to be 95 percent lower then the national norm. . . .

Parental Authority and Family Unity

The standards for adolescents growing up in today's society should be
set by the family and reinformed by the school. Parents are, and always have
been, the primary educators of their children. Having conferred life on them
in God's presence, they have the right and responsibility to guide the growth
and development of their sons and daughters and to instill in them the values
they wish to inculcate. . . .

7: Anencephaly

DOCUMENT 1:

Source: NCCB Doctrine Committee, "Moral Principles Concerning Infants with Anencephaly," *Origins* 26: no. 17 (Oct. 10, 1996), p. 276.

Anencephaly is a congenital anomaly characterized by failure of development of the cerebral hemispheres and overlying skull and scalp, exposing the brain stem. This condition exists in varying degrees of severity. Most infants who have anencephaly do not survive for more than a few days after birth. Modern medical techniques usually can determine this condition with a high degree of certainty before birth. When anencephaly is detected, some physicians recommend that the pregnancy be terminated in order to free the mother from the psychological anxiety and possible physical complications throughout the remainder of the pregnancy.

According to the well-established teaching of the Catholic Church, the rights of a mother and her unborn child deserve equal protection because they are based on the dignity of the human person whatever the condition of that person. Consequently, it can never be morally justified directly to cause the death of an innocent person no matter the age or condition of that person.

Some have attempted to argue that anencephalic children may be prematurely delivered, even when this would be inappropriate for other children. This argument is based on the opinion that because of their apparent lack of cognitive function and in view of the probable brevity of their lives, these infants are not the subject of human rights or at least have lives of less meaning or purpose than others. Doubts about the human dignity of the anencephalic infant, however, have no solid ground, and the benefit of any doubt must be in the child's favor. As a general rule, conditions of the human body, regardless of severity, in no way compromise human dignity or human rights.

The "Ethical and Religious Directives for Catholic Health Care Services," Directive 45, states:

"Abortion (that is, the directly intended termination of pregnancy before viability or the directly intended destruction of a viable fetus) is never permitted. Every procedure whose sole immediate effect is the termination of pregnancy before viability is an abortion, which in its moral content includes the interval between conception and implantation of the embryo."

The phrase sole immediate effect is further explained by Directive 47 which states:

"Operations, treatments, and medications that have as their direct purpose the cure of a proportionately serious pathological condition of a pregnant

woman are permitted when they cannot be safely postponed until the unborn   **61**
child is viable, even if they will result in the death of the unborn child."

In other words, it is permitted to treat directly a pathology of the mother even when this has the unintended side effect of causing the death of her child, if this pathology left untreated would have life-threatening effects on both mother and child, but it is not permitted to terminate or gravely risk the child's life as a means of treating or protecting the mother.

Hence, it is clear that before "viability" it is never permitted to terminate the gestation of an anencephalic child as the means of avoiding psychological or physical risks to the mother. Nor is such termination permitted after "viability" if early delivery endangers the child's life due to complications of prematurity. In such cases it cannot reasonably be maintained that such a termination is simply a side effect of the treatment of a pathology of the mother (as described in Directive 47). Anencephaly is not a pathology of the mother, but of the child, and terminating her pregnancy cannot be a treatment of a pathology she does not have. Only if the complications of the pregnancy result in a life-threatening pathology of the mother may the treatment of this pathology be permitted even at a risk to the child, and then only if the child's death is not a means to treating the mother.

The fact that the life of a child suffering from anencephaly will probably be brief cannot excuse directly causing death before "viability" or gravely endangering the child's life after "viability" as a result of the complications of prematurity.

The anencephalic child, during his or her probably brief life after birth, should be given the comfort and palliative care appropriate to all the dying. This failing life need not be further troubled by using extraordinary means to prolong it (see "Ethical and Religious Directives," Directives 57 and 58). It is most commendable for parents to wish to donate the organs of an anencephalic child for transplants that may assist other children, but this may never be permitted before the donor child is certainly dead.

The profound and personal suffering of the parents of an anencephalic child gives us cause for concern and calls for compassionate pastoral and medical care as the parents prepare for the pain and emptiness that the certain death of their newborn child will bring. The mother who carries to term a child who will soon die deserves our every possible support. The baptism of the child assures the parents of the child's eternal happiness, and the provision of Christian burial of the deceased infant gives witness to the Church's unconditional respect for human life and the recognition that in the face of every human being is an encounter with God.

8: Artificial Insemination

DOCUMENT 1:

SOURCE: Congregation for the Doctrine of the Faith, "Instruction on Respect for Human Life in Its Origin and on the Dignity of Procreation" (Feb. 22, 1987), *Origins* 16: no. 40, Mar. 19, 1987, pp. 698–711.

II. Interventions upon Human Procreation

By artificial procreation or artificial fertilization are understood here the different technical procedures directed toward obtaining a human conception in a manner other than the sexual union of man and woman. This instruction deals with fertilization of an ovum in a test tube (in vitro fertilization) and artificial insemination through transfer into the woman's genital tracts of previously collected sperm.

A preliminary point for the moral evaluation of such technical procedures is constituted by the consideration of the circumstances and consequences which those procedures involve in relation to the respect due the human embryo. Development of the practice of in vitro fertilization has required innumerable fertilizations and destructions of human embryos. Even today, the usual practice presupposes a hyperovulation on the part of the woman: a number of ova are withdrawn, fertilized and then cultivated in vitro for some days. Usually not all are transferred into the genital tracts of the woman; some embryos, generally called "spare," are destroyed or frozen. On occasion, some of the implanted embryos are sacrificed for various eugenic, economic, or psychological reasons. Such deliberate destruction of human beings or their utilization for different purposes to the detriment of their integrity and life is contrary to the doctrine on procured abortion already recalled.

The connection between in vitro fertilization and the voluntary destruction of human embryos occurs too often. This is significant: through these procedures, with apparently contrary purposes, life and death are subjected to the decision of man, who thus sets himself up as the giver of life and death by decree. This dynamic of violence and domination may remain unnoticed by those very individuals who, in wishing to utilize this procedure, become subject to it themselves. The facts recorded and the cold logic which links them must be taken into consideration for a moral judgment on in vitro fertilization and embryo transfer: the abortion mentality which has made this procedure possible thus leads, whether one wants it or not, to man's domination over the life and death of his fellow human beings and can lead to a system of radical eugenics.

Nevertheless, such abuses do not exempt one from a further and thorough ethical study of the techniques of artificial procreation considered in them-

selves, abstracting as far as possible from the destruction of embryos produced   **63**
in vitro.

1. Why must human procreation take place in marriage?

Every human being is always to be accepted as a gift and blessing of
God. However, from the moral point of view a truly responsible procreation
vis-à-vis the unborn child must be the fruit of marriage.

For human procreation has specific characteristics by virtue of the personal
dignity of the parents and of the children: the procreation of a new person,
whereby the man and the woman collaborate with the power of the Creator,
must be the fruit and the sign of the mutual self-giving of the spouses, of their
love, and of their fidelity. The fidelity of the spouses in the unity of marriage
involves reciprocal respect of their right to become a father and a mother only
through each other.

The child has the right to be conceived, carried in the womb, brought
into the world, and brought up within marriage: it is through the secure and
recognized relationship to his own parents that the child can discover his own
identity and achieve his own proper human development.

The parents find in their child a confirmation and completion of their
reciprocal self-giving: the child is the living image of their love, the permanent
sign of their conjugal union, the living and indissoluble concrete expression of
their paternity and maternity.

By reason of the vocation and social responsibilities of the person, the
good of the children and of the parents contributes to the good of civil society;
the vitality and stability of society require that children come into the world
within a family and that the family be firmly based on marriage.

The tradition of the Church and anthropological reflection recognize in
marriage and in its indissoluble unity the only setting worthy of truly responsible procreation.

2. Does heterologous artificial fertilization conform to the dignity of the couple and to the truth of marriage?

Through in vitro fertilization and embryo transfer and heterologous artificial insemination, human conception is achieved through the fusion of gametes
of at least one donor other than the spouses who are united in marriage.
Heterologous artificial fertilization is contrary to the unity of marriage, to the
dignity of the spouses, to the vocation proper to parents, and to the child's
right to be conceived and brought into the world in marriage and from marriage.

Respect for the unity of marriage and for conjugal fidelity demands that
the child be conceived in marriage; the bond existing between husband and
wife accords the spouses, in an objective and inalienable manner, the exclusive
right to become father and mother solely through each other. Recourse to the
gametes of a third person in order to have sperm or ovum available constitutes
a violation of the reciprocal commitment of the spouses and a grave lack in
regard to that essential property of marriage which is its unity.

Heterologous artificial fertilization violates the rights of the child; it deprives him of his filial relationship with his parental origins and can hinder

64   the maturing of his personal identity. Furthermore, it offends the common vocation of the spouses who are called to fatherhood and motherhood: it objectively deprives conjugal fruitfulness of its unity and integrity; it brings about and manifests a rupture between genetic parenthood, gestational parenthood, and responsibility for upbringing. Such damage to the personal relationships within the family has repercussions on civil society: what threatens the unity and stability of the family is a source of dissension, disorder, and injustice in the whole of social life.

These reasons lead to a negative moral judgment concerning heterologous artificial fertilization. Consequently, fertilization of a married woman with the sperm of a donor different from her husband and fertilization with the husband's sperm of an ovum not coming from his wife are morally illicit. Furthermore, the artificial fertilization of a woman who is unmarried or a widow, whoever the donor may be, cannot be morally justified.

The desire to have a child and the love between spouses who long to obviate a sterility which cannot be overcome in any other way constitute understandable motivations; but subjectively good intentions do not render heterologous artificial fertilization conformable to the objective and inalienable properties of marriage or respectful of the rights of the child and of the spouses. . . .

6. How is homologous artificial insemination to be evaluated from the moral point of view?

Homologous artificial insemination within marriage cannot be admitted except for those cases in which the technical means is not a substitute for the conjugal act but serves to facilitate and to help so that the act attains its natural purpose.

The teaching of the Magisterium on this point has already been stated. This teaching is not just an expression of particular historical circumstances, but is based on the Church's doctrine concerning the connection between the conjugal union and procreation and on a consideration of the personal nature of the conjugal act and of human procreation. "In its natural structure, the conjugal act is a personal action, a simultaneous and immediate cooperation on the part of the husband and wife, which by the very nature of the agents and the proper nature of the act is the expression of the mutual gift which, according to the words of Scripture, brings about union 'in one flesh.' " Thus moral conscience "does not necessarily proscribe the use of certain artificial means destined solely either to the facilitating of the natural act or to ensuring that the natural act normally performed achieves its proper end." If the technical means facilitates the conjugal act or helps it to reach its natural objectives, it can be morally acceptable. If, on the other hand, the procedure were to replace the conjugal act, it is morally illicit.

Artificial insemination as a substitute for the conjugal act is prohibited by reason of the voluntarily achieved dissociation of the two meanings of the conjugal act. Masturbation, through which the sperm is normally obtained, is another sign of this dissociation. Even when it is done for the purpose of procreation the act remains deprived of its unitive meaning: "It lacks the sexual

relationship[1] called for by the moral order, namely the relationship which   **65**
realizes 'the full sense of mutual self-giving and human procreation in the
context of true love.'. . ."

---

[1]*By the term *heterologous artificial fertilization* or *procreation*, the instruction means
techniques used to obtain a human conception artificially by the use of gametes coming
from at least one donor other than the spouses who are joined in marriage. Such
techniques can be of two types:

a) *Heterologous "in vitro" fertilization and embryo transfer*: the technique used to
obtain a human conception through the meeting in vitro of gametes taken from at least
one donor other than the two spouses joined in marriage;

b) *Heterologous artificial insemination*: the technique used to obtain a human conception through the transfer into the genital tracts of the woman of the sperm previously
collected from a donor other than the husband.

**By *artificial homologous fertilization* or *procreation*, the instruction means the tech-
nique used to obtain a human conception using the gametes of the two spouses joined in
marriage. Homologous artificial fertilization can be carried out by two different methods:

a) *Homologous "in vitro" fertilization and embryo transfer*: the technique used to
obtain a human conception through the meeting in vitro of the gametes of the spouses
joined in marriage;

b) *Homologous artificial insemination*: the technique used to obtain a human conception through the transfer into the genital tracts of a married woman of the sperm
previously collected from her husband.

DOCUMENT 2 / Artificial Insemination

SOURCE: Pope Pius XII, "Christian Norms of Morality" (Sept. 29, 1949), *The Human Body: Papal Teachings*, pp. 117–19.

Now there has arisen another pressing problem, which demands, no less urgently than the rest, the light of Catholic moral doctrine: the problem of artificial insemination. We cannot let this occasion pass without indicating, at least in its broad lines, the moral judgment which governs this matter.

1. When dealing with man, the question of artificial insemination cannot be considered either exclusively—nor yet principally—under its biological and medical aspect, leaving aside the moral and juridical point of view.

2. Artificial insemination outside matrimony must be condemned as immoral purely and simply.

In fact the natural law and divine positive law state that the procreation of new life cannot take place except in marriage. Only matrimony safeguards the dignity of the partners—in the present case principally that of the woman—their personal well-being, and guarantees at the same time the well-being of the child and his upbringing.

It follows that there cannot be any difference of opinion among Catholics regarding the condemnation of artificial insemination outside the conjugal union. The child born under these conditions would be by that very fact illegitimate.

3. Artificial insemination in matrimony, but produced by means of the active element of a third person, is equally immoral, and as such is to be condemned without right of appeal.

Only the husband and wife have the reciprocal right on the body of the other for the purpose of generating new life: an exclusive, inalienable, incommunicable right. And that is as it should be, also for the sake of the child. To whoever gives life to the tiny creature, nature imposes, in virtue of that very bond, the duty of protecting and educating the child. But when the child is the fruit of the active elements of a third person—even granting the husband's consent—between the legitimate husband and the child there is no such bond of origin, nor the moral and juridical bond of conjugal procreation.

4. What of the liceity of artificial insemination in matrimony? For the moment let it suffice to recall these principles of the natural law: the mere fact that the means reaches the goal intended does not justify the use of such a means. Nor does the desire for a child—a completely legitimate desire of the married couple—suffice to prove that recourse to artificial fecundation is legitimate because it would satisfy such a desire.

. . . Though new methods cannot be excluded a priori simply because they are new, in the case of artificial insemination one should not only keep a very cautious reserve, but must exclude it altogether. This does not necessarily forbid the use of certain artificial means destined simply either to facilitate the natural act, or to enable the natural act, normally carried out, to attain its proper end.

Let it not be forgotten that only procreation of a new life according to the will and the plan of the Creator carries with it, to an amazing degree of perfection, the realization of intended aims. It is at the same time in conformity with the corporal and spiritual nature and the dignity of the marriage partners, and with the normal and happy development of the child.

DOCUMENT 3 / Artificial Insemination

SOURCE: Pope Pius XII, "Fundamental Laws Governing Conjugal Relations" (Oct. 29, 1951), *The Human Body: Papal Teachings*, pp. 171–72.

To consider unworthily the cohabitation of husband and wife, and the marital act as a simple organic function for the transmission of seed, would be the same as to convert the domestic hearth, which is the family sanctuary, into a mere biological laboratory. For this reason, in our address of September 29, 1949, made to the International Congress of Catholic Doctors, we formally rejected artificial insemination in marriage. The marital act, in its natural setting, is a personal action. It is the simultaneous and direct cooperation of husband and wife which, by the very nature of the agents and the propriety of the act, is the expression of the mutual giving which, in the words of Scripture, results in the union "in one flesh."

This is much more than the union of two life-germs, which can be brought about even artificially, that is, without the cooperation of the husband and wife. The marital act, in the order of and by nature's design, consists of a personal cooperation which the husband and wife exchange as a right when they marry.

9: Artificial Reproduction

DOCUMENT 1:

SOURCE: Pope John Paul II, "The Gospel of Life" (Mar. 25, 1995), *Origins* 24: no. 42, Apr. 6, 1995, pp. 695, 711.

14. . . . The various techniques of artificial reproduction, which would seem to be at the service of life and which are frequently used with this intention, actually open the door to new threats against life. Apart from the fact that they are morally unacceptable since they separate procreation from the fully human context of the conjugal act, these techniques have a high rate of failure: not just failure in relation to fertilization, but with regard to the subsequent development of the embryo, which is exposed to the risk of death, generally within a very short space of time. Furthermore, the number of embryos produced is often greater than that needed for implantation in the woman's womb, and these so-called "spare embryos" are then destroyed or used for research which, under the pretext of scientific or medical progress, in fact reduces human life to the level of simple "biological material" to be freely disposed of.

Prenatal diagnosis, which presents no moral objections if carried out in order to identify the medical treatment which may be needed by the child in the womb, all too often becomes an opportunity for proposing and procuring an abortion. This is eugenic abortion, justified in public opinion on the basis of a mentality—mistakenly held to be consistent with the demands of "therapeutic interventions"—which accepts life only under certain conditions and rejects it when it is affected by any limitation, handicap or illness. . . .

63. . . . Special attention must be given to evaluating the morality of prenatal diagnostic techniques which enable the early detection of possible anomalies in the unborn child. In view of the complexity of these techniques, an accurate and systematic moral judgment is necessary. When they do not involve disproportionate risks for the child and the mother, and are meant to make possible early therapy or even to favor a serene and informed acceptance of the child not yet born, these techniques are morally licit. But since the possibilities of prenatal therapy are today still limited, it not infrequently happens that these techniques are used with a eugenic intention which accepts selective abortion in order to prevent the birth of children affected by various types of anomalies. Such an attitude is shameful and utterly reprehensible, since it presumes to measure the value of a human life only within the parameters of "normality" and physical well-being, thus opening the way to legitimizing infanticide and euthanasia as well. . . .

10: Assisted Suicide

DOCUMENT 1:

SOURCE: Pope John Paul II, "The Gospel of Life" (Mar. 25, 1995), *Origins* 24: no. 42, Apr. 6, 1995, p. 712.

66. . . . Suicide is always as morally objectionable as murder. The Church's tradition has always rejected it as a gravely evil choice. Even though a certain psychological, cultural, and social conditioning may induce a person to carry out an action which so radically contradicts the innate inclination to life, thus lessening or removing subjective responsibility, suicide, when viewed objectively, is a gravely immoral act. In fact, it involves the rejection of love of self and the renunciation of the obligation of justice and charity toward one's neighbor, toward the communities to which one belongs, and toward society as a whole. In its deepest reality, suicide represents a rejection of God's absolute sovereignty over life and death as proclaimed in the prayer of the ancient sage of Israel: "You have power over life and death; you lead men down to the gates of Hades and back again" (Wis 16:13; cf. Tb 13:2). . . .

DOCUMENT 2 / Assisted Suicide

SOURCE: Michigan Bishops, "Living and Dying According to the Voice of Faith," *Origins* 27: no. 19 (Oct. 23, 1997), pp. 318–321.

The Church's teaching on human life is based on the voice of faith which echoes in every human heart, the truth that we have been created in God's image and likeness and are stewards of his gift of life. For us Christians, this voice of faith is reinforced by the teaching of Jesus Christ and his Church over the centuries. This divine and human wisdom provides the answers we seek to the challenging and troubling questions about how we are to die.

The prospect of our own inevitable dying and watching our loved ones die naturally raises anxieties and fears about our capacity to bear the physical pain and psychological stress that might be connected to the dying process. We fear the possibility of being alone and forgotten. We perhaps lack the appropriate information about the proper steps to take in planning for our future death and that of our loved ones. We worry about the financial resources required for long-term care.

For many people the dying process is especially frightening because it seems to be the final and most complete moment of isolation, separation, and loneliness. We imagine being caught in unending physical agony, with no one who could possibly understand, much less comfort us. Following the voice of fear, we run away from death and desperately try to put it out of mind and sight—as far and as long as possible. And when it seems that death can no longer be avoided, we are naturally tempted to consider a quick escape or exit.

In the face of these questions and struggles, as a Church we have the good news of our faith in the death-resurrection of Jesus. We proclaim a message of hope: no one has to die alone or unwanted, in terrible physical pain or psychological distress. We put our faith and hope into concrete expression by promising to share our life journey with one another. As brothers and sisters in a family of faith, we live and die together.

As we all struggle to live and die well, we, your shepherds, want to offer consolation and guidance through this pastoral letter and related resources published by the Michigan Catholic Conference. These educational materials cover in greater detail the Catholic understanding of dying and death and the related questions which we raise in our letter.

This pastoral letter is divided into two parts: first, we present the teaching of the Catholic Church on dying and death; then we explain why we profess these beliefs and how we can find peace for ourselves and our family by living and dying according to the voice of faith.

72   **What We Believe About Dying and Death**

We often think that death is the end of the story. We forget that it is foreshadowed throughout our life; dying is woven into the very fiber of our life from its inception. The voice of faith reassures us that we need not fear death, but at the same time, because we are human, we can still be anxious about the circumstances of our death. Not knowing what the future may hold, we do not want to give up all the opportunities and gifts around us. When it is time for us to leave this world, it is fitting that we should want to die in a way that is meaningful, even beautiful and inspiring, for us and for all those we love.

In the dying process there is still a great scope for personal choice and responsibility: how we face the mysteries of suffering, dying, and death makes a critical difference for us and for our loved ones who wish to offer us compassionate support. As stewards of the gift of life, we see every aspect of life and death as part of a larger picture and part of our ongoing relationship with God and neighbor.

Choosing death by one's own hand contradicts our deepest identity as sons and daughters of God. Such an action also conveys a tragic message to our family and friends—that we reject their genuine love and our solidarity with them.

Suicide—the conscious choice to destroy one's own life—is always morally wrong. Concurring with someone's intention to commit suicide and cooperating in the process can never be condoned. Such assisted suicide is a perversion of genuine mercy. It is especially tragic when undertaken by physicians, whose very professional code charges them never to harm but always to respect life.

For several years there has been a continuing debate about the legality and practice of assisted suicide in Michigan. On the national scene, the U.S. Supreme Court upheld laws banning assisted suicide in the states of Washington and New York and said there is no constitutional right to assisted suicide. We need such a statutory ban in our own state: to protect the vulnerable, to prevent unscrupulous and unethical medical practices, to guarantee the best possible care for all and to affirm the value of human life.

Above and beyond what civil laws may say, we Christians are ultimately responsible to God our Creator. As a Church, we definitively say no to assisted suicide because we say yes to life—from the first moment of conception until your last natural breath. Suicide in any form prevents us from fulfilling the plan God intended for us when we were given life.

Euthanasia, or so-called "mercy killing," may at first sound like an appealing form of death because it proposes to eliminate all suffering. Yet it is not at all what it seems! By definition, euthanasia is any action that of itself and by intention causes death so as to relieve suffering. As Catholics, we believe euthanasia is morally wrong because it is the destruction of life. It also opens the door to other potential crimes against life, especially against those who are chronically ill or disabled. Euthanasia is unnecessary as well as wrong, because suffering and pain can be relieved in many morally acceptable ways.

No human being has absolute control over his or her own life; God alone **73** has dominion over all creation. Since many aspects of life exceed our immediate control, we have to learn to accept gracefully the limitations imposed by time and circumstances, relationships and commitments, economic realities and other factors. We find peace of mind and heart precisely when we come to terms with the fact that life is a mystery, a gift from God, a blessing over which we do not have complete control.

We are born into a social network, a family of one kind or another, and various communities. Our life story is interwoven and those of our families and communities; we are accountable to them as well as to God. Our individual identity and rights do not separate us from others but should call us into greater communion and solidarity with them.

Every right brings with it responsibilities for the good of all. Our decisions about life and death are never purely private matters for many other persons are necessarily involved—doctors, nurses, family, and friends. Our choices in dying have a profound impact on those we leave behind. They also influence others who are suffering in body or spirit, especially the elderly, the dying, the chronically ill, and persons who are physically or mentally challenged. By the way we live and die we can inspire and console them—or we can add to the voices that tell them their lives are burdensome and without value.

11: Autonomy

DOCUMENT 1:

SOURCE: Congregation for the Doctrine of the Faith, "Pastoral Constitution on the Church in the Modern World" (Dec. 7, 1965) *Vatican Council II,* Vol. 1, 1975, pp. 913–28.

THE DIGNITY OF THE HUMAN PERSON

MAN AS THE IMAGE OF GOD

12. . . . For Sacred Scripture teaches that man was created "to the image of God," as able to know and love his Creator, and as set by him over all earthly creatures that he might rule them, and make use of them, while glorifying God. "What is man that thou art mindful of him, and the son of man that thou dost care for him? Yet thou hast made him little less than God, and dost crown him with glory and honor. Thou hast given him dominion over the works of thy hands; thou hast put all things under his feet" (Ps 8:5–8).

But God did not create man a solitary being. From the beginning "male and female he created them" (Gn 1:27). This partnership of man and woman constitutes the first form of communion between persons. For by his innermost nature man is a social being; and if he does not enter into relations with others he can neither live nor develop his gifts.

So God, as we read again in the Bible, saw "all the things that he had made, and they were very good" (Gn 1:31).

THE ESSENTIAL NATURE OF MAN

14. Man, though made of body and soul, is a unity. Through his very bodily condition he sums up in himself the elements of the material world. Through him they are thus brought to their highest perfection and can raise their voice in praise freely given to the creator. For this reason man may not despise his bodily life. Rather he is obliged to regard his body as good and to hold it in honor since God has created it and will raise it up on the last day. Nevertheless man has been wounded by sin. He finds by experience that his body is in revolt. His very dignity therefore requires that he should glorify God in his body, and not allow it to serve the evil inclinations of his heart. . . .

DIGNITY OF THE INTELLECT, OF TRUTH, AND OF WISDOM

15. Man, as sharing in the light of the divine mind, rightly affirms that by his intellect he surpasses the world of mere things. By diligent use of his talents through the ages he has indeed made progress in the empirical sciences,

in technology, and in the liberal arts. In our time his attempts to search out the secrets of the material universe and to bring it under his control have been extremely successful. Yet he has always looked for, and found, truths of a higher order. For his intellect is not confined to the range of what can be observed by the senses. It can, with genuine certainty, reach to realities known only to the mind, even though, as a result of sin, its vision has been clouded and its powers weakened.

The intellectual nature of man finds at last its perfection, as it should, in wisdom, which gently draws the human mind to look for and to love what is true and good. Filled with wisdom man is led through visible realities to those which cannot be seen. . . .

DIGNITY OF MORAL CONSCIENCE

16. Deep within his conscience man discovers a law which he has not laid upon himself but which he must obey. Its voice, ever calling him to love and to do what is good and to avoid evil, tells him inwardly at the right moment: do this, shun that. For man has in his heart a law inscribed by God. His dignity lies in observing this law, and by it he will be judged. His conscience is man's most secret core, and his sanctuary. There he is alone with God whose voice echoes in his depths. By conscience, in a wonderful way, that law is made known which is fulfilled in the love of God and of one's neighbor. Through loyalty to conscience Christians are joined to other men in the search for truth and for the right solution to so many moral problems which arise both in the life of individuals and from social relationships. Hence, the more a correct conscience prevails, the more do persons and groups turn aside from blind choice and try to be guided by the objective standards of moral conduct. Yet it often happens that conscience goes astray through ignorance which it is unable to avoid without thereby losing its dignity. This cannot be said of the man who takes little trouble to find out what is true and good, or when conscience is by degrees almost blinded through the habit of committing sin.

THE EXCELLENCE OF FREEDOM

17. It is, however, only in freedom that man can turn himself towards what is good. The people of our time prize freedom very highly and strive eagerly for it. In this they are right. Yet they often cherish it improperly, as if it gave them leave to do anything they like, even when it is evil. But that which is truly freedom is an exceptional sign of the image of God in man. For God willed that man should "be left in the hand of his own counsel" so that he might of his own accord seek his Creator and freely attain his full and blessed perfection by cleaving to him. Man's dignity therefore requires him to act out of conscious and free choice, as moved and drawn in a personal way from within, and not by blind impulses in himself or by mere external constraint. Man gains such dignity when, ridding himself of all slavery to the passions, he presses forward towards his goal by freely choosing what is good and, by his diligence and skill, effectively secures for himself the means suited to this end. Since human freedom has been weakened by sin it is only by the help of

76   God's grace that man can give his actions their full and proper relationship to God. Before the judgment seat of God an account of his own life will be rendered to each one according as he has done either good or evil.

THE COMMUNITY OF MANKIND

RESPECT FOR THE HUMAN PERSON

27. Wishing to come down to topics that are practical and of some urgency, the Council lays stress on respect for the human person: everyone should look upon his neighbor (without any exception) as another self, bearing in mind above all his life and the means necessary for living it in a dignified way lest he follow the example of the rich man who ignored Lazarus, the poor man.

Today there is an inescapable duty to make ourselves the neighbor of every man, no matter who he is, and if we meet him, to come to his aid in a positive way, whether he is an aged person abandoned by all, a foreign worker despised without reason, a refugee, an illegitimate child wrongly suffering for a sin he did not commit, or a starving human being who awakens our conscience by calling to mind the words of Christ: "As you did it to one of the least of these my brethren, you did it to me" (Mt 25:40).

The varieties of crime are numerous: all offenses against life itself, such as murder, genocide, abortion, euthanasia and willful suicide; all violations of the integrity of the human person, such as mutilation, physical and mental torture, undue psychological pressures; all offenses against human dignity, such as subhuman living conditions, arbitrary imprisonment, deportation, slavery, prostitution, the selling of women and children, degrading working conditions where men are treated as mere tools for profit rather than free and responsible persons: all these and the like are criminal: they poison civilization; and they debase the perpetrators more than the victims and militate against the honor of the creator.

12: Autopsy

DOCUMENT 1:

SOURCE: Pope Pius XII, "Moral Problems in Medicine" (Sept. 30, 1954), *The Human Body: Papal Teachings*, pp. 316–17.

With respect to the question of removing a dead man's bodily parts to further therapeutic objectives, no doctor should be given the right to do with a corpse as he pleases. It is up to public authority to enact appropriate legislation regarding such matters. But public authority, on the other hand, does not have the right to proceed arbitrarily. There are certain provisions of the law to which it is possible to have serious objections. A norm, such as that which would permit a doctor in a sanatorium to remove parts of a body for therapeutic purposes—all thought of personal profit being duly foresworn—cannot be honored because of the existent possibility that it might be interpreted too freely. Then, too, the rights and duties of those whose obligation it is to assume responsibility for the body of the deceased must also be taken into consideration. And, finally, the demands of natural morality, which forbid us to consider and treat the body of a human being merely as a thing, or as that of an animal, must at all times be dutifully respected.

13: Brain Death

DOCUMENT 1:

Source: Pontifical Academy of Sciences, "Report on Prolonging Life and Determining Death" (Oct. 30, 1985), *Health Progress*, Dec. 1985, p. 31.

I. Definition of Death

A person is dead when he has irreversibly lost all capacity to integrate and coordinate the physical and mental functions of the body.

Death has occurred when: A. The spontaneous cardiac and respiratory functions have definitively ceased; or B. An irreversible cessation of every brain function is verified.

From the debate it emerged that cerebral death is the true criterion of death, since the definitive arrest of the cardiorespiratory functions leads very quickly to cerebral death.

The group then analyzed the various clinical and instrumental methods that enable one to ascertain the irreversible arrest of cerebral functions. To be certain—by means of the electroencephalogram—that the brain has become flat, that is, that it no longer displays electric activity, it is necessary that the examination be carried out at least twice within a six-hour interval.

II. Medical Guidelines

By "treatment" the group understands all the medical interventions, however technically complex, which are available and appropriate for a given case.

If the patient is in permanent coma, irreversible as far as it is possible to predict, treatment is not required, but all care should be lavished on him, including feeding.

If it is clinically established that there is a possibility of recovery, treatment is required.

If treatment is of no benefit to the patient, it may be withdrawn, while continuing with the care of the patient.

By "care" the group understands ordinary help due to sick patients, such as compassion and affective and spiritual support due to every human being in danger.

III. Artificial prolongation of vegetative functions

In case of cerebral death, artificial respiration can prolong the cardiac function for a limited time. This induced survival of the organs is indicated in the case of a foreseen removal of organs for a transplant.

This eventually is possible only in the case of total and irreversible brain   79
damage occurring in a young person, essentially as a result of a very severe
injury.

Taking into consideration the important advances made in surgical techniques and in the means to increase tolerance to transplants, the group holds
that transplants deserve the support of the medical profession, of the law, and
of people in general. The donation of organs should, in all circumstances,
respect the last will of the donor or the consent of the family, if present.

DOCUMENT 2 / Brain Death

Source: Pope Pius XII, "The Prolongation of Life" (Nov. 24, 1957), *The Pope Speaks* 4: no. 4, 1958, pp. 396–98.

THE FACT OF DEATH

The question of the fact of death and that of verifying the fact itself ("de facto") or its legal authenticity ("de jure") have, because of their consequences, even in the field of morals and of religion, an even greater importance. What we have just said about the presupposed essential elements for the valid reception of a sacrament has shown this. But the importance of the question extends also to effects in matters of inheritance, marriage and matrimonial processes, benefices (vacancy of a benefice), and to many other questions of private and social life.

It remains for the doctor, and especially the anesthesiologist, to give a clear and precise definition of "death" and the "moment of death" of a patient who passes away in a state of unconsciousness. Here one can accept the usual concept of complete and final separation of the soul from the body; but in practice one must take into account the lack of precision of the terms "body" and "separation." One can put aside the possibility of a person being buried alive, for removal of the artificial respiration apparatus must necessarily bring about stoppage of blood circulation and therefore death within a few minutes.

In case of insoluble doubt, one can resort to presumptions of law and of fact. In general, it will be necessary to presume that life remains, because there is involved here a fundamental right received from the Creator, and it is necessary to prove with certainty that it has been lost. . . .

WHEN IS ONE "DEAD"?

3. "When the blood circulation and the life of a patient who is deeply unconscious because of a central paralysis are maintained only through artificial respiration, and no improvement is noted after a few days, at what time does the Catholic Church consider the patient 'dead,' or when must he be declared dead according to natural law (questions 'de facto' and 'de jure')?"

(Has death already occurred after grave trauma of the brain, which has provoked deep unconsciousness and central breathing paralysis, the fatal consequences of which have nevertheless been retarded by artificial respiration? Or does it occur, according to the present opinion of doctors, only when there is complete arrest of circulation despite prolonged artificial respiration?)

Where the verification of the fact in particular cases is concerned, the answer cannot be deduced from any religious and moral principle and, under this aspect, does not fall within the competence of the Church. Until an answer can be given, the question must remain open. But considerations of a general nature allow us to believe that human life continues for as long as its vital

functions—distinguished from the simple life of organs—manifest themselves 81
spontaneously or even with the help of artificial processes. A great number of these cases are the object of insoluble doubt, and must be dealt with according to the presumptions of law and of fact of which we have spoken.

May these explanations guide you and enlighten you when you must solve delicate questions arising in the practice of your profession. As a token of divine favors which we call upon you and all those who are dear to you, we heartily grant you our apostolic blessing.

DOCUMENT 3 / Brain Death

SOURCE: United States Catholic Conference Advisory Committee on Ethical and Religious Directives for Catholic Health Facilities, "Guidelines for the Determination of Brain Death," *Hospital Progress*, Dec. 1975, p. 26.

INTRODUCTION

In issuing guidelines on the determination of brain death, the Committee of Health Affairs of the United States Catholic Conference offers to Catholic health facilities the present state of the art for assisting the patient's physician in making his decision that brain death has occurred. These guidelines are consonant with the Church's teaching that life is sacred and that death marks a person's entry into a fuller life.

The Committee on Health Affairs affirms the precept that the traditional medical criteria that have been used for determining death (the permanent cessation of the heartbeat and respiration) should remain as the standard criteria and will be sufficient in the great majority of instances when death is to be pronounced. The committee appreciates, however, that there are certain clinical circumstances when these criteria may be insufficient particularly in the course of maintenance of cardiopulmonary function and when considering the procurement of donor organs for transplantation. Under these circumstances an additional set of criteria, which provides a moral certainty of brain death, may be more suitable. It is important to emphasize that these are additional means of determining the same end point. These are not meant to imply different kinds or degrees of death.

After considerable research and discussion, the Advisory Committee on the Ethical and Religious Directives has proposed "Guidelines for the Determination of Brain Death." The Committee on Health Affairs considers that these criteria, medically sound, are also morally sound and acceptable.

GUIDELINES

Recent advances in technologic methods for maintaining certain physiologic functions have frequently made it difficult to determine at what point death has occurred. The determination of clinical death can be a problem particularly in those cases relating to certain illnesses of the central nervous system. These criteria are recommended only as a guide in those cases in which a diagnosis of death may be questionable after the usual methods for determining clinical death have been employed.

1. There is total unawareness to externally applied stimuli. Even the most intensely painful stimuli evoke no vocal or other response, not even a groan, withdrawal of a limb, or spontaneous respiration.

2. Observations covering a period of at least one hour by physicians are adequate to satisfy the criteria of no spontaneous muscular movements or spontaneous respiration or response to stimuli such as pain, touch, sound, or light. After the patient is on a mechanical respirator, the total absence of spontaneous breathing may be established by turning off the respirator for three minutes and observing whether there is any effort on the part of the subject to breathe spontaneously. (The respirator may be turned off for this time provided that at the start of the trial period the patient's carbon dioxide tension is within the normal range, and provided also that the patient has been ventilated with room air for a least 10 minutes prior to the trial.)

3. Irreversible coma with abolition of central nervous system activity is evidenced in part by the absence of elicitable reflexes. The pupil will be fixed and dilated and will not respond to a direct source of bright light or to pinching the neck. Ocular movement (to head turning and to irrigation of the ears with ice water) and blinking are absent. There is no evidence of postural activity (decerebrate or other). Swallowing, yawning, vocalization are in abeyance. Corneal and pharyngeal reflexes are absent.

As a rule the stretch or tendon reflexes cannot be elicited; i.e., tapping the tendons of the biceps, triceps, and pronator muscles, quadriceps and gastrocnemius muscles with the reflex hammer elicits no contraction of the respective muscles. Plantar or noxious stimulation gives no response.

All of the above tests shall have been repeated at a 24-hour interval with no change.

4. Of great confirmatory value is the flat or isoelectric EEG. A flat electroencephalogram is not an essential determination but may be used if desired by the individual physician. We must assume that the electrodes have been properly applied, that the apparatus is functioning normally, and that the personnel in charge are competent. We consider it prudent to have one channel of the apparatus used for an electrocardiogram. This channel will monitor the ECG so that, if it appears in the electroencephalographic leads because of high resistance, it can be readily identified. It also establishes the presence of the active heart in the absence of the EEG. We recommend that another channel be used for a noncephalic lead. This will pick up space-borne or vibration-borne artifacts and identify them. The simplest form of such a monitoring noncephalic electrode has two leads over the dorsum of the hand, so the ECG will be minimal or absent. Since one of the requirements of this state is that there be no muscle activity, these two dorsal hand electrodes will not be bothered by muscle artifact. The apparatus should be run at standard gains 10 uv/mm, 50 uv/5 mm. Also it should be isoelectric at double this standard gain which is 5 uv/5 mm or 25 uv/5mm. At least 10 full minutes of recording are desirable, but twice that would be better.

It is also suggested that the gains at some point be opened to their full amplitude for a brief period (five to 100 seconds) to see what is going on. Usually in an intensive care unit artifacts will dominate the picture, but these are readily identifiable. There shall be no electroencephalographic response to noise or to pinch.

The validity of such data as indications of irreversible cerebral damage depends on the exclusion of two conditions: hypothermia (temperature below 90° [12.2°]) or central nervous system depressants, such as barbiturates.

14: Capital Punishment

DOCUMENT 1:

Source: Pope John Paul II, "The Gospel of Life," (Mar. 25, 1995), *Origins* 24: no. 42, Apr. 6, 1995, p, 709.

56. This is the context in which to place the problem of the death penalty. On this matter there is a growing tendency, both in the Church and in civil society, to demand that it be applied in a very limited way or even that it be abolished completely. The problem must be viewed in the context of a system of penal justice ever more in line with human dignity and thus, in the end, with God's plan for man and society. The primary purpose of the punishment which society inflicts is "to redress the disorder caused by the offense." Public authority must redress the violation of personal and social rights by imposing on the offender an adequate punishment for the crime, as a condition for the offender to regain the exercise of his or her freedom. In this way authority also fulfills the purpose of defending public order and ensuring people's safety, while at the same time offering the offender an incentive and help to change his or her behavior and be rehabilitated.

It is clear that for these purposes to be achieved, the nature and extent of the punishment must be carefully evaluated and decided upon, and ought not go to the extreme of executing the offender except in cases of absolute necessity. In other words, when it would not be possible otherwise to defend society. Today, however, as a result of steady improvements in the organization of the penal system, such cases are very rare if not practically nonexistent.

In any event, the principle set forth in the new Catechism of the Catholic Church remains valid: "If bloodless means are sufficient to defend human lives against an aggressor and to protect public order and the safety of persons, public authority must limit itself to such means, because they better correspond to the concrete conditions of the common good and are more in conformity to the dignity of the human person" (Catechism of the Catholic Church, no. 2267).

DOCUMENT 2 / Capital Punishment

SOURCE: New Mexico Bishops, "An Opportune Time to Review the Correctional System," *Origins* 26: no. 36 (Feb. 27, 1997), pp. 586–88.

In the context of protecting the public order and contributing to the common good, the state has both the right and the responsibility to punish wrongdoers. Some of those in our prisons and jails have done horrible things and have caused undue suffering. They have hurt the innocent and the defenseless, such as women and children, and have destroyed the security in our neighborhoods and communities. We support the mission of public safety which is committed to the reduction of criminal acts in our society. Of special concern to us as ministers of compassion are victims of violent crimes and their families. We pledge our solidarity to these and offer the healing outreach of our ministry.

On Sept. 19, 1995, we issued a statement opposing capital punishment. Today we wish to reiterate our opposition to the death penalty. In solidarity with the U.S. Catholic bishops, we view our commitment to the value and dignity of human life. We believe that a return to the use of the death penalty is only leading to further erosion of respect for life in our society.

In light of the above, we offer the following practical recommendations:

1. Expand treatment for low-risk offenders in a community-based setting wherever possible.

2. We recommend that there be a separation between the violent and nonviolent offenders as well as a separation of those inmates committed to rehabilitation from those who show no interest in reform. Models of therapeutic communities should be fostered.

3. Viable education, as well as behavior modification and treatment programs, need to be made available to those who are willing to commit themselves to them.

4. Effective drug and alcohol rehabilitation programs need to be in place if we are to lessen the rate of recidivism. Twelve-step programs have proven effective around the country, and we urge that these programs be made available to all inmates.

5. The state needs to commit itself to contribute to a successful transition of a released inmate to his or her family and community. Included in this are would-be considerations regarding employments, housing, and further education.

6. The Corrections Department should seriously consider developing a victim-awareness program inside the prisons as well as in our communities. Victim awareness programs respond to the needs of victims and contribute to the process of healing for the victim and reformation of the offender.

86   7. We call for a dialogue between officials of the New Mexico Department of Corrections and religious leaders of the state in order to promote a more collaborative relationship. The exchange would include such areas as sensitivity for religious diversity and other issues of mutual concern.

15: Catholic Health Care

DOCUMENT 1:

Source: New Jersey Bishops, "The Rationale of Catholic Health Care," *Origins* 25: no. 27 (Dec. 21, 1995), pp. 450–52.

. . . The New Jersey bishops said November 27 in a pastoral statement on health care.

. . . Health involves not only a scientific concept but a moral judgment. It addresses the interconnected array of the elements of body, mind, spirit, and emotion in which and through which human life is identified and experienced. Likewise, health care is not simply scientific but has specific moral dimensions. Catholic health care also involves primary moral judgments. It is delivered and received within a particular Christian religious community, which community is dedicated to faith and specific moral principles. In the tradition of Catholic health care, affirmation of human dignity guides the manner of treatment and care. The community is characterized by compassion, sustenance, companionship, prayer, and sacraments. Care of the poor and the rejected is part of our Catholic commitment to reflect how God has acted to save us.

What kind of community are we which creates a system of health care which is precisely moral, particularly Christian, and specifically Catholic? We are a community of faith and worship and fraternal love and care, who know who we are and become who we are through the life, death, and resurrection of Jesus. In the life of Jesus, God reveals himself in the flesh not as a wonder worker who eradicated all human sickness, fear and confusion, but as the God who endured sickness, fear and confusion along with us. In the life of Jesus we recognize not only a man who suffered, but also the God who suffered along with us. In Jesus we encounter the God who did not escape death but died a human death. In his resurrection we acknowledge not only the power of God, but also the new life given by God—in fullness to Jesus, and in truth and in promise to us. God is still with us really, truly, and personally. God dwells with us and within us through the power of his Holy Spirit, and that makes us really and truly different: It makes us Christlike. We who have been touched and saved and changed by God must make all this visible not only by our grateful faith-filled praise of God, but also by our loving presence with each other and our compassionate care for one another. Catholic health care exists as a practical sign of living faith; it exists "to be Jesus' love for the other in the health care setting."

Catholic health care shares a number of aims with health care generally: to cure disease whenever possible, to relieve pain and anxiety, to offer programs

88 of preventive medicine, and to offer palliative care to the terminal and dying. But we require even more from health care which is genuinely Catholic. As Catholics we journey in faith and love with the living, and we keep watch with the dying. Moreover, we offer hope based on our conviction that all life exists under the ordinance of God, who is a trustworthy creator and a faithful savior. Contained within this hope is our certainty that suffering need not be absurd and that death need not be tragic. In all of our efforts the dignity of the person created in the image of God and re-created in the image of Christ is paramount. While we make no claim that such aims are exclusively Catholic, we insist that Catholic health care must embrace these components.

Grateful faith and responsive Christian love have always characterized Catholic health care. In faithful imitation of Jesus Christ, the Church has served the sick, suffering, and dying in various ways throughout history. The zealous service of individuals and communities has provided shelter for the traveler, infirmaries for the sick, and homes for children, adults, and the elderly. In the United States, the many religious communities as well as dioceses that sponsor and staff this country's Catholic health care institutions and services have established an effective Catholic presence in health care. Modeling their efforts on the Gospel parable of the good Samaritan, these communities of women and men have exemplified authentic neighborliness to those in need (cf. Lk 10:25–37). The Church seeks to ensure that the service offered in the past will be continued into the future.

Catholic health care acknowledges that human life is a gift from God over which we exercise stewardship, not dominion. Catholic health care also witnesses to the saving love of God, extending special concern to the helpless. For these reasons we are zealous in our protection of unborn life and in our defense of incompetent and dying patients. For these same reasons we work to ensure that adequate health care be given to the poor.

We cannot ignore that there are forces which imperil the identity and integrity of Catholic health care. Some of these influences are external, some are internal; some are structural, some are personal. There are, for example, market forces which gauge the effectiveness of health care delivery solely in terms of profitability.

There are mergers, integrated delivery networks, and managed-care organizations which have the potential of jeopardizing the identity of Catholic health care institutions. Then too, health insurance providers run the risk of exercising undue control over medical treatment options, of rationing care even when resources are readily available and putting the poor, the uninsured, and the underinsured at risk. Among some who work in or support Catholic health care delivery systems, there may be a tendency to believe that the overriding purpose of health care in a Catholic system is to cure sickness and to forestall death. This leads to a lack of sympathy for the rationale of Catholic health care and a lack of appreciation of its specific Catholic identity. . . .

DOCUMENT 2 / Catholic Health Care

SOURCE: Pope John Paul II, "Health Care: Ministry in Transition" (Sept. 14, 1987), *Origins* 17: no. 17, Oct. 8, 1987, pp. 292–94.

... This is the high dignity to which you and your colleagues are called. This is your vocation, your commitment, and the path of your specific witness to the presence of God's kingdom in the world. Your health care ministry, pioneered and developed by congregations of women religious and by congregations of brothers, is one of the most vital apostolates of the ecclesial community and one of the most significant services which the Catholic Church offers to society in the name of Jesus Christ. ...

2. Because of your dedication to caring for the sick and the poor, the aged and the dying, you know from your own daily experience how much illness and suffering are basic problems of human existence. When the sick flocked to Jesus during his earthly life, they recognized in him a friend whose deeply compassionate and loving heart responded to their needs. He restored physical and mental health to many. These cures, however, involved more than just healing sickness. They were also prophetic signs of his own identity and of the coming of the kingdom of God, and they very often caused a new spiritual awakening in the one who had been healed.

The power that went out from Jesus and cured people of his own time (cf. Lk 6:19) has not lost its effect in the 2,000-year history of the Church. This power remains, in the life and prayer of the Church, a source of healing and reconciliation. Ever active, this power confirms the identity of the Church today, authenticates her proclamation of the Kingdom of God, and stands as a sign of triumph over evil.

With all Catholic health care, the immediate aim is to provide for the well-being of the body and mind of the human person, especially in sickness or old age. By his example, Christ teaches the Christian "to do good by his or her suffering and to do good to those who suffer" (John Paul II, Apostolic Exhortation *On Human Suffering*, 30). This latter aspect naturally absorbs the greater part of the energy and attention of health care ministry.

Today in the United States Catholic health care extends the mission of the Church in every state of the union, in major cities, small towns, rural areas, on the campuses of academic institutions, in remote outposts, and in inner-city neighborhoods. By providing health care in all these places, especially to the poor, the neglected, the needy, the newcomer, your apostolate penetrates and transforms the very fabric of American society. And sometimes you yourselves, like those you serve, are called to bow, in humble and loving resignation, to the experience of sickness—or to other forms of pain and suffering.

90   **3.** All concern for the sick and suffering is part of the Church's life and mission. The Church has always understood herself to be charged by Christ with the care of the poor, the weak, the defenseless, the suffering, and those who mourn. This means that as you alleviate suffering and seek to heal you also bear witness to the Christian view of suffering and to the meaning of life and death as taught by your Christian faith.

In the complex world of modern health care in industrialized society, this witness must be given in a variety of ways. First, it requires continual efforts to ensure that everyone has access to health care. I know that you have already examined this question in the report of your task force on health care of the poor. In seeking to treat patients equally, regardless of social and economic status, you proclaim to your fellow citizens and to the world Christ's special love for the neglected and powerless. This particular challenge is a consequence of your Christian dedication and conviction, and it calls for great courage on the part of Catholic bodies and institutions operating in the field of health care. It is a great credit to your zeal and efficiency when, despite formidable costs, you still succeed in preventing the economic factor from being the determinant factor in human and Christian service.

Similarly, the love with which Catholic health care is performed and its professional excellence have the value of a sign testifying to the Christian view of the human person. The inalienable dignity of every human being is, of course, fundamental to all Catholic health care. All who come to you for help are worthy of respect and love, for all have been created in the image and likeness of God. All have been redeemed by Christ and, in their sufferings, bear his cross. It is fitting that our meeting is taking place on the feast of the Triumph of the Cross. Christ took upon himself the whole of human suffering and radically transformed it through the paschal mystery of his passion, death, and resurrection. The triumph of the cross gives human suffering a new dimension, a redemptive value (cf. ibid., 24). It is your privilege to bear constant witness to this profound truth in so many ways.

The structural changes which have been taking place within Catholic health care in recent years have increased the challenge of preserving and even strengthening the Catholic identity of the institutions and the spiritual quality of the services given. The presence of dedicated women and men religious in hospitals and nursing homes has ensured in the past, and continues to ensure in the present, that spiritual dimension so characteristic of Catholic health care centers. The reduced number of religious and new forms of ownership and management should not lead to a loss of a spiritual atmosphere or to a loss of a sense of vocation in caring for the sick. This is an area in which the Catholic laity, at all levels of health care, have an opportunity to manifest the depth of their faith and to play their own specific part in the Church's mission of evangelization and service.

4. As I have said, Catholic health care must always be carried out within the framework of the Church's saving mission. This mission she has received from her divine founder, and she has accomplished it down through the ages

with the help of the Holy Spirit, who guides her into the fullness of truth (cf. **91**
Jn 16:13; *Dogmatic Constitution on the Church*, 4). Your ministry therefore must
also reflect the mission of the Church as the teacher of moral truth, especially in
regard to the new frontiers of scientific research and technological achievement.
Here too you face great challenges and opportunities.

Many times in recent years the Church has addressed issues related to
the advances of biomedical technology. She does so not in order to discourage
scientific progress or to judge harshly those who seek to extend the frontiers
of human knowledge and skill, but in order to affirm the moral truths which
must guide the application of this knowledge and skill. Ultimately, the purpose
of the Church's teaching in this field is to defend the innate dignity and fundamental rights of the human person. In this regard the Church cannot fail to
emphasize the need to safeguard the life and integrity of the human embryo
and fetus.

5. The human person is a unique composite—a unity of spirit and matter,
soul and body, fashioned in the image of God and destined to live forever.
Every human life is sacred, because every human person is sacred. It is in the
light of this fundamental truth that the Church constantly proclaims and defends the dignity of human life from the moment of conception to the moment
of natural death. It is also in the light of this fundamental truth that we see
the great evil of abortion and euthanasia. . . .

6. In the exercise of your professional activities you have a magnificent
opportunity, by your constant witness to moral truth, to contribute to the
formation of society's moral vision. As you give the best of yourselves in
fulfilling your Christian responsibilities, you will also be aware of the important
contribution you must make to building a society based on truth and justice.
Your service to the sick enables you with great credibility to proclaim to the
world the demands and values of the Gospel of Jesus Christ, and to foster
hope and renewal of heart. In this respect, your concern with the Catholic
identity of your work and your institutions is not only timely and commendable,
it is essential for the success of your ecclesial mission.

You must always see yourselves and your work as part of the Church's
life and mission. You are indeed a very special part of the people of God.
You and your institutions have precise responsibilities toward the ecclesial
community, just as that community has responsibilities toward you. It is important at every level—national, state, and local—that there be close and harmonious links between you and the bishops, who "preside in place of God over the
flock whose shepherds they are, as teachers of doctrine, priests of sacred worship, and officers of good order" (*Dogmatic Constitution on the Church*, 20). They,
for their part, wish to support you in your witness and service.

. . . Today you are faced with new challenges, new needs. One of these
is the present crisis of immense proportions which is that of AIDS and AIDS-
related complex. Besides your professional contribution and your human sensitivities toward all affected by this disease, you are called to show the love
and compassion of Christ and his Church. As you courageously affirm and

92   implement your moral obligation and social responsibility to help those who suffer, you are individually and collectively living out the parable of the good Samaritan (cf. Lk 10:30–32).

The good Samaritan of the parable showed compassion to the injured man. By taking him to the inn and giving of his own material means, he truly gave of himself. This action, a universal symbol of human concern, has become one of the essential elements of moral culture and civilization. How beautifully the Lord speaks of the Samaritan! He "was neighbor to the man who fell in with the robbers" (Lk 10:36). To be "neighbor" is to express love, solidarity, and service, and to exclude selfishness, discrimination, and neglect. The message of the parable of the good Samaritan echoes a reality connected with today's feast of the Triumph of the Cross: "The kindness and love of God our Savior appeared . . . that we might be justified by his grace and become heirs, in hope, of eternal life" (Ti 3:4–7). In the changing world of health care, it is up to you to ensure that this "kindness and love of God our Savior" remains the heart and soul of Catholic health services. . . .

16: Children and the Family

DOCUMENT 1:

SOURCE: Pope John Paul II, "The Christian Family in the Modern World" (Nov. 22, 1981), *Vatican Council II*, Vol. 2, pp. 827–37.

THE ROLE OF THE CHRISTIAN FAMILY

17. The family finds in the plan of God the Creator and Redeemer not only its identity, what it is, but also its mission, what it can and should do. The role that God calls the family to perform in history derives from what the family is; its role represents the dynamic and existential development of what it is. Each family finds within itself a summons that cannot be ignored and that specifies both its dignity and its responsibility: family become what you are.

Accordingly, the family must go back to the "beginning" of God's creative act, if it is to attain self-knowledge and self-realization in accordance with the inner truth not only of what it is but also of what it does in history. And since in God's plan it has been established as an "intimate community of life and love," the family has the mission to become more and more what it is, that is to say, a community of life and love, in an effort that will find fulfillment, as will everything created and redeemed, in the Kingdom of God. Looking at it in such a way as to reach its very roots, we must say that the essence and role of the family are in the final analysis specified by love. Hence the family has the mission to guard, reveal, and communicate love, and this is a living reflection of and a real sharing in God's love for humanity and the love of Christ the Lord for the Church his bride.

Every particular task of the family is an expression and concrete actuation of that fundamental mission. We must therefore go deeper into the unique riches of the family's mission and probe its contents, which are both manifold and unified.

Thus, with love as its point of departure and making constant reference to it, the recent Synod emphasized four general tasks for the family: 1) forming a community of persons; 2) serving life; 3) participating in the development of society; 4) sharing in the life and mission of the Church.

I—FORMING A COMMUNITY OF PERSONS

22. In that it is, and ought always to become, a communion and community of persons, the family finds in love the source and the constant impetus for welcoming, respecting, and promoting each one of its members in his or her lofty dignity as a person, that is, as a living image of God. As the Synod Fathers rightly stated, the moral criterion for the authenticity of conjugal and family

94 relationships consists in fostering the dignity and vocation of the individual persons, who achieve their fullness by sincere self-giving.

In this perspective the Synod devoted special attention to women, to their rights and role within the family and society. In the same perspective are also to be considered men as husbands and fathers, and likewise children and the elderly.

Above all it is important to underline the equal dignity and responsibility of women with men. This equality is realized in a unique manner in that reciprocal self-giving by each one to the other and by both to the children which is proper to marriage and the family. What human reason intuitively perceives and acknowledges is fully revealed by the word of God: the history of salvation, in fact, is a continuous and luminous testimony to the dignity of women.

In creating the human race "male and female," God gives man and woman an equal personal dignity, endowing them with the inalienable rights and responsibilities proper to the human person. God then manifests the dignity of women in the highest form possible, by assuming human flesh from the Virgin Mary, whom the Church honors as the Mother of God, calling her the new Eve and presenting her as the model of redeemed woman. The sensitive respect of Jesus towards the women that he called to his following and his friendship, his appearing on Easter morning to a woman before the other disciples, the mission entrusted to women to carry the good news of the resurrection to the Apostles—these are all signs that confirm the special esteem of the Lord Jesus for women. The Apostle Paul will say: "In Christ Jesus you are all children of God through faith. . . . There is neither Jew nor Greek, there is neither slave nor free, there is neither male nor female; for you are all one in Christ Jesus."

23. Without intending to deal with all the various aspects of the vast and complex theme of the relationships between women and society, and limiting these remarks to a few essential points, one cannot but observe that in the specific area of family life a widespread social and cultural tradition has considered women's role to be exclusively that of wife and mother, without adequate access to public functions, which have generally been reserved for men.

. . . This will come about more easily if, in accordance with the wishes expressed by the Synod, a renewed "theology of work" can shed light upon and study in depth the meaning of work in the Christian life and determine the fundamental bond between work and the family and therefore the original and irreplaceable meaning of work in the home and in rearing children. Therefore the Church can and should help modern society by tirelessly insisting that the work of women in the home be recognized and respected by all in its irreplaceable value. This is of particular importance in education: for possible discrimination between the different types of work and professions is eliminated at its very root once it is clear that all people, in every area, are working with equal rights and equal responsibilities. The image of God in man and in woman will thus be seen with added luster.

While it must be recognized that women have the same right as men to **95** perform various public functions, society must be structured in such a way that wives and mothers are not in practice compelled to work outside the home, and that their families can live and prosper in a dignified way even when they themselves devote their full time to their own family.

Furthermore, the mentality which honors women more for their work outside the home than for their work within the family must be overcome. This requires that men should truly esteem and love women with total respect for their personal dignity, and that society should create and develop conditions favoring work in the home.

With due respect to the different vocation of men and women, the Church must in her own life promote as far as possible their equality of rights and dignity: and this for the good of all, the family, the Church, and society.

But clearly all of this does not mean for women a renunciation of their femininity or an imitation of the male role, but the fullness of true feminine humanity which should be expressed in their activity, whether in the family or outside of it, without disregarding the differences of customs and cultures in this sphere.

24. Unfortunately the Christian message about the dignity of women is contradicted by that persistent mentality which considers the human being not as a person but as a thing, as an object of trade, at the service of selfish interest and mere pleasure; the first victims of this mentality are women.

This mentality produces very bitter fruits, such as contempt for men and for women, slavery, oppression of the weak, pornography, prostitution— especially in an organized form—and all those various forms of discrimination that exist in the fields of education, employment, wages, etc.

. . . The Synod Fathers deplored these and other forms of discrimination as strongly as possible. I therefore ask that vigorous and incisive pastoral action be taken by all to overcome them definitively so that the image of God that shines in all human beings without exception may be fully respected.

26. In the family, which is a community of persons, special attention must be devoted to the children, by developing a profound esteem for their personal dignity and a great respect and generous concern for their rights. This is true for every child, but it becomes all the more urgent the smaller the child is and the more it is in need of everything, when it is sick, suffering, or handicapped.

By fostering and exercising a tender and strong concern for every child that comes into this world, the Church fulfills a fundamental mission: for she is called upon to reveal and put forward anew in history the example and the commandment of Christ the Lord, who placed the child at the heart of the Kingdom of God: "Let the children come to me, and do not hinder them; for to such belongs the kingdom of heaven."

I repeat once again what I said to the General Assembly of the United Nations on Oct. 2, 1979: "I wish to express the joy that we all find in children, the springtime of life, the anticipation of the future history of each of our present earthly homelands. No country on earth, no political system can think

96 of its own future otherwise than through the image of these new generations that will receive from their parents the manifold heritage of values, duties, and aspirations of the nation to which they belong and of the whole human family. Concern for the child, even before birth, from the first moment of conception and then throughout the years of infancy and youth, is the primary and fundamental test of the relationship of one human being to another. And so, what better wish can I express for every nation and for the whole of mankind, and for all the children of the world than a better future in which respect for human rights will become a complete reality throughout the third millennium, which is drawing near."

Acceptance, love, esteem, many-sided and united material, emotional, educational, and spiritual concern for every child that comes into this world should always constitute a distinctive, essential characteristic of all Christians, in particular of the Christian family: thus children, while they are able to grow "in wisdom and in stature, and in favor with God and man," offer their own precious contribution to building up the family community and even to the sanctification of their parents.

II—SERVING LIFE
1. The transmission of life

28. With the creation of man and woman in his own image and likeness, God crowns and brings to perfection the work of his hands: he calls them to a special sharing in his love and in his power as Creator and Father, through their free and responsible cooperation in transmitting the gift of human life: "God blessed them, and God said to them, 'Be fruitful and multiply, and fill the earth and subdue it.' "

Thus the fundamental task of the family is to serve life, to actualize in history the original blessing of the Creator—that of transmitting by procreation the divine image from person to person.

Fecundity is the fruit and the sign of conjugal love, the living testimony of the full reciprocal self-giving of the spouses: "While not making the other purposes of matrimony of less account, the true practice of conjugal love, and the whole meaning of the family life which results from it, have this aim: that the couple be ready with stout hearts to cooperate with the love of the Creator and the Savior, who through them will enlarge and enrich his own family day by day."

However, the fruitfulness of conjugal love is not restricted solely to the procreation of children, even understood in its specifically human dimension: it is enlarged and enriched by all those fruits of oral, spiritual, and supernatural life which the father and mother are called to hand on to their children, and through the children to the Church and to the world.

DOCUMENT 2 / Children and the Family

SOURCE: Congregation for the Doctrine of the Faith, "Instruction on Respect for Human Life in Its Origin and on the Dignity of Procreation" (Feb. 22, 1987), *Origins* 16: no. 40, Mar. 19, 1987, p. 706.

4, c) Only respect for the link between the meanings of the conjugal act and respect for the unity of the human beings make possible procreation in conformity with the dignity of the person. In his unique and irrepeatable origin, the child must be respected and recognized as equal in personal dignity to those who give him life. The human person must be accepted in his parents' act of union and love; the generation of a child must therefore be the fruit of that mutual giving which is realized in the conjugal act wherein the spouses cooperate as servants and not as masters in the work of the Creator, who is love.

In reality, the origin of a human person is the result of an act of giving. The one conceived must be the fruit of his parents' love. He cannot be desired or conceived as the product of an intervention of medical or biological techniques; that would be equivalent to reducing him to an object of scientific technology. No one may subject the coming of a child into the world to conditions of technical efficiency which are to be evaluated according to standards of control and dominion.

The moral relevance of the link between the meanings of the conjugal act and between the goods of marriage, as well as the unity of the human being and the dignity of his origin, demand that the procreation of a human person be brought about as the fruit of the conjugal act specific to the love between spouses. The link between procreation and the conjugal act is thus shown to be of great importance on the anthropological and moral planes, and it throws light on the positions of the Magisterium with regard to homologous artificial fertilization.

8. The suffering caused by infertility in marriage. The suffering of spouses who cannot have children or who are afraid of bringing a handicapped child into the world is a suffering that everyone must understand and properly evaluate.

On the part of the spouses, the desire for a child is natural: it expresses the vocation to fatherhood and motherhood inscribed in conjugal love. This desire can be even stronger if the couple is affected by sterility which appears incurable. Nevertheless, marriage does not confer upon the spouses the right to have a child, but only the right to perform those natural acts which are per se ordered to procreation.

A true and proper right to a child would be contrary to the child's dignity and nature. The child is not an object to which one has a right, nor can he be considered as an object of ownership: rather, a child is a gift, "the supreme gift" and the most gratuitous gift of marriage, and is a living testimony of the mutual giving of his parents. For this reason, the child has the right, as already

98   mentioned, to be the fruit of the specific act of the conjugal love of his parents; and he also has the right to be respected as a person from the moment of his conception.

Nevertheless, whatever its cause or prognosis, sterility is certainly a difficult trial. The community of believers is called to shed light upon and support the suffering of those who are unable to fulfill their legitimate aspiration to motherhood and fatherhood. Spouses who find themselves in this sad situation are called to find in it an opportunity for sharing in a particular way in the Lord's cross, the source of spiritual fruitfulness. Sterile couples must not forget that "even when procreation is not possible, conjugal life does not for this reason lose its value. Physical sterility in fact can be for spouses the occasion for other important services to the life of the human person, for example, adoption, various forms of educational work, and assistance to other families and to poor or handicapped children."

Many researchers are engaged in the fight against sterility. While fully safeguarding the dignity of human procreation, some have achieved results which previously seemed unattainable. Scientists therefore are to be encouraged to continue their research with the aim of preventing the causes of sterility and of being able to remedy them so that sterile couples will be able to procreate in full respect for their own personal dignity and that of the child to be born.

DOCUMENT 3 / Children and the Family

SOURCE: Pope John Paul II, "The Transmission of Life" (Aug. 22, 1984), *The Pope Speaks* 29: no. 4, 1984, pp. 349–51.

What is the essence of the Church's doctrine on the transmission of life in the community of married persons? It is a doctrine we are reminded of by the council's pastoral constitution, *Gaudium et Spes,* and by Pope Paul VI's encyclical *Humanae Vitae.*

The problem consists in maintaining a suitable relationship between what is defined as "domination . . . of the forces of nature" and the "mastery of self," which is indispensable for the human person. Modern man tends to use for the latter, the methods proper to the former. "Man has made stupendous progress in the domination and rational organization of the forces of nature," as we read in the encyclical, "to the point that he is endeavoring to extend this control over every aspect of his own life—over his body, over his mind and emotions, over his social life, and even over the laws that regulate the transmission of life."

Extending our sphere of "domination over the forces of nature" threatens the human person, for whom the method of "self-mastery" is and remains specific. The mastery of self, in fact, corresponds to the fundamental constitution of the person. It is indeed a "natural" method. On the contrary, resorting to "artificial means" destroys the constitutive dimension of the person, by depriving man of the subjectivity proper to him and by making him an object of manipulation.

"BODY LANGUAGE"

The human body is not merely an organism of sexual reactions, but it is, at the same time, the means of expressing the entire man, the person, which reveals itself by means of the "language of the body." This "language" has an important interpersonal meaning, especially in mutual relationships between man and woman. Moreover, our previous analysis shows that in this case the "language of the body" should express the truth of the sacrament. Participating in the eternal plan of love ("a sacrament hidden in God"), the "language of the body" becomes, in fact, a kind of "prophecy for the body."

It may be said that the encyclical *Humanae Vitae* carries to its extreme consequences—not merely logical and moral, but also practical and pastoral— this truth concerning the human body in its masculinity and femininity.

DEMANDS OF TRUTH

The unity of the two aspects of the problem—of the sacramental (or theological) dimension and of the personalistic one—corresponds to the overall **99**

100 "revelation of the body." From this derives also the connection between the strictly theological vision and the ethical one, which appeals to the "natural law."

The subject of the natural law, in fact, is man not only in his "natural existence but also in the whole truth of his personal subjectivity. He is shown to us, in revelation, as male and female, in his full temporal and eschatological vocation. He is called by God to be a witness and interpreter of the eternal plan of love, by becoming the minister of the sacrament that "from the beginning" was constituted by the sign of the "union of flesh."

As ministers of a sacrament that is constituted by consent and perfected by conjugal union, man and woman are called to express that mysterious "language" of their bodies in all the truth that is proper to it. By means of gestures and reactions, by means of the whole mutually conditioned dynamism of tension and enjoyment—whose direct source is the body in its masculinity and its femininity, the body in its action and interaction—by means of all this, man, the person, "speaks."

LOVE AND PROCREATION

In the "language of the body," man and woman carry on that dialogue, which according to Genesis, began on the day of creation. Precisely on the level of this "language of the body"—which is something more than mere sexual reaction and which, as an authentic language of the persons, is subject to the demands of truth (that is, to objective moral norms)—man and woman mutually express themselves in the fullest and most profound way possible to them by the very corporeal dimension of masculinity and femininity: man and woman express themselves in the measure of the whole truth of the human person.

Man is a person precisely because he is master of himself and has self-control. Indeed, insofar as he is master of himself, he can "give himself" to the other. And it is this dimension—the dimension of a free gift—that becomes essential and decisive for that "language of the body," in which man and woman mutually express themselves in the conjugal union. Granted that this is a communion of person, the "language of the body" should be judged according to the criterion of truth. It is precisely this criterion which the encyclical *Humanae Vitae* recalls, as we saw in the passages quoted earlier.

According to the criterion of this truth, the conjugal act, which is expressed in the "language of the body," "signifies" not only love, but also potential fruitfulness, and therefore it cannot be deprived of its full and proper significance by artificial means. In the conjugal act, it is not licit to separate artificially the unitive aspect from the procreative aspect, because both the one and the other pertain to the intimate truth of the conjugal act. The one is activated together with the other and, in a certain sense, the one by means of the other. This is what the encyclical teaches. Therefore, in such a case the conjugal act, deprived of its interior truth because it is artificially deprived of its procreative capacity, also ceases to be an act of love.

It can be said that when these two aspects are artificially separated, the conjugal act may be a real bodily union, but it does not correspond to the interior

truth and to the dignity of personal communion, communion of persons. Such   **101**
communion, in fact, demands that the "language of the body" mutually express
the whole truth of its meaning. If this truth is lacking, one can speak neither
of the truth of self-mastery, nor of the truth of the reciprocal gift and of the
reciprocal acceptance of self on the part of the persons. Such a violation of the
interior order of conjugal union, which is rooted in the very order of the person,
constitutes the essential evil of the contraceptive act.

REFLECTIONS ON "SIGN"

The above-given interpretation of moral doctrine expressed in the encyclical *Humanae Vitae* is set against a vast background of reflections on the theology
of the body. Of special validity for understanding this are the reflections on
"sign" in connection with marriage understood as a sacrament. The essence of
the violation that upsets the interior order of the conjugal act cannot be understood in a theologically adequate way without the reflections on the theme of
the "concupiscence of the flesh."

17: Confidentiality

DOCUMENT 1:

SOURCE: Pope Pius XII, "Christian Principles and the Medical Profession" (Nov. 12, 1944), *The Human Body: Papal Teachings*, p. 63.

THE PROFESSIONAL SECRET

Another of the duties which derive from the eighth commandment is the observance of the professional secret, which must serve and serves the good of the individual and even more of society. In this sector, too, there can arise conflicts between the public and private interests, or between different elements and aspects pertaining to the common good. In these conflicts it will often be very difficult indeed to measure and weigh justly the pros and cons for speaking out or keeping silent. In such a dilemma, the conscientious doctor seeks his norm in the basic tenets of Christian ethics, which will help him to pick the right course. These norms, in fact, while they clearly affirm the obligation on the physician to preserve the professional secret, above all in the interest of the common good, do not concede to this an absolute value. For that very common good would suffer were the professional secret placed at the service of crime or injustice.

DOCUMENT 2 / Confidentiality

Source: Pope Pius XII, "The Intangibility of the Human Person" (Sept. 13, 1952), *The Human Body: Papal Teachings*, pp. 196–97.

MEDICAL SCIENCE

Scientific knowledge has its own value in the domain of medical science—not less than in the domains of the other sciences, such as, for example, physics, chemistry, cosmology, psychology—a value which should by no means be minimized, and is imposed quite independently of the usefulness and of the use made of the acquired knowledge. Moreover, knowledge as such and the fullness of knowledge of all truth are the occasion of no moral objection. In virtue of the same principle, research and the acquisition of truth with a view to arriving at new knowledge and a new, more vast, more profound comprehension of this same truth, are in themselves in harmony with the moral order.

This does not mean, however, that every method, even a method well established by scientific research and technique, offers a moral guarantee, or further, that every method becomes lawful by the fact that it increases and deepens our knowledge. Sometimes it happens that one method cannot be put into operation without infringing on the rights of another, or violating some absolute moral value. In this case, advancement of knowledge is the goal seen and aimed at—all well and good; but this method is not morally admissible. Why is this? Because science is not the highest value to which all the other orders of values—or in a single scale of values, all the particular values—should be subjected. Science itself then, along with its researches and attainments, must be inserted in the order of values. Here, well-defined frontiers present themselves, which even medical science cannot transgress without violating higher moral rules. The relationship of confidence between doctor and patient, the right of the patient to life, physical and spiritual, in its psychic or moral integrity—here, amongst others, are values which rule scientific interests.

18: Contraception

DOCUMENT 1:

SOURCE: Pope Pius XI, Encyclical Letter "On Christian Marriage" (Dec. 31, 1930), *The Human Body, Papal Teachings*, pp. 27–29.

IV. VICES OPPOSED TO CHRISTIAN MARRIAGE

. . . We shall explain in detail the evils opposed to each of the benefits of matrimony. First consideration is due to the offspring, which many have the boldness to call the disagreeable burden of matrimony and which they say is to be carefully avoided by married people not through virtuous continence (which Christian law permits in matrimony when both parties consent) but by frustrating the marriage act. Some justify this criminal abuse on the ground that they are weary of children and wish to gratify their desires without their consequent burden. Others say that they cannot on the one hand remain continent nor on the other can they have children because of the difficulties whether on the part of the mother or on the part of family circumstances.

But no reason, however grave, may be put forward by which anything intrinsically against nature may become conformable to nature and morally good. Since, therefore, the conjugal act is destined primarily by nature for the begetting of children, those who in exercising it deliberately frustrate its natural power and purpose sin against nature and commit a deed which is shameful and intrinsically vicious.

. . . Since, therefore, openly departing from the uninterrupted Christian tradition some recently have judged it possible solemnly to declare another doctrine regarding this question, the Catholic Church, to whom God has entrusted the defense of the integrity and purity of morals, standing erect in the midst of the moral ruin which surrounds her, in order that she may preserve the chastity of the nuptial union from being defiled by this foul stain, raises her voice in token in her divine ambassadorship and through our mouth proclaims anew: any use whatsoever of matrimony exercised in such a way that the act is deliberately frustrated in its natural power to generate life is an offense against the law of God and of nature, and those who indulge in such are branded with the guilt of a grave sin.

DOCUMENT 2 / Contraception

SOURCE: Pope Paul VI, Encyclical Letter "On the Regulation of Births" (July 25, 1968), *Vatican Council II*, Vol. 2, pp. 397–408.

NEW ASPECTS OF THE PROBLEM AND COMPETENCY OF THE MAGISTERIUM

New Formulation of the Problem

2. The changes that have taken place [in society] are in fact of considerable importance and concern different problems. In the first place there is the question of the rapid increase in population which has made many fear that world population is going to grow faster than available resources, with the consequence that many families and developing countries are being faced with greater hardships. This fact can easily induce public authorities to be tempted to take radical measures to avert this danger. There is also the fact that not only working and housing conditions, but the greater demands made both in the economic and educational field require that kind of life in which it is frequently extremely difficult these days to provide for a large family.

It is also apparent that, with the new understanding of the dignity of woman and her place in society, there has been an appreciation of the value of love in marriage and of the meaning of intimate married life in the light of that love.

But the most remarkable development of all is to be seen in man's stupendous progress in the domination and rational organization of the forces of nature to the point that he is endeavoring to extend this control over every aspect of his own life—over his body, over his mind and emotions, over his social life, and even over the laws that regulate the transmission of life.

New Questions

3. This new state of things gives rise to new questions. Granted the conditions of life today and taking into account the relevance of married love to the harmony and mutual fidelity of husband and wife, would it not be right to review the moral norms in force till now, especially when it is felt that these can be observed only with the gravest difficulty, sometimes only by heroic effort?

Moreover, if one were to apply here the so-called principle of totality, could it not be accepted that the intention to have a less prolific but more rationally planned family might not transform an action which renders natural processes infertile into a licit and provident control of birth? Could it not be admitted, in other words, that procreative finality applies to the totality of married life rather than to each single act? It is being asked whether, because people are more conscious today of their responsibilities, the time has not come

106 when the transmission of life should be regulated by their intelligence and will rather than through the specific rhythms of their own bodies.

DOCTRINAL QUESTIONS
A Total Vision of Man

7. The question of the birth of children, like every other question which touches human life, is too large to be resolved by limited criteria, such as are provided by biology, psychology, demography, or sociology. It is the whole man and the whole complex of his responsibilities that must be considered, not only what is natural and limited to this earth, but also what is supernatural and eternal. And since in the attempt to justify artificial methods of birth control many appeal to the demands of married love or of "responsible parenthood," these two important realities of married life must be accurately defined and analyzed. This is what we mean to do, with special reference to what the Second Vatican Council taught with the highest authority in its Pastoral Constitution *Gaudium et Spes.*

Marriage Is a Sacrament

8. Married love particularly reveals its true nature and nobility when we realize that it derives from God and finds its supreme origin in him who "is Love," the Father "from whom every family in heaven and on earth is named."

Marriage, then, is far from being the effect of chance or the result of the blind evolution of natural forces. It is in reality the wise and provident institution of God the Creator, whose purpose was to establish in man his loving design. As a consequence, husband and wife, through that mutual gift of themselves which is specific and exclusive to them alone, seek to develop that kind of personal union in which they complement one another in order to cooperate with God in the generation and education of new lives.

Furthermore, the marriage of those who have been baptized is invested with the dignity of a sacramental sign of grace, for it represents the union of Christ and his Church.

Married Love

9. In the light of these facts the characteristic features and exigencies of married love are clearly indicated, and it is of the highest importance to evaluate them exactly.

This love is above all fully human, a compound of sense and spirit. It is not, then, merely a question of natural instinct or emotional drive. It is also, and above all, an act of the free will, whose dynamism ensures that not only does it endure through the joys and sorrows of daily life, but also that it grows, so that husband and wife become in a way one heart and one soul, and together attain their human fulfillment.

Then it is a love which is total—that very special form of personal friendship in which husband and wife generously share everything, allowing no unreasonable exceptions or thinking just of their own interests. Whoever really

loves his partner loves not only for what he receives, but loves that partner **107**
for her own sake, content to be able to enrich the other with the gift of himself.

Again, married love is faithful and exclusive of all other, and this until
death. This is how husband and wife understood it on the day on which, fully
aware of what they were doing, they freely vowed themselves to one another
in marriage. Though this fidelity of husband and wife sometimes presents
difficulties, no one can assert that it is impossible, for it is always honorable
and worthy of the highest esteem. The example of so many married persons
down through the centuries shows not only that fidelity is conatural to marriage,
but also that it is the source of profound and enduring happiness.

And finally this love is creative of life, for it is not exhausted by the loving
interchange of husband and wife, but also contrives to go beyond this to bring
new life into being. "Marriage and married love are by their character ordained
to the procreation and bringing up of children. Children are the outstanding
gift of marriage, and contribute in the highest degree to the parents' welfare."

Responsible Parenthood

10. Married love, therefore, requires of husband and wife the full awareness of their obligations in the matter of responsible parenthood, which today,
rightly enough, is much insisted upon, but which, at the same time, should be
rightly understood. Hence, this must be studied in the light of the various
interrelated arguments which are its justification.

If first we consider it in relation to the biological processes involved,
responsible parenthood is to be understood as the knowledge and observance
of their specific functions. Human intelligence discovers in the faculty of procreating life the biological laws which involve human personality.

If, on the other hand, we examine the innate drives and emotions of man,
responsible parenthood expresses the domination which reason and will must
exert over them.

But if we then attend to relevant physical, economic, psychological, and
social conditions, those are considered to exercise responsible parenthood who
prudently and generously decide to have a large family, or who, for serious
reasons and with due respect to the moral law, choose to have no more children
for the time being or even for an indeterminate period.

Responsible parenthood, moreover, in the terms in which we use the
phrase, retains a further and deeper significance of paramount importance
which refers to the objective moral order instituted by God—the order of which
a right conscience is the true interpreter. As a consequence the commitment to
responsible parenthood requires that husband and wife, keeping a right order
of priorities, recognize their own duties towards God, themselves, their families,
and human society.

From this it follows that they are not free to do as they like in the service
of transmitting life, on the supposition that it is lawful for them to decide
independently of other considerations what is the right course to follow. On
the contrary, they are bound to ensure that what they do corresponds to the

108 will of God the Creator. The very nature of marriage and its use makes this
clear, while the constant teaching of the Church affirms it.

Respect for the Nature and Purpose of the Marriage Act

11. The sexual activity, in which husband and wife are intimately and
chastely united with one another, through which human life is transmitted, is,
and the recent Council recalled, "honorable and good." It does not, moreover,
cease to be legitimate even when, for reasons independent of their will, it
is foreseen to be infertile. For its natural adaptation to the expression and
strengthening of the union of husband and wife is not thereby suppressed. The
facts are, as experience shows, that new life is not the result of each and every
act of sexual intercourse. God has wisely ordered the laws of nature and the
incidence of fertility in such a way that successive births are already naturally
spaced through the inherent operation of these laws. The Church, nevertheless,
in urging men to the observance of the doctrine, teaches as absolutely required
that in any use whatever of marriage there must be no impairment of its natural
capacity to procreate human life.

Teaching in Harmony With Human Reason

12. This particular doctrine, often expounded by the Magisterium of the
Church, is based on the inseparable connection, established by God, which
man on his own initiative may not break, between the unitive significance and
the procreative significance which are both inherent to the marriage act.

The reason is that the marriage act, because of its fundamental structure,
while it unites husband and wife in the closest intimacy, also brings into
operation laws written into the actual nature of man and of woman for the
generation of new life. And if each of these essential qualities, the unitive and
the procreative, is preserved, the use of marriage fully retains its sense of true
mutual love and its ordination to the supreme responsibility of parenthood to
which man is called. We believe that our contemporaries are particularly capable
of seeing that this teaching is in harmony with human reason.

Faithfulness to God's Design

13. For men rightly observe that to force the use of marriage on one's
partner without regard to his or her condition or personal and reasonable
wishes in that matter, is no true act of love, and therefore offends the moral
order in its particular application to the intimate relationship of husband and
wife. In the same way, if they reflect, they must also recognize that an act of
mutual love which impairs the capacity to transmit life which God the Creator,
through specific laws, has built into it, frustrates his design which constitutes
the norms of marriage, and contradicts the will of the Author of life. Hence,
to use this divine gift while depriving it, even if only partially, of its meaning
and purpose, is equally repugnant to the nature of man and of woman, strikes
at the heart of their relationship, and is consequently in opposition to the plan
of God and his holy will. But to experience the gift of married love while
respecting the laws of conception is to acknowledge that one is not the master

of the sources of life but rather the minister of the design established by the
Creator. Just as man does not have unlimited dominion over his body in general,
so also, and with more particular reason, he has no such dominion over his
specifically sexual faculties, for these are concerned by their very nature with
the generation of life, of which God is the source. For human life is sacred—
all men must recognize that fact, our predecessor, Pope John XXIII, recalled,
"since from its first beginnings it calls for the creative action of God."

Unlawful Ways of Regulating Birth

14. Therefore we base our words on the first principles of a human and
Christian doctrine of marriage when we are obliged once more to declare that
the direct interruption of the generative process already begun and, above all,
direct abortion, even for therapeutic reasons, are to be absolutely excluded as
lawful means of controlling the birth of children.

Equally to be condemned, as the Magisterium of the Church has affirmed
on various occasions, is direct sterilization, whether of the man or the woman,
whether permanent or temporary.

Similarly excluded is any action which either before, at the moment of,
or after sexual intercourse is specifically intended to prevent procreation—
whether as an end or as a means.

Neither is it valid to argue, as a justification for sexual intercourse which
is deliberately contraceptive, that a lesser evil is to be preferred to a greater
one, or that such intercourse would merge with the normal relations of past
and future to form a single entity, and so be qualified by exactly the same
moral goodness as these. Though it is true that sometimes it is lawful to tolerate
a lesser moral evil in order to avoid a greater or in order to promote a greater
good, it is never lawful, even for the gravest reasons, to do evil that good may
come of it—in other words, to intend positively something which intrinsically
contradicts the moral order, and which must therefore be judged unworthy of
man, even though the intention is to protect or promote the welfare of an
individual, of a family, or of society in general. Consequently it is a serious
error to think that a whole married life of otherwise normal relations can justify
sexual intercourse which is deliberately contraceptive and so intrinsically
wrong.

Lawfulness of Therapeutic Means

15. But the Church in no way regards as unlawful therapeutic means
considered necessary to cure organic diseases, even though they also have a
contraceptive effect, and this is foreseen—provided that this contraceptive effect
is not directly intended for any motive whatsoever.

Lawfulness of Recourse to Infertile Periods

16. However, as we noted earlier (n. 3), some people today raise the
objection against this particular doctrine of the Church concerning the moral
laws governing marriage, that human intelligence has both the right and the
responsibility to control those forces of irrational nature which come within its

110 ambit and to direct them towards ends beneficial to man. Others ask on the same point whether it is not reasonable in so many cases to use artificial birth control if by so doing the harmony and peace of a family are better served and more suitable conditions are provided for the education of children already born. To this question we must give a clear reply. The Church is the first to praise and commend the application of human intelligence to an activity in which a rational creature such as man is so closely associated with his Creator. But she affirms that this must be done within the limits of the order of reality established by God.

If, therefore, there are reasonable grounds for spacing births, arising from the physical or psychological condition of husband or wife, or from external circumstances, the Church teaches that then married people may take advantage of the natural cycles immanent in the reproductive system and use their marriage at precisely those times that are infertile, and in this way control birth, a way which does not in the least offend the moral principles which we have just explained.

Neither the Church nor her doctrine is inconsistent when she considers it lawful for married people to take advantage of the infertile period but condemns as always unlawful the use of means which directly exclude conception, even when the reasons given for the latter practice are neither trivial nor immoral. In reality, these two cases are completely different. In the former married couples rightly use a facility provided them by nature. In the latter they obstruct the natural development of the generative process. It cannot be denied that in each case married couples, for acceptable reasons, are both perfectly clear in their intention to avoid children and mean to make sure that none will be born. But it is equally true that it is exclusively in the former case that husband and wife are ready to abstain from intercourse during the fertile period as often as for reasonable motives the birth of another child is not desirable. And when the infertile period recurs, they use their married intimacy to express their mutual love and safeguard their fidelity towards one another. In doing this they certainly give proof of a true and authentic love.

Grave Consequences of Artificial Birth Control

17. Responsible men can become more deeply convinced of the truth of the doctrine laid down by the Church on this issue if they reflect on the consequences of methods and plans for the artificial restriction of increases in the birth-rate. Let them first consider how easily this course of action can lead to the way being wide open to marital infidelity and a general lowering of moral standards. Not much experience is needed to be fully aware of human weakness and to understand that man—and especially the young, who are so exposed to temptation—need incentives to keep the moral law, and it is an evil thing to make it easy for them to break that law. Another effect that gives cause for alarm is that a man who grows accustomed to the use of contraceptive methods may forget the reverence due to a woman, and, disregarding her physical and emotional equilibrium, reduce her to being a mere instrument for

the satisfaction of his own desires, no longer considering her as his partner **111**
whom he should surround with care and affection.

Finally, grave consideration should be given to the danger of this power
passing into the hands of those public authorities who care little for the precepts
of the moral law. Who will blame a government which in its attempt to resolve
the problems affecting an entire country resorts to the same measures as are
regarded as lawful by married people in the solution of a particular family
difficulty? Who will prevent public authorities from favoring those contraceptive methods which they consider more effective? Should they regard this as
necessary, they may even impose their use on everyone. It could well happen,
therefore, that when people, either individually or in family or social life,
experience the inherent difficulties of the divine law and are determined to
avoid them, they may be giving into the hands of public authorities the power to
intervene in the most personal and intimate responsibility of husband and wife.

Consequently, unless we are willing that the responsibility of procreating
life should be left to the arbitrary decision of men, we must accept that there
are certain limits, beyond which it is wrong to go, to the power of man over
his own body and its natural functions—limits, let it be said, which no one,
whether as a private individual or as a public authority, can lawfully exceed.
These limits are expressly imposed because of the reverence due to the whole
human organism and its natural functions, in the light of the principles, which
we stated earlier, and according to a correct understanding of the so-called
"principle of totality," enunciated by our predecessor, Pope Pius XII.

19. Our words would ill reflect the thought and loving care of the Church,
who is the Mother and Teacher of all nations, did they not also sustain men
in the proper ordering of the number of their children at a time when living
conditions are harsh and press heavily on families and nations. Yet it is these
men and women whom we have just urged to observe and honor the law of
God concerning marriage. For the Church cannot adopt towards mankind a
different attitude from that of the divine Redeemer. She knows their weakness;
she has compassion on the multitudes; she welcomes sinners. But at the same
time she cannot do otherwise than teach the law. For it is in fact the law of
human life restored to its native truth and led by the Spirit of God.

DOCUMENT 3 / Contraception

SOURCE: Pope John Paul II, "The Christian Family in the Modern World" (Nov. 22, 1981), *Vatican Council II*, Vol. 2, pp. 837–44.

II—SERVING LIFE

1. The Transmission of Life

29. Precisely because the love of husband and wife is a unique participation in the mystery of life and of the love of God himself, the Church knows that she has received the special mission of guarding and protecting the lofty dignity of marriage and the most serious responsibility of the transmission of human life.

Thus, in continuity with the living tradition of the ecclesial community throughout history, the recent Second Vatican Council and the Magisterium of my predecessor Paul VI, expressed above all in the encyclical *Humanae Vitae*, have handed on to our times a truly prophetic proclamation, which reaffirms and reproposes with clarity the Church's teaching and norm, always old yet always new, regarding marriage and regarding the transmission of human life.

For this reason the Synod Fathers made the following declaration at their last assembly: "This sacred Synod, gathered together with the successor of Peter in the unity of faith, firmly holds what has been set forth in the Second Vatican Council (cf. *Gaudium et Spes*, 50) and afterwards in the encyclical *Humanae Vitae*, particularly that love between husband and wife must be fully human, exclusive, and open to new life (HV, 11; cf. 9, 12)."

30. The teaching of the Church in our day is placed in a social and cultural context which renders it more difficult to understand and yet more urgent and irreplaceable for promoting the true good of men and women.

Scientific and technical progress, which contemporary man is continually expanding in his dominion over nature, not only offers the hope of creating a new and better humanity, but also causes ever greater anxiety regarding the future. Some ask themselves if it is a good thing to be alive or if it would be better never to have been born; they doubt therefore if it is right to bring others into life when perhaps they will curse their existence in a cruel world with unforeseeable terrors. Others consider themselves to be the only ones for whom the advantages of technology are intended and they exclude others by imposing on them contraceptives or even worse means. Still others, imprisoned in a consumer mentality and whose sole concern is to bring about a continual growth of material goods, finish by ceasing to understand, and thus by refusing, the spiritual riches of a new human life. The ultimate reason for these mentalities is the absence in people's hearts of God, whose love alone is stronger than all the world's fears and can conquer them.

Thus an anti-life mentality is born, as can be seen in many current issues: one thinks, for example, of a certain panic deriving from the studies of ecologists

and futurologists on population growth, which sometimes exaggerate the danger of demographic increase to the quality of life.

But the Church firmly believes that human life, even if weak and suffering, is always a splendid gift of God's goodness. Against the pessimism and selfishness which cast a shadow over the world, the Church stands for life: in each human life she sees the splendor of that "Yes," that "Amen," who is Christ himself. To the "No" which assails and afflicts the world, she replies with this living "Yes," thus defending the human person and the world from all who plot against and harm life.

The Church is called upon to manifest anew to everyone, with clear and stronger conviction, her will to promote human life by every means and to defend it against all attacks, in whatever condition or state of development it is found.

Thus the Church condemns as a grave offense against human dignity and justice all those activities of government or other public authorities which attempt to limit in any way the freedom of couples in deciding about children. Consequently any violence applied by such authorities in favor of contraception or, still worse, of sterilization and procured abortion, must be altogether condemned and forcefully rejected. Likewise to be denounced as gravely unjust are cases where, in international relations, economic help given for the advancement of people is made conditional on programs of contraception, sterilization, and procured abortion.

32. In the context of a culture which seriously distorts or entirely misinterprets the true meaning of human sexuality, because it separates it from its essential reference to the person, the Church more urgently feels how irreplaceable is her mission of presenting sexuality as a value and task of the whole person, created male and female in the image of God.

In this perspective the Second Vatican Council clearly affirmed that "when there is a question of harmonizing conjugal love with the responsible transmission of life, the moral aspect of any procedure does not depend solely on sincere intentions or on an evaluation of motives. It must be determined by objective standards. These, based on the nature of the human person and his or her acts, preserve the full sense of mutual self-giving and human procreation in the context of true love. Such a goal cannot be achieved unless the virtue of conjugal chastity is sincerely practiced."

It is precisely by moving from "an integral vision of man and of his vocation, not only his natural and earthly, but also his supernatural and eternal vocation," that Paul VI affirmed that the teaching of the Church "is founded upon the inseparable connection, willed by God and unable to be broken by man on his own initiative, between the two meanings of the conjugal act: the unitive meaning and the procreative meaning." And he concluded by reemphasizing that there must be excluded as intrinsically immoral "every action which, either in anticipation of the conjugal act, or in its accomplishment, or in the development of its natural consequences, proposes, whether as an end or as a means, to render procreation impossible."

When couples, by means of recourse to contraception, separate these two

114   meanings that God the Creator has inscribed in the being of man and woman and in the dynamism of their sexual communion, they act as "arbiters" of the divine plan and they "manipulate" and degrade human sexuality—and with it themselves and their married partner—by altering its value of "total" self-giving. Thus the innate language that expresses the total reciprocal self-giving of husband and wife is overlaid, through contraception, by an objectively contradictory language, namely, that of not giving oneself totally to the other. This leads not only to a positive refusal to be open to life but also to a falsification of the inner truth of conjugal love, which is called upon to give itself in personal totality.

When, instead, by means of recourse to periods of infertility, the couple respect the inseparable connection between the unitive and procreative meanings of human sexuality, they are acting as "ministers" of God's plan and they "benefit from" their sexuality according to the original dynamism of "total" self-giving, without manipulation or altercation.

In the light of the experience of many couples and of the data provided by the different human sciences, theological reflection is able to perceive and is called to study further the difference, both anthropological and moral, between contraception and recourse to the rhythm of the cycle: it is a difference which is much wider and deeper than is usually thought, one which involves in the final analysis two irreconcilable concepts of the human person and of human sexuality. The choice of the natural rhythms involves accepting the cycle of the person, that is the woman, and thereby accepting dialogue, reciprocal respect, shared responsibility, and self-control. To accept the cycle and to enter into dialogue means to recognize both the spiritual and corporal character of conjugal communion, and to live personal love with its requirement of fidelity. In this context the couple comes to experience how conjugal communion is enriched with those values of tenderness and affection which constitute the inner soul of human sexuality, in its physical dimension also. In this way sexuality is respected and promoted in its truly and fully human dimension, and is never "used" as an "object" that, by breaking the personal unity of soul and body, strikes at God's creation itself at the level of the deepest interaction of nature and person.

34. It is always very important to have a right notion of the moral order, its values, and its norms; and the importance is all the greater when the difficulties in the way of respecting them become more numerous and serious.

Since the moral order reveals and sets forth the plan of God the Creator, for this very reason it cannot be something that harms man, something impersonal. On the contrary, by responding to the deepest demands of the human being created by God, it places itself at the service of that person's full humanity with the delicate and binding love whereby God himself inspires, sustains, and guides every creature towards its happiness.

But man, who has been called to live God's wise and loving design in a responsible manner, is an historical being who day by day builds himself up through his many free decisions; and so he knows, loves, and accomplishes moral good by stages of growth.

Married people too are called upon to progress unceasingly in their moral **115** life, with the support of a sincere and active desire to gain ever better knowledge of the values enshrined in and fostered by the law of God. They must also be supported by an upright and generous willingness to embody these values in their concrete decisions. They cannot, however, look on the law as merely an ideal to be achieved in the future: they must consider it as a command of Christ the Lord to overcome difficulties with constancy. "And so what is known as 'the law of gradualness' or step-by-step advance cannot be identified with 'gradualness of the law,' as if there were different degrees or forms of precept in God's law for different individuals and situations. In God's plan, all husbands and wives are called in marriage to holiness, and this lofty vocation is fulfilled to the extent that the human person is able to respond to God's command with serene confidence in God's grace and in his or her own will." On the same lines, it is part of the Church's pedagogy that husbands and wives should first of all recognize clearly the teaching of *Humanae Vitae* as indicating the norm for the exercise of their sexuality, and that they should endeavor to establish the conditions necessary for observing that norm. . . .

DOCUMENT 4 / Contraception

SOURCE: National Conference of Catholic Bishops Committee for Pro-Life Activities, "Human Sexuality From God's Perspective," *Origins* 23: no. 10 (Aug. 12, 1993), pp. 164–66.

. . . Due to our world's increasing technological ability to prevent conception, many today view human sexuality in a purely pragmatic way. They believe that we are simply sexual beings who instinctively seek to be sexually active. From a physiological and psychological point of view, sexual intercourse is looked on as solely a natural response to human instinct and human need. Science is often called upon to help people divorce sexual activity from the prospect of unwanted pregnancy and free them from religious teachings which are thought to inhibit freedom. This is a secular perspective about human sexuality which has become pervasive and dominant in our culture. But it is a very limited perspective, a perspective devoid of God's revelation about the uniqueness of human life, a perspective unmindful of the data gathered from our observations about the true nature of human sexuality.

. . . In *Humanae Vitae*, Pope Paul recognized conjugal love as eminently human, but rooted in God's love for his people. He saw it as the dynamic element in every marriage, bringing permanence to the marriage and enabling the couple to make wise, generous, and responsible decisions about the spacing of births and the size of their family. *Humanae Vitae* provides a positive and dignified understanding of sexuality as a gift from God which ennobles, enriches, and reconciles married couples. Through sexual union, couples strengthen their marital relationship and participate in a special way in God's creation of new life. From this follows the profound meaning of a life of intimacy, that communion of two persons who must be open to each other in a mutual self-donation that reaches its apex in the loving union that bears fruit in children.

Sexuality, then, is not merely a matter of biology nor is it simply a source of personal pleasure. Rather, it concerns, as Pope John Paul II reminds us in the apostolic exhortation *Familiaris Consortio*, "the innermost being of the human person as such. It is realized in a truly human way only if it is an integral part of the love by which a man and woman commit themselves totally to one another until death" (FC, 11).

Spouses are called to celebrate their conjugal love by becoming one flesh in the Lord and to see their sexual intimacy in the context of God's creative role and the nature of marriage itself. By remaining open to life each time they come together in the conjugal embrace, by preserving "the two meanings of the conjugal act: the unitive meaning and the procreative meaning" (*Humanae Vitae*, 12), married couples reverence the presence of God in their union. In truth, the Church teaches that there are two aspects of marital intercourse—the strengthening of interpersonal unity between the spouses and the procreation of

new life. These two goods are inseparable—not in the sense that both must be **117**
achieved in every act of conjugal intimacy, but in the sense that one may not
deliberately act against either good in any act of conjugal intimacy.

RESPONSIBLE PARENTHOOD

Complementing its teaching on conjugal love, Paul VI reaffirmed the
Church's tradition that responsible parenthood flows from the intimate communion that is at the heart of the meaning of marriage. Too often childbearing is
characterized as burdensome, risky, destructive of personal aspirations and
dangerous for a world thought by some to be already overpopulated. But in
reality married couples also experience a profound desire to share their life
and love by cooperating with God in creating new life and building a family.

The teaching of *Humanae Vitae* reminds us that parenthood is a privilege
as well as a responsibility. Couples are able to associate themselves in the
deepest and closest way with God in the work of procreation. They are able,
in John Paul II's words, "to serve life, to actualize in history the original blessing
of the Creator—that of transmitting by procreation the divine image from
person to person" (FC, 28). Today it is especially important to remember that
each child is a unique and unrepeatable person and a testimony to the love of
his or her parents as well as a testimony to the love of God. Too often the
personal joys of parenthood and the promise that children hold for the future
are overlooked or denigrated. All who follow Christ must see each child as a
creature of God endowed with inestimable dignity who is called to accomplish
his or her human destiny and to take an active role in the Church's missionary vocation.

Responsible parenthood, then, implies a positive openness to life. It is a
decision that couples make mutually and prayerfully, confident that God's
grace will complement their generosity. Couples should make decisions about
spacing births and the size of their families free of coercion or pressure. Taking
into account their mutual responsibilities to God, themselves, their family, and
the society of which they are a part, in a correct hierarchy of values a couple
may responsibly decide to delay childbearing. Or a husband or wife may
conclude that they are unable to have more children. In the formation of their
consciences, however, the couple must be well-instructed in and guided "by
objective standards . . . that preserve the full sense of mutual self-giving and
human procreation in the context of true love" (*Gaudium et Spes*, 51).

We recognize the problems and difficulties couples face in making decisions about parenthood. Concerns about economic stability, employment, health
care, education of children, or fulfilling existing responsibilities must be taken
into account; and these concerns may suggest the avoidance, at least for the
time being, of another birth. But we also recognize that unsubstantiated claims
about population growth and cultural attitudes that diminish the value of the
child may induce fear of having more than one or two children. These pressures
compromise the freedom of the couple. We recall the teaching of the Second
Vatican Council that "children are really the supreme gift of marriage and
contribute very substantially to the welfare of their parents" (*Gaudium et Spes*,

118   50). We also recognize that for some couples, despite their intense desire, childbearing does not occur. At the same time, "Those merit special mention who with a gallant heart, and with wise and common deliberation, undertake to bring up suitably even a relatively large family" (*Gaudium et Spes*, 50).

DOCUMENT 5 / Contraception

Source: Pontifical Council for the Family, "Vade Mecum for Confessors Concerning Some Aspects of the Morality of Conjugal Life," *Origins* 26: no. 38 (Mar. 13, 1997), pp. 618–25.

... The family, which the Second Vatican Council has defined as the domestic sanctuary of the Church and as "the primary vital cell of society," constitutes a privileged object of the Church's pastoral attention. "At a moment of history in which the family is the object of numerous forces that seek to destroy it or in some way to deform it, and aware that the well-being of society and her own good are intimately tied to the good of the family, the Church perceives in a more urgent and compelling way her mission of proclaiming to all people the plan of God for marriage and the family."

... Christian tradition has always upheld the goodness and honesty of the marital union and of the family against numerous heresies which arose from the very beginnings of the Church. Willed by God with creation itself, brought back to its primal origin and elevated to the dignity of a sacrament by Christ, marriage consists of an intimate communion of the spouses of love and life, intrinsically ordered to the good of the children that God wishes to entrust to them. Both for the good of the spouses and of the children as well as for the good of society itself, the natural bond no longer depends on human decision.

... By means of the sacrament of marriage, married couples receive from Christ the Redeemer the gift of grace that confirms and elevates the communion of faithful and fruitful love. The holiness to which they are called is above all a grace given.

The persons called to live in the married state realize their vocation to love in the full gift of self which adequately expresses the language of the body. From the mutual gift of the spouses comes as its fruit the gift of life to the children, who are a sign and crowning of their spousal love.

Contraception, directly opposed to the transmission of life, betrays and falsifies the self-sacrificing love proper to marriage, "altering its value of total self-giving" and contradicting God's design of love, in which it has been granted to married couples to participate.

... This vade mecum consists of a set of positions which confessors are to keep in mind while administering the sacrament of reconciliation in order to better help married couples to live their vocation to fatherhood or motherhood in a Christian way within their own personal and social circumstances.

... All Christians must be fittingly made "aware of their call to holiness." The invitation to follow Christ, addressed, in fact, to each and every member of the faithful, must tend toward the fullness of the Christian life and to the perfection of charity in each one's own state.

120 . . . The Church has always taught the intrinsic evil of contraception, that is, of every marital act intentionally rendered unfruitful. This teaching is to be held as definitive and irreformable. Contraception is gravely opposed to marital chastity; it is contrary to the good of the transmission of life (the procreative aspect of matrimony) and to the reciprocal self-giving of the spouses (the unitive aspect of matrimony); it harms true love and denies the sovereign role of God in the transmission of human life.

A specific and more serious moral evil is present in the use of means which have an abortive effect, impeding the implantation of the embryo which has just been fertilized or even causing its expulsion in an early state of pregnancy.

However, profoundly different from any contraceptive practice is the behavior of married couples who, always remaining fundamentally open to the gift of life, live their intimacy only in the unfruitful periods, when they are led to this course by serious motives of responsible parenthood. This is true both from the anthropological and moral points of view, because it is rooted in a different conception of the person and of sexuality.

. . . In dealing with penitents on the matter of responsible procreation, the confessor should keep four aspects in mind: a) the example of the Lord, who "is capable of reaching down to every prodigal son, to every human misery and above all to every form of moral misery, to sin"; b) a prudent reserve in inquiring into these sins; c) help and encouragement to the penitents so that they may be able to reach sufficient repentance and accuse themselves fully of grave sins; d) advice which would inspire all, in a gradual way, to embrace the path of holiness.

The minister of reconciliation should always keep in mind that the sacrament has been instituted for men and women who are sinners. Therefore, barring manifest proof to the contrary, he will receive the penitents who approach the confessional taking for granted their good will to be reconciled with the merciful God, a good will that is born, although in different degrees, of a contrite and humbled heart (cf. Ps 50:19).

. . . The confessor is bound to penitents regarding objectively grave transgressions of God's law and to ensure that they truly desire absolution and God's pardon, with the resolution to re-examine and correct their behavior. Frequent relapse into sins of contraception does not in itself constitute a motive for denying absolution; absolution cannot be imparted, however, in the absence of sufficient repentance or of the resolution not to fall again into sin.

. . . The principle according to which it is preferable to let penitents remain in good faith in cases of error due to subjectively invincible ignorance is certainly to be considered always valid, even in matters of conjugal chastity. And this applies whenever it is foreseen that the penitent, although oriented toward living within the bounds of a life of faith, would not be prepared to change his own conduct, but rather would begin formally to sin. Nonetheless, in these cases the confessor must try to bring such penitents ever closer to accepting God's plan in their own lives even in these demands by means of prayer, admonition, and exhorting them to form their consciences, and by the teaching of the Church.

The pastoral "law of gradualness not to be confused with the gradualness of the law" which would tend to diminish the demands it places on us, consists of requiring a decisive break with sin together with a progressive path toward total union with the will of God and with his loving demands.

. . . Sacramental absolution is not to be denied to those who, repentant after having gravely sinned against conjugal chastity, demonstrate the desire to strive to abstain from sinning again, notwithstanding relapses. In accordance with the approved doctrine and practice followed by the holy doctors and confessors with regard to habitual penitents, the confessor is to avoid demonstrating lack of trust either in the grace of God or in the dispositions of the penitent by exacting humanly impossible absolute guarantees of an irreproachable future conduct.

. . . Special difficulties are presented by cases of cooperation in the sin of a spouse who voluntarily renders the unitive act infecund. In the first place, it is necessary to distinguish cooperation in the proper sense from violence or unjust imposition on the part of one of the spouses, which the other spouse in fact cannot resist. This cooperation can be licit when the three following conditions are jointly met:

1. when the action of the cooperating spouse is not already illicit in itself;
2. when proportionally grave reasons exist for cooperating in the sin of the other spouse;
3. when one is seeking to help the other spouse to desist from such conduct (patiently, with prayer, charity, and dialogue; although not necessarily in that moment nor on every single occasion).

Furthermore, it is necessary to evaluate carefully the question of cooperation in evil when recourse is made to means which can have an abortifacient effect. . . .

19: Embryo Research

DOCUMENT 1:

SOURCE: Congregation for the Doctrine of the Faith, "Instruction on Respect for Human Life in Its Origin and on the Dignity of Procreation" (Feb. 22, 1987), *Origins* 16: no. 40, Mar. 19, 1987, pp. 701–02.

I. RESPECT FOR HUMAN EMBRYOS

1. What respect is due to the human embryo, taking into account his nature and identity?

The human being must be respected—as a person—from the very first instant of his existence.

The implementation of procedures of artificial fertilization has made possible various interventions upon embryos and human fetuses. The aims pursued are of various kinds: diagnostic and therapeutic, scientific and commercial. From all of this, serious problems arise. Can one speak of a right to experimentation upon human embryos for the purpose of scientific research? What norms or laws should be worked out with regard to this matter? The response to these problems presupposes a detailed reflection on the nature and specific identity—the word status is used—of the human embryo itself.

At the Second Vatican Council, the Church for her part presented once again to modern man her constant and certain doctrine according to which: "Life, once conceived, must be protected with the utmost care; abortion and infanticide are abominable crimes." More recently, the Charter of the Rights of the Family, published by the Holy See, confirmed that "human life must be absolutely respected and protected from the moment of conception."

This Congregation is aware of the current debates concerning the beginning of human life, concerning the individuality of the human being, and concerning the identity of the human person. The Congregation recalls the teachings found in the Declaration on Procured Abortion:

"From the time that the ovum is fertilized, a new life is begun which is neither that of the father nor of the mother; it is rather the life of a new human being with his own growth. It would never be made human if it were not human already. To this perpetual evidence . . . modern genetic science brings valuable confirmation. It has demonstrated that, from the first instant, the program is fixed as to what this living being will be: a man, this individual man with his characteristic aspects already well determined. Right from fertilization is begun the adventure of a human life, and each of its great capacities requires time . . . to find its place and to be in a position to act."

This teaching remains valid and is further confirmed, if confirmation were needed, by recent findings of human biological science which recognize that in the zygote (the cell produced when the nuclei of the two gametes have fused) resulting from fertilization the biological identity of a new human individual is already constituted.

Certainly no experimental datum can be in itself sufficient to bring us to the recognition of a spiritual soul; nevertheless, the conclusions of science regarding the human embryo provide a valuable indication for discerning by the use of reason a personal presence at the moment of this first appearance of a human life. How could a human individual not be a human person? The Magisterium has not expressly committed itself to an affirmation of a philosophical nature, but it constantly reaffirms the moral condemnation of any kind of procured abortion. This teaching has not been changed and is unchangeable.

Thus the fruit of human generation from the first moment of its existence, that is to say, from the moment the zygote has formed, demands the unconditional respect that is morally due to the human being in his bodily and spiritual totality. The human being is to be respected and treated as a person from the moment of conception and therefore from that same moment his rights as a person must be recognized, among which in the first place is the inviolable right of every innocent human being to life.

This doctrinal reminder provides the fundamental criterion for the solution of the various problems posed by the development of the biomedical sciences in this field. Since the embryo must be treated as a person, it must also be defended in its integrity, tended and cared for, to the extent possible, in the same way as any other human being as far as medical assistance is concerned.

4. How is one to evaluate morally research and experimentation on human embryos and fetuses?

Medical research must refrain from operations on live embryos, unless there is a moral certainty of not causing harm to the life or integrity of the unborn child and the mother, and on condition that the parents have given their free and informed consent to the procedure. It follows that all research, even when limited to the simple observation of the embryo, would become illicit were it to involve risk to the embryo's physical integrity or life by reason of the methods used or the effects induced.

As regards experimentation, and presupposing the general distinction between experimentation for purposes which are not directly therapeutic and experimentation which is clearly therapeutic for the subject himself, in the case in point one must also distinguish between experimentation carried out on embryos which are still alive and experimentation carried out on embryos which are dead. If the embryos are living, whether viable or not, they must be respected just like any other human person; experimentation on embryos which is not directly therapeutic is illicit.

No objective, even though noble in itself such as a foreseeable advantage to science, to other human beings, or to society, can in any way justify

124   experimentation on living human embryos or fetuses, whether viable or not, either inside or outside the mother's womb. The informed consent ordinarily required for clinical experimentation on adults cannot be granted by the parents, who may not freely dispose of the physical integrity or life of the unborn child. Moreover, experimentation on embryos and fetuses always involves risk, and indeed in most cases it involves the certain expectation of harm to their physical integrity or even their death.

To use human embryos or fetuses as the object or instrument of experimentation constitutes a crime against their dignity as human beings having a right to the same respect that is due to the child already born and to every human person.

The Charter of the Rights of the Family published by the Holy See affirms: "Respect for the dignity of the human being excludes all experimental manipulation or exploitation of the human embryo." The practice of keeping alive human embryos in vivo or in vitro for experimental or commercial purposes is totally opposed to human dignity.

In the case of experimentation that is clearly therapeutic, namely, when it is a matter of experimental forms of therapy used for the benefit of the embryo itself in a final attempt to save its life and in the absence of other reliable forms of therapy, recourse to drugs or procedures not yet fully tested can be licit.

The corpses of human embryos and fetuses, whether they have been deliberately aborted or not, must be respected just as the remains of other human beings. In particular, they cannot be subjected to mutilation or to autopsies if their death has not yet been verified and without the consent of the parents or of the mother. Furthermore, the moral requirements must be safeguarded that there be no complicity in deliberate abortion and that the risk of scandal be avoided. Also, in the case of dead fetuses, as for the corpses of adult persons, all commercial trafficking must be considered illicit and should be prohibited.

5. How is one to evaluate morally the use for research purposes of embryos obtained by fertilization "in vitro?"

Human embryos obtained in vitro are human beings and subjects with rights. Their dignity and right to life must be respected from the first moment of their existence. It is immoral to produce human embryos destined to be exploited as disposable "biological material."

In the usual practice of in vitro fertilization, not all of the embryos are transferred to the woman's body; some are destroyed. Just as the Church condemns induced abortion, so she also forbids acts against the life of these human beings. It is a duty to condemn the particular gravity of the voluntary destruction of human embryos obtained "in vitro" for the sole purpose of research, either by means of artificial insemination or by means of "twin fission." By acting in this way the researcher usurps the place of God; and, even though he may be unaware of this, he sets himself up as the master of the destiny of others inasmuch as he arbitrarily chooses whom he will allow to live and whom he will send to death and kills defenseless human beings.

Methods of observation or experimentation which damage or impose grave and disproportionate risks upon embryos obtained in vitro are morally illicit for the same reasons. Every human being is to be respected for himself and cannot be reduced in worth to a pure and simple instrument for the advantage of others. It is therefore not in conformity with the moral law deliberately to expose to death human embryos obtained "in vitro." In consequence of the fact that they have been produced in vitro, those embryos which are not transferred into the body of the mother and are called "spare" are exposed to an absurd fate, with no possibility of their being offered safe means of survival which can be licitly pursued.

DOCUMENT 2 / Embryo Research

SOURCE: Pope John Paul II, "Biological Experimentation" (Oct. 23, 1982), *The Pope Speaks* 28: no. 1, 1983, pp. 75–76.

. . . The substantial unity between spirit and body, and indirectly with the cosmos, is so essential that every human activity, even the most spiritual one, is in some way permeated and colored by the bodily condition; at the same time the body must in turn be directed and guided to its final end by the spirit. There is no doubt that the spiritual activities of the human person proceed from the personal center of the individual, who is predisposed by the body to which the spirit is substantially united.

Hence the great importance, for the life of the spirit, of the sciences which promote the knowledge of corporeal reality and activity.

Consequently, I have no reason to be apprehensive for those experiments in biology that are performed by scientists who, like you, have a profound respect for the human person, since I am certain that they will contribute to the integral well-being of man.

On the other hand, I condemn in the most explicit and formal way experimental manipulations of the human embryo, since the human being, from conception to death, cannot be exploited for any purpose whatsoever. Indeed, as the Second Vatican Council teaches, man is "the only creature on earth which God willed for itself."

Worthy of esteem is the initiative of those scientists who have expressed their disapproval of experiments which violate human freedom, and I praise those who have endeavored to establish, with full respect for man's dignity and freedom, guidelines and limits for experiments concerning man.

The experimentation which you have been discussing is directed to a greater knowledge of the most intimate mechanisms of life, by means of artificial models, such as the cultivation of tissues, and experimentation on some species of animals genetically selected. Moreover, you have indicated some experiments to be accomplished on animal embryos, which will permit you to know better how cellular differences are determined.

DOCUMENT 3 / Embryo Research

SOURCE: Pope John Paul II, "The Gospel of Life" (Mar. 25, 1995), *Origins* 24: no. 42 Apr. 6, 1995, p. 711.

63. This evaluation of the morality of abortion is to be applied also to the recent forms of intervention on human embryos which, although carried out for purposes legitimate in themselves, inevitably involve the killing of those embryos. This is the case with experimentation on embryos, which is becoming increasingly widespread in the field of biomedical research and is legally permitted in some countries. Although "one must uphold as licit procedures carried out on the human embryo which respect the life and integrity of the embryo and do not involve disproportionate risks for it, but rather are directed to its healing, the improvement of its condition of health or its individual survival, "it must nonetheless be stated that the use of human embryos or fetuses as an object of experimentation constitutes a crime against their dignity as human beings who have a right to the same respect owed to a child born, just as to every person.

This moral condemnation also regards procedures that exploit living human embryos and fetuses—sometimes specifically "produced" for this purpose by in vitro fertilization—either to be used as "biological material" or as providers of organs or tissue for transplants in the treatment of certain diseases. The killing of innocent human creatures, even if carried out to help others, constitutes an absolutely unacceptable act.

20: Ethical and Religious Directives

DOCUMENT 1:

Source: National Conference of Catholic Bishops, "Ethical and Religious Directives for Catholic Health Care Services," *Origins* 24: no. 27 (Dec. 15, 1994), pp. 450–462.

"A contemporary understanding of the Catholic health care ministry must take into account the new challenges presented by transitions both in the Church and in American society," say the "Ethical and Religious Directives for Catholic Health Care Services" approved by the U.S. bishops Nov. 17 during their meeting in Washington and made public by their Committee on Doctrine Dec. 1. The text revises and updates directives approved by the U.S. bishops in 1971 and revised in 1975. The directives "are concerned primarily with institutionally based Catholic health care services. They address the sponsors, trustees, administrators, chaplains, physicians, health care personnel, and patients or residents of these institutions and services," says the text. But, it is added, the directives "also will be helpful to Catholic professionals engaged in health care services in other settings." The document includes six parts, each divided into two sections. The first section "serves as an introduction and provides the context in which concrete issues can be discussed from the perspective of the Catholic faith. The second section is in prescriptive form." The six parts cover: social responsibility; pastoral and spiritual responsibility; the professional-patient relationship; the beginning of life; the dying; new partnerships with health care organizations and providers. The directives discuss abortion, euthanasia, treatment of rape victims, advance directives for health care decisions, care for the poor, medical or genetic experimentation, treatment for infertility, prenatal diagnosis, experiments on a living embryo or fetus, surrogate motherhood, in vitro fertilization, nutrition and hydration for the terminally ill, pain treatment, organ donation, employee rights and responsibilities, and many other issues. The text is accompanied by a note explaining that "at the annual meeting of the National Conference of Catholic Bishops the directives were approved as the national code, recommended for implementation by the diocesan bishop." The text of the directives follows.

PREAMBLE

Health care in the United States is marked by extraordinary change. Not only is there continuing change in clinical practice due to technological advances, but the health care system in the United States is being challenged by both institutional and social factors. At the same time, there are a number of developments within the Catholic Church affecting the ecclesial mission of health care. Among these are significant changes in religious orders and congregations, the increased involvement of lay men and women, a heightened awareness of the Church's social role in the world and developments in moral theology since the Second Vatican Council. A contemporary understanding of the Catholic health care ministry must take into account the new challenges presented by transitions both in the Church and in American society.

Throughout the centuries, with the aid of other sciences a body of moral principles has emerged that expresses the Church's teaching on medical and moral matters and has proven to be pertinent and applicable to the ever-changing circumstances of health care and its delivery. In response to today's challenges, these same moral principles of Catholic teaching provide the rationale and direction for this revision of the "Ethical and Religious Directives for Catholic Health Care Services."

These directives presuppose our statement "Health and Health Care," published in 1981. There we presented the theological principles that guide the Church's vision of health care, called for all Catholics to share in the healing mission of the Church, expressed our full commitment to the health care ministry, and offered encouragement to all those who are involved in it. Now, with American health care facing even more dramatic changes, we reaffirm the Church's commitment to health care ministry and the distinctive Catholic identity of the Church's institutional health care services. The purpose of these ethical and religious directives then is twofold: first, to reaffirm the ethical standards of behavior in health care which flow from the Church's teaching about the dignity of the human person; second, to provide authoritative guidance on certain moral issues which face Catholic health care today.

The ethical and religious directives are concerned primarily with institutionally based Catholic health care services. They address the sponsors, trustees, administrators, chaplains, physicians, health care personnel, and patients or residents of these institutions and services. Since they express the Church's moral teaching, these directives also will be helpful to Catholic professionals engaged in health care services in other settings. The moral teachings that we profess here flow principally from the natural law, understood in the light of the revelation Christ has entrusted to his Church. From this source the Church has derived its understanding of the nature of the human person, of human acts, and of the goals that shape human activity.

The directives have been refined through an extensive process of consultation with bishops, theologians, sponsors, administrators, physicians and other health care providers. While providing standards and guidance, the directives do not cover in detail all of the complex issues that confront Catholic health care today. Moreover, the directives will be reviewed periodically by the National Conference of Catholic Bishops, in the light of authoritative Church teaching, in order to address new insights from theological and medical research or new requirements of public policy.

The directives begin with a general introduction that presents a theological basis for the Catholic health care ministry. Each of the six parts that follows is

130 divided into two sections. The first section is in expository form; it serves as an introduction and provides the context in which concrete issues can be discussed from the perspective of the Catholic faith. The second section is in prescriptive form; the directives promote and protect the truths of the Catholic faith as those truths are brought to bear on concrete issues in health care.

GENERAL INTRODUCTION

The Church has always sought to embody our Savior's concern for the sick. The Gospel accounts of Jesus' ministry draw special attention to his acts of healing: he cleansed a man with leprosy (cf. Mt 8:1–4; Mk 1:40–42); he gave sight to two people who were blind (cf. Mt 20:29–34; Mk 10:46–52); he enabled one who was mute to speak (cf. Lk 11:14); he cured a woman who was hemorrhaging (cf. Mt 9:20–22; Mk 5:25–34); and he brought a young girl back to life (cf. Mt 9:18, 23–25; Mk 5:35–42). Indeed, the Gospels are replete with examples of how the Lord cured every kind of ailment and disease (cf. Mt 9:35). In the account of Matthew, Jesus' mission fulfilled the prophecy of Isaiah: "He took away our infirmities and bore our diseases" (Mt 8:17; cf. Is 53:4).

Jesus' healing mission went further than caring only for physical affliction. He touched people at the deepest level of their existence; he sought their physical, mental and spiritual healing (cf. Jn 6:35; 11:25–27). He "came so that they might have life and have it more abundantly" (Jn 10:10).

The mystery of Christ casts light on every facet of Catholic health care: to see Christian love as the animating principle of health care; to see healing and compassion as a continuation of Christ's mission; to see suffering as a participation in the redemptive power of Christ's passion, death and resurrection; and to see death, transformed by the resurrection, as an opportunity for a final act of communion with Christ.

For the Christian, our encounter with suffering and death can take on a positive and distinctive meaning through the redemptive power of Jesus' suffering and death. As St. Paul says, we are "always carrying about in the body the dying of Jesus, so that the life of Jesus may also be manifested in our body" (2 Cor 4:10). This does not lessen the pain and fear, but gives confidence and grace for bearing suffering rather than being overwhelmed by it. Catholic health care ministry bears witness to the truth that, for those who are in Christ, suffering and death are the birth pangs of the new creation. "God himself will always be with them. He will wipe every tear in their eyes and there shall be no more death or mourning, wailing or pain, for the old order has passed away" (Rv 21:3–4).

In faithful imitation of Jesus Christ, the Church has served the sick, suffering and dying in glorious ways throughout history. The zealous service of individuals and communities has provided shelter for the traveler, infirmaries for the sick and homes for children, adults and the elderly. In the United States, the many religious communities as well as dioceses that sponsor and staff this country's Catholic health care institutions and services have established an effective Catholic presence in health care. Modeling their efforts on the Gospel parable of the good Samaritan, these communities of women and men have **131** exemplified authentic neighborliness to those in need (cf. Lk 10:25–37). The Church seeks to ensure that the service offered in the past will be continued into the future.

While many religious communities continue their commitment to the health care ministry, lay Catholics increasingly have stepped forward to collaborate in this ministry. Inspired by the example of Christ and mandated by the Second Vatican Council, lay faithful are invited to broader and more intense fields of ministries than in the past. By virtue of their baptism, lay faithful are called to participate actively in the Church's life and mission. Their participation and leadership in the health care ministry, through new forms of sponsorship and governance of institutional Catholic health care, are essential for the Church to continue her ministry of healing and compassion. They are joined in the Church's health care mission by many men and women who are not Catholic.

Catholic health care expresses the healing ministry of Christ in a specific way within the local Church. Here the diocesan bishop exercises responsibilities that are rooted in his office as pastor, teacher, and priest. As the center of unity in the diocese and coordinator of ministries in the local Church, the diocesan bishop fosters the mission of Catholic health care in a way that promotes collaboration among health care leaders, providers, medical professionals, theologians and other specialists. As pastor, the diocesan bishop is in a unique position to encourage the faithful to greater responsibility in the healing ministry of Church. As teacher, the diocesan bishop ensures the moral and religious identity of the health care ministry in whatever setting it is carried out in the diocese. As priest, the diocesan bishop oversees the sacramental care of the sick. These responsibilities will require that Catholic health care providers and diocesan bishops engage in ongoing communication on ethical and pastoral matters that require his attention.

In a time of new medical discoveries, rapid technological developments, and social change, what is new can either be an opportunity for genuine advance in human culture or it can lead to policies and actions that are contrary to the true dignity and vocation of the human person. In consultation with medical professionals, Church leaders review these developments, judge them according to the principles of right reason and the ultimate standard of revealed truth, and offer authoritative teaching and guidance about the moral and pastoral responsibilities entailed by the Christian faith. While the Church cannot furnish a ready answer to every moral dilemma, there are many questions about which she provides normative guidance and direction. In the absence of a determination by the Magisterium, but never contrary to Church teaching, the guidance of approved authors can offer appropriate guidance for ethical decision making.

Created in God's image and likeness, the human family shares in the dominion which Christ manifested in his healing ministry. This sharing involves a stewardship over all material creation (cf. Gn 1:26) that should neither abuse nor squander nature's resources. Through science the human race comes to understand God's wonderful work; and through technology it must conserve,

132 protect, and perfect nature in harmony with God's purposes. Health care professionals pursue a special vocation to share in carrying forth God's life-giving and healing work.

The dialogue between medical science and Christian faith has for its primary purpose the common good of all human persons. It presupposes that science and faith do not contradict each other. Both are grounded in respect for truth and freedom. As new knowledge and new technologies expand, each person must form a correct conscience based on the moral norms for proper health care.

PART I
THE SOCIAL RESPONSIBILITY OF
CATHOLIC HEALTH CARE SERVICES

Introduction

Their embrace of Christ's healing mission has led institutionally based Catholic health care services in the United States to become an integral part of the nation's health care system. Today this complex health care system confronts a range of economic, technological, social, and moral challenges. The response of Catholic health care institutions and services to these challenges is guided by normative principles that inform the Church's healing ministry.

First, Catholic health care ministry is rooted in a commitment to promote and defend human dignity; this is the foundation of its concern to respect the sacredness of every human life from the moment of conception until death. The first right of the human person, the right to life, entails a right to the means for the proper development of life such as adequate health care.

Second, the biblical mandate to care for the poor requires us to express this in concrete action at all levels of Catholic health care. This mandate prompts us to work to ensure that our country's health care delivery system provides adequate health care for the poor. In Catholic institutions, particular attention should be given to the health care needs of the poor, the uninsured, and the underinsured.

Third, Catholic health care ministry seeks to contribute to the common good. The common good is realized when economic, political, and social conditions ensure protection for the fundamental rights of all individuals, and enable all to fulfill their common purpose and reach their common goals.

Fourth, Catholic health care ministry exercises responsible stewardship of available health care resources. A just health care system will be concerned both with promoting equity of care to assure that the right of each person to basic health care is respected and with promoting the good health of all in the community. The responsible stewardship of health care resources can be accomplished best in dialogue with people from all levels of society, in accordance with the principle of subsidiarity and with respect for the moral principles which guide institutions and persons.

Fifth, within a pluralistic society Catholic health care services will encounter requests for medical procedures contrary to the moral teachings of the

Church. Catholic health care does not offend the rights of individual conscience **133** by refusing to provide or permit medical procedures that are judged morally wrong by the teaching authority of the Church.

Directives

1. A Catholic institutional health care service is a community which provides health care to those in need of it. This service must be animated by the Gospel of Jesus Christ and guided by the moral tradition of the Church.

2. Catholic health care should be marked by a spirit of mutual respect among caregivers which disposes them to deal with those it serves and their families with the compassion of Christ, sensitive to their vulnerability at a time of special need.

3. In accord with its mission, Catholic health care should distinguish itself by service to and advocacy for those people whose social condition puts them at the margins of our society and makes them particularly vulnerable to discrimination: the poor, the uninsured, and the underinsured; children, the unborn, single parents and the elderly; those with incurable diseases and chemical dependencies; and racial minorities, immigrants, and refugees. In particular, the person with mental or physical disabilities, regardless of the cause or severity, must be treated as a unique person of incomparable worth, with the same right to life and to adequate health care as all other persons.

4. A Catholic health care institution, especially a teaching hospital, will promote medical research consistent with its mission of providing health care and with concern for the responsible stewardship of health care resources. Such medical research must adhere to Catholic moral principles.

5. Catholic health care services must adopt these directives as policy, require adherence to them within the institution as a condition for medical privileges and employment, and provide appropriate instruction regarding the directives for administration, medical and nursing staff, and other personnel.

6. A Catholic health care organization should be a responsible steward of the health care resources available to it. Collaboration with other health care providers in ways that do not compromise Catholic social and moral teaching can be an effective means of such stewardship.

7. A Catholic health care institution must treat its employees respectfully and justly. This responsibility includes: equal employment opportunities for anyone qualified for the task, irrespective of a person's race, sex, age, national origin, or disability; a workplace that promotes employee participation; a work environment that ensures employee safety and well-being; just compensation and benefits; and recognition of the rights of employees to organize and bargain collectively without prejudice to the common good.

8. Catholic health care institutions have a unique relationship to both the Church and the wider community they serve. Because of the ecclesial nature of this relationship, the relevant requirements of canon law will be observed with regard to the foundation of a new Catholic health care institution, the substantial revision of the mission of an institution, and the sale, sponsorship, transfer, or the closure of an existing institution.

134   **9.** Employees of a Catholic health care institution must respect and uphold the religious mission of the institution and adhere to these directives. They should maintain professional standards and promote the institution's commitment to human dignity and the common good.

PART 2

PASTORAL AND SPIRITUAL RESPONSIBILITY
OF CATHOLIC HEALTH CARE

Introduction

The dignity of human life flows from creation in the image of God (cf. Gn 1:26), from redemption by Jesus Christ (cf. Eph 1: 10; 1 Tm 2:46), and from our common destiny to share a life with God beyond all corruption (cf. 1 Cor 15:42–57). Catholic health care has the responsibility to treat those in need in a way that respects the human dignity and eternal destiny of all. The words of Christ have provided inspiration for Catholic health care: "I was ill and you cared for me" (Mt 25:36). The care provided assists those in need to experience their own dignity and value, especially when these are obscured by the burdens of illness or the anxiety of imminent death.

Since a Catholic health care institution is a community of healing and compassion, the care offered is not limited to the treatment of a disease or bodily ailment but embraces the physical, psychological, social, and spiritual dimensions of the human person. The medical expertise offered through Catholic health care is combined with other forms of care to promote health and relieve human suffering. For this reason, Catholic health care extends to the spiritual nature of the person.

"Without health of the spirit, high technology used strictly on the body offers limited hope for healing the whole person." Directed to spiritual needs that are often appreciated more deeply during times of illness, pastoral care is an integral part of Catholic health care. Pastoral care encompasses the full range of spiritual services, including a listening presence, help in dealing with powerlessness, pain, and alienation, and assistance in recognizing and responding to God's will with greater joy and peace. It should be acknowledged, of course, that technological advances in medicine have reduced the length of hospital stays dramatically. It follows, therefore, that the pastoral care of patients, especially administration of the sacraments, will be provided more often than not at the parish level, both before and after one's hospitalization. For this reason, it is essential that there be very cordial and cooperative relationships between the personnel of pastoral care departments and the local clergy and ministers of care.

Priests, deacons, religious, and laity exercise diverse but complementary roles in this pastoral care. Since many areas of pastoral care call upon the creative response of these pastoral caregivers to the particular needs of patients or residents, the following directives address only a limited number of specific pastoral activities.

10. A Catholic health care organization should provide pastoral care to minister to the religious and spiritual needs of all those it serves. Pastoral care personnel, clergy, religious, and lay alike, should have appropriate professional preparation, including an understanding of these directives.

11. Pastoral care personnel should work in close collaboration with local parishes and community clergy. Appropriate pastoral services and/or referrals should be available to all in keeping their religious beliefs or affiliation.

12. For Catholic patients or residents, provision for the sacraments is an especially important of Catholic health care ministry. Every effort should be made to have priests assigned to hospitals and health care institutions to celebrate the Eucharist and provide the sacraments to patients and staff.

13. Particular care should be taken to provide and to publicize opportunities for patients or residents to receive the sacrament of penance.

14. Properly prepared lay Catholics can be appointed to serve as extraordinary ministers of holy communion, in accordance with canon law and the policies of the local diocese. They should assist pastoral care personnel—clergy, religious and laity–by providing supportive visits, advising patients regarding the availability of priests for the sacrament of penance and distributing holy communion to the faithful who request it.

15. Responsive to a patient's desires and condition, all involved in pastoral care should facilitate the availability of priests to provide the sacrament of anointing of the sick, recognizing that through this sacrament Christ provides grace and support to those who are seriously ill or weakened by advanced age. Normally, the sacrament is celebrated when the sick person is fully conscious. It may be conferred upon the sick who have lost consciousness or the use of reason if there is reason to believe that they would have asked for the sacrament while in control of their faculties.

16. All Catholics who are capable of receiving communion should receive viaticum when they are in danger of death, while still in full possession of their faculties.

17. Except in cases of emergency (i.e., danger of death), any request for baptism made by adults or for infants should be referred to the chaplain of the institution. Newly born infants in danger of death, including those miscarried, should be baptized if this is possible. 'I In case of emergency, if a priest or deacon is not available, anyone can validly baptize. In the case of emergency baptism, the chaplain or the director of pastoral care is to be notified.

18. When a Catholic who has been baptized but not yet confirmed is in danger of death, any priest may confirm the person."

19. A record of the conferral of baptism or confirmation should be sent to the parish in which the institution is located and posted in its baptism/confirmation registers.

20. Catholic discipline generally reserves the reception of the sacraments to Catholics. In accord with Canon 844.3, Catholic ministers may administer the sacraments of eucharist, penance and anointing of the sick to members of

136 the Oriental churches which do not have full communion with the Catholic Church or of other churches that in the judgment of the Holy See are in the same condition as the Oriental churches, if such persons ask for the sacraments on their own and are properly disposed.

With regard to other Christians not in full communion with the Catholic Church, when the danger of death or other grave necessity is present, the four conditions of Canon 844.4 also must be present, namely, they cannot approach a minister of their own community, they ask for the sacraments on their own, they manifest Catholic faith in these sacraments and they are properly disposed. The diocesan bishop has the responsibility to oversee this pastoral practice.

21. The appointment of priests and deacons to the pastoral care staff of a Catholic institution must have the explicit approval or confirmation of the local bishop in collaboration with the administration of the institution. The appointment of the director of the pastoral care staff should be made in consultation with the diocesan bishop.

22. For the sake of appropriate ecumenical and interfaith relations, a diocesan policy should be developed with regard to the appointment of non-Catholic members to the pastoral care staff of a Catholic health care institution. The director of pastoral care at a Catholic institution should be a Catholic; any exception to this norm should be approved by the diocesan bishop.

PART 3
THE PROFESSIONAL-PATIENT RELATIONSHIP

Introduction

A person in need of health care and the professional health care provider who accepts that person as a patient enter into a relationship that requires, among other things, mutual respect, trust, honesty, and appropriate confidentiality. The resulting free exchange of information must avoid manipulation, intimidation, or condescension. Such a relationship enables the patient to disclose personal information needed for effective care and permits the health care provider to use his or her professional competence most effectively to maintain or restore the patient's health. Neither the health care professional nor the patient acts independently of the other; both participate in the healing process.

Today, a patient often receives health care from a team of providers, especially in the setting of the modem acute-care hospital. But the resulting multiplication of relationships does not alter the personal character of the interaction between health care providers and the patient. The relationship of the persons seeking health care and the professionals providing that care is an important part of the foundation on which diagnosis and care are provided. Diagnosis and care therefore entail a series of decisions with ethical as well as medical dimensions. The health care professional has the knowledge and experience to pursue the goals of healing, the maintenance of health, and the compassionate care of the dying, taking into account the patient's convictions and spiritual needs and the moral responsibilities of all concerned. The person in need of health care depends on the skill of the health care provider to assist in preserving life and promoting health of body, mind, and spirit. The patient, in turn, has a responsibility to use these physical and mental resources in the service of moral and spiritual goals to the best of his or her ability.

When the health care professional and the patient use institutional Catholic health care, they also accept its public commitment to the Church's understanding of and witness to the dignity of the human person. The Church's moral teaching on health care nurtures a truly interpersonal professional-patient relationship. This professional-patient relationship is never separated, then, from the Catholic identity of the health care institution. The faith that inspires Catholic health care guides medical decisions in ways that fully respect the dignity of the person and the relationship with the health care professional.

Directives

23. The inherent dignity of the human person must be respected and protected regardless of the nature of the person's health problem or social status. The respect for human dignity extends to all persons who are served by Catholic health care.

24. In compliance with federal law, a Catholic health care institution will make available to patients information about their rights, under the laws of their state, to make an advance directive for their medical treatment. The institution, however, will not honor an advance directive that is contrary to Catholic teaching. If the advance directive conflicts with Catholic teaching, an explanation should be provided as to why the directive cannot be honored.

25. Each person may identify in advance a representative to make health care decisions as his or her surrogate in the event that the person loses the capacity to make health care decisions. Decisions by the designated surrogate should be faithful to Catholic moral principles and to the person's intentions and values or, if the person's intentions are unknown, to the person's best interests. In the event that an advance directive is not executed, those who are in a position to know best the patient's wishes—usually family members and loved ones—should participate in the treatment decisions for the person who has lost the capacity to make health care decisions.

26. The free and informed consent of the person or the person's surrogate is required for medical treatments and procedures, except in an emergency situation when consent cannot be obtained and there is no indication that the patient would refuse consent to the treatment.

27. Free and informed consent requires that the person or the person's surrogate receive all reasonable information about the essential nature the proposed treatment and its benefits; its risks, side effects, consequences and cost; and reasonable and morally legitimate alternatives including no treatment at all.

28. Each person or the person's surrogate should have access to medical and moral information and counseling so as to be able to form his or her conscience. The free and informed health decision of the person or the person's surrogate is to be followed so long as it does not contradict Catholic principles.

138   **29.** All persons served by Catholic health have the right and duty to protect and preserve their bodily and functional integrity. The functional integrity of the person may be sacrificed to maintain the health or life of the person when no other morally permissible means is available.

30. The transplantation of organs from living donors is morally permissible when such a donation will not sacrifice or seriously impair any essential bodily function and the anticipated benefit to the recipient is proportionate to the harm done to the donor. Furthermore, the freedom of the prospective donor must be respected, and economic advantages should not accrue to the donor.

31. No one should be the subject of medical or genetic experimentation, even if it is therapeutic, unless the person or surrogate first has given free and informed consent. In instances of nontherapeutic experimentation, the surrogate can give this consent only if the experiment entails no significant risk to the person's well-being. Moreover, the greater the person's incompetency and vulnerability, the greater the reasons must be to perform any medical experimentation, especially nontherapeutic.

32. While every person is obliged to use ordinary means to preserve his or her health, no person should be obliged to submit to a health care procedure that the person has judged, with a free and informed conscience, not to provide a reasonable hope of benefit without imposing excessive risks and burdens on the patient, or excessive expense to family or community.

33. The well-being of the whole person must be taken into account in deciding about any therapeutic intervention or use of technology. Therapeutic procedures that are likely to cause harm or undesirable side effects can be justified only by a proportionate benefit to the patient.

34. Health care providers are to respect each person's privacy and confidentiality regarding information related to the person's diagnosis, treatment and care.

35. Health care professionals should be educated to recognize the symptoms of abuse and violence, and are obliged to report cases of abuse to the proper authorities in accordance with local statutes.

36. Compassionate and understanding care should be given to a person who is the victim of sexual assault. Health care providers should cooperate with law enforcement officials, offer the person psychological and spiritual support, and accurate medical information. A female who has been raped should be able to defend herself against a potential conception from the sexual assault. If, after appropriate testing, there is no evidence that conception has occurred already, she may be treated with medications that would prevent ovulation, sperm capacitation or fertilization. It is not permissible, however, to initiate or to recommend treatments that have as their purpose or direct effect the removal, destruction or interference with the implantation of a fertilized ovum.

37. An ethics committee or some alternate form of ethical consultation should be available to assist by advising on particular ethical situations, by offering educational opportunities, and by reviewing and recommending policies. To these ends there should be appropriate standards for medical ethical

consultation within a particular diocese that will respect the diocesan bishop's
pastoral responsibility as well as assist members of ethics committees to be
familiar with Catholic medical ethics and, in particular, these directives.

PART 4
ISSUES IN CARE FOR THE BEGINNING OF LIFE

Introduction

The church's commitment to human dignity inspires an abiding concern
for the sanctity of human life from its very beginning, and with the dignity of
marriage and of the marriage act by which human life is transmitted. The
church cannot approve medical practices that undermine the biological, psychological and moral bonds on which the strength of marriage and the family depends.

Catholic health care ministry witnesses to the sanctity of life "from the
moment of conception until death." The church's defense of life encompasses
the unborn, and the care of women and their children during and after pregnancy. The church's commitment to life is seen in its willingness to collaborate
with others to alleviate the causes of the high infant mortality rate and to provide
adequate health care to mothers and their children before and after birth.

The church has the deepest respect for the family, for the marriage covenant and for the love that binds a married couple together. This includes respect
for the marriage act by which husband and wife express their love and cooperate
with God in the creation of a new human being. The Second Vatican Council
affirms: "This love is an eminently human one. . . . It involves the good of the
whole person. . . . The actions within marriage by which the couple are united
intimately and chastely are noble and worthy ones. Expressed in a manner
which is truly human, these actions signify and promote that mutual self-giving
by which spouses enrich each other with a joyful and thankful will. Marriage
and conjugal love are by their nature ordained toward the begetting and educating of children. Children are really the supreme gift of marriage and contribute
very substantially to the welfare of their parents. . . . Parents should regard as
their proper mission the task of transmitting human life and educating those
to whom it has been transmitted. . . . They are thereby cooperators with the
love of God the Creator, and are, so to speak, the interpreters of that love."

For legitimate reasons of responsible parenthood, married couples may
limit the number of their children by natural means. The church cannot approve
contraceptive interventions which "either in anticipation of the marital act, or
in its accomplishment or in the development of its natural consequences have
the purpose, whether as an end or a means, to render procreation impossible."
Such interventions violate "the inseparable connection, willed by God . . . between the two meanings of the conjugal act: the unitive and procreative
meaning."

With the advance of the biological and medical sciences, society has at
its disposal new technologies for responding to the problem of infertility. While
we rejoice in the potential for good inherent in many of these technologies,

140   we cannot assume that what is technically possible is always morally right. Reproductive technologies that substitute for the marriage act are not consistent with human dignity. Just as the marriage act is joined naturally to procreation, so procreation is joined naturally to the marriage act. As Pope John XXIII observed: "The transmission of human life is entrusted by nature to a personal and conscious act and as such is subject to all the holy laws of God: the immutable and inviolable laws which must be recognized and observed. For this reason, one cannot use means and follow methods which could be licit in the transmission of the life of plants and animals. Because the moral law is rooted in the whole of human nature, human persons, through intelligent reflection on their own spiritual destiny, can discover and cooperate in the plan of the Creator.

Directives

38. When the marital act of sexual intercourse is not able to attain its procreative purpose, assistance that does not separate the unitive and procreative ends of the act, and does not substitute for the marital act itself, may be used to help married couples conceive.

39. Those techniques of assisted conception that respect the unitive and procreative meanings of sexual intercourse and do not involve the destruction of human embryos or their deliberate generation in such numbers that it is clearly envisaged that all cannot implant and some are simply being used to maximize the chances of others implanting, may be used as therapies for infertility.

40. Heterologous fertilization (that is, any technique used to achieve conception by the use of gametes coming from at least one donor other than the spouses) is prohibited because it is contrary to the covenant of marriage, the unity of the spouses and the dignity proper to parents and the child.

41. Homologous artificial fertilization (that is, any technique used to achieve conception using the gametes of the two spouses joined in marriage) is prohibited when it separates procreation from the marital act in its unitive significance, e.g., any technique used to achieve extracorporal conception.

42. Because of the dignity of the child and of marriage, and because of the uniqueness of the mother-child relationship, participation in contracts or arrangements for surrogate motherhood is not permitted. Moreover, the commercialization of such surrogacy denigrates the dignity of women, especially the poor.

43. A Catholic health care institution that provides treatment for infertility should offer not only technical assistance to infertile couples but also should help couples pursue other solutions, e.g. counseling, adoption.

44. A Catholic health care institution should provide prenatal, obstetric and postnatal services for mothers and their children in a manner consonant with its mission.

45. Abortion, that is, the directly intended termination of pregnancy before viability or the directly intended destruction of a viable fetus, is never permitted.

Every procedure whose sole immediate effect is the termination of pregnancy before viability is an abortion, which, in its moral context, includes the interval between conception and implantation of the embryo. Catholic health care institutions are not to provide abortion services even based upon the principle of material cooperation. In this context, Catholic health care institutions need to be concerned about the danger of scandal in any association with abortion providers.

46. Catholic health care providers should be ready to offer compassionate physical, psychological, moral and spiritual care to those persons who have suffered from the trauma of abortion.

47. Operations, treatments and medications that have as their direct purpose the cure of a proportionately serious pathological condition of a pregnant woman are permitted when they cannot be safely postponed until the unborn child is viable, even if they will result in the death of the unborn child.

48. In case of extrauterine pregnancy, no intervention is morally licit which constitutes a direct abortion.

49. For a proportionate reason, labor may be induced after the fetus is viable.

50. Prenatal diagnosis is permitted when the procedure does not threaten the life or physical integrity of the unborn child or the mother and does not subject them to disproportionate risks, when the diagnosis can provide information to guide preventative care for the mother or pre- or postnatal care for the child and when the parents, or at least the mother, give free and informed consent. Prenatal diagnosis is not permitted when undertaken with the intention of aborting an unborn child with a serious defect.

51. Nontherapeutic experiments on a living embryo or fetus are not permitted, even with the consent of the parents. Therapeutic experiments are permitted for a proportionate reason with the free and informed consent of the parents or, if the father cannot be contacted, at least of the mother. Medical research that will not harm the life or physical integrity of an unborn child is permitted with parental consent.

52. Catholic health institutions may not promote or condone contraceptive practices, but should provide, for married couples and the medical staff who counsel them, instruction both about the church's teaching on responsible parenthood and in methods of natural family planning.

53. Direct sterilization of either men or women, whether permanent or temporary, is not permitted in a Catholic health care institution when its sole immediate effect is to prevent conception. Procedures that induce sterility are permitted when their direct effect is the cure or alleviation of a present pathology and a simpler treatment is not available.

54. Genetic counseling may be provided in order to promote responsible parenthood and to prepare for the proper treatment and care of children with genetic defects, in accordance with Catholic moral teaching and the intrinsic rights and obligations of married couples regarding the transmission of life.

142

PART 5
ISSUES IN CARE FOR THE DYING

Introduction

Christ's redemption and saving grace embrace the whole person, especially in his or her illness, suffering and death. The Catholic health care ministry faces the reality of death with the confidence of faith. In the face of death—for many, a time when hope seems lost—the church witnesses to her belief that God has created each person for eternal life.

Above all, as a witness to its faith, a Catholic health care institution will be a community of respect, love and support to patients or residents and their families as they face the reality of death. What is hardest to face is the process of dying itself, especially the dependency, helplessness and the pain that so often accompany terminal illness. One of the primary purposes of medicine in caring for the dying is the relief of pain and the suffering caused by it. Effective management of pain in all its forms is critical in the appropriate care of the dying.

The truth that life is a precious gift from God has profound implications for the question of stewardship over human life. We are not the owners of our lives and hence do not have absolute power over life. We have a duty to preserve our life and to use it for the glory of God; but the duty to preserve life is not absolute, for we may reject life-prolonging procedures that are insufficiently beneficial or excessively burdensome. Suicide and euthanasia are never morally acceptable options.

The task of medicine is to care even when it cannot cure. Physicians and their patients must evaluate the use of the technology at their disposal. Reflection on the innate dignity of human life in all its dimensions and on the purpose of medical care is indispensable for formulating a true moral judgment about the use of technology to maintain life. The use of life-sustaining technology is judged in light of the Christian meaning of life, suffering and death. Only in this way are two extremes avoided: on the one hand, an insistence on useless or burdensome technology even when a patient may legitimately wish to forgo it and, on the other hand, the withdrawal of technology with the intention of causing death.

Some state Catholic conferences, individual bishops and the NCCB Committee on ProLife Activities have addressed the moral issues concerning medically assisted hydration and nutrition. The bishops are guided by the church's teaching forbidding euthanasia, which is "an action or an omission which of itself or by intention causes death, in order that all suffering may in this way be eliminated." These statements agree that hydration and nutrition are not morally obligatory either when they bring no comfort to a person who is imminently dying or when they cannot be assimilated by a person's body. The NCCB Committee on Pro-Life Activities report, in addition, points out the necessary distinctions between questions already resolved by the magisterium and those requiring further reflection, as, for example, the morality of withdrawing medically assisted hydration and nutrition from a person who is in the condition which is recognized by physicians as the "persistent vegetative state."

Directives

55. Catholic health care institutions offering care to persons in danger of death from illness, accident, advanced age or similar condition should provide them with appropriate opportunities to prepare for death. Persons in danger of death should be provided with whatever information is necessary to help them understand their condition, and have the opportunity to discuss their condition with their family members and care providers. They should also be offered the appropriate medical information which would make it possible to address the morally legitimate choices available to them. They should be provided the spiritual support as well as the opportunity to receive the sacraments in order to prepare well for death.

56. A person has a moral obligation to use ordinary or proportionate means of preserving his or her life. Proportionate means are those that in the judgment of the patient offer a reasonable hope of benefit and do not entail an excessive burden or impose excessive expense on the family or the community.

57. A person may forgo extraordinary or disproportionate means of preserving life. Disproportionate means are those that in the patient's judgment do not offer a reasonable hope of benefit or entail an excessive burden or impose excessive expense on the family or the community.

58. There should be a presumption in favor of providing nutrition and hydration to all patients, including patients who require medically assisted nutrition and hydration, as long as this is of sufficient benefit to outweigh the burdens involved to the patient.

59. The free and informed judgment made by a competent adult patient concerning the use or withdrawal of life-sustaining procedures should always be respected and normally complied with, unless it is contrary to Catholic moral teaching.

60. Euthanasia is an action or omission which of itself or by intention causes death, in order to alleviate suffering. Catholic health care institutions may never condone or participate in euthanasia or assisted suicide in any way. Dying patients who request euthanasia should receive loving care, psychological and spiritual support, and appropriate remedies for pain and other symptoms so that they can live with dignity until the time of natural death.

61. Patients should be kept as free of pain as possible so that they may die comfortably and with dignity, and in the place where they wish to die. Since a person has the right to prepare for his or her death while fully conscious, he or she should not be deprived of consciousness without a compelling reason. Medicines capable of alleviating or suppressing pain may be given to a dying person even if this therapy may indirectly shorten the person's life, so long as the intent is not to hasten death. Patients experiencing suffering that cannot be alleviated should be helped to appreciate the Christian understanding of redemptive suffering.

62. The determination of death should be made by the physician or competent medical authority in accordance with responsible and commonly accepted scientific criteria.

144   **63.** Catholic health care institutions should encourage and provide the means whereby those who wish to do so may arrange for the donation of their organs and bodily tissue for ethically legitimate purposes, so that they may be used for donation and research after death.

64. Such organs should not be removed until it has been medically determined that the patient has died. In order to prevent any conflict of interest, the physician who determines death should not be a member of the transplant team.

65. The use of tissue or organs from an infant may be permitted after death has been determined and with the informed consent of the parents or guardians.

66. Catholic health care institutions should not make use of human tissue obtained by direct abortions, even for research and therapeutic purposes.

PART 6
FORMING NEW PARTNERSHIPS
WITH HEALTH CARE ORGANIZATIONS AND PROVIDERS

Introduction

Until recently, most health care providers enjoyed a degree of independence from one another. In ever-increasing ways, Catholic health care providers have become involved with other health care organizations and providers. For instance, many Catholic health care systems and institutions share in the joint purchase of technology and services with other local facilities or physicians' groups. Another phenomenon is the growing number of Catholic health care systems and institutions joining or co-sponsoring integrated delivery networks or managed-care organizations in order to contract with insurers and other health care payers. In some instances, Catholic health care systems sponsor a health care plan or health maintenance organization. In many dioceses new partnerships will result in a decrease in the number of health care providers, at times leaving the Catholic institution as the sole provider of health care services. At whatever level, new partnerships forge a variety of interwoven relationships: between the various institutional partners, between health care providers and the community, between physicians and health care services, and between health care services and payers.

On the one hand, new partnerships can be viewed as opportunities for Catholic health care institutions and services to witness to their religious and ethical commitments and so influence the healing profession. For example, new partnerships can help to implement the church's social teaching. New partnerships can be opportunities to realign the local delivery system in order to provide a continuum of health care to the community; they can witness to a responsible stewardship of limited health care resources; and they can be opportunities to provide to poor and vulnerable persons a more equitable access to basic care.

On the other hand, new partnerships can pose serious challenges to the viability of the identity of Catholic health care institutions and services, and their ability to implement these directives in a consistent way, especially when partnerships are formed with those who do not share Catholic moral principles. The risk of scandal cannot be underestimated when partnerships are not built upon common values and moral principles. Partnership opportunities for some Catholic health care providers may even threaten the continued existence of other Catholic institutions and services, particularly when partnerships are driven by financial considerations alone. Because of the potential dangers involved in the new partnerships that are emerging, an increased collaboration among Catholic-sponsored health care institutions is essential and should be sought before other forms of partnerships.

The significant challenges that new partnerships may pose, however, do not necessarily prelude their possibility on moral grounds. The potential dangers require that new partnerships undergo systematic and objective moral analysis which takes into account the various factors that often pressure institutions and services into new partnerships that can diminish the autonomy and ministry of the Catholic partner. The following directives are offered to assist institutionally based Catholic health care services in this process of analysis. To this end the National Conference of Catholic Bishops has established the Ad Hoc committee on Health Care Issues and the Church as a resource for bishops and health care leaders. An appendix at the end offers a clarification of the terms relative to the principles governing cooperation and their application to concrete situations.

Directives

67. Decisions that may lead to serious consequences for the identity or reputation of Catholic health care services or entail the high risk of scandal should be made in consultation with the diocesan bishop or his health care liaison.

68. Any partnership that will affect the mission or religious and ethical identity of Catholic health care institutional services must respect church teaching and discipline. Diocesan bishops and other church authorities should be involved as such partnerships are developed, and the diocesan bishop should give the appropriate authorization before they are completed. The diocesan bishop's approval is required for partnerships sponsored by institutions subject to his governing authority; for partnerships sponsored by religious institutes of pontifical right, his *nihil obstat* should be obtained.

69. When a Catholic health care institution is participating in a partnership which may be involved in activities judged morally wrong by the church, the Catholic institution should limit its involvement in accord with the moral principles governing cooperation.

70. The possibility of scandal, e.g. generating a confusion about Catholic moral teaching, is an important factor that should be considered when applying the principles governing cooperation. Cooperation, which in all other respects is morally appropriate, may be refused because of the scandal that would be caused in the circumstances.

CONCLUSION

Sickness speaks to us of our limitations and human frailty. It can take the form of infirmity resulting from the simple passing of years or injury from the exuberance of youthful energy. It can be temporary or chronic, debilitating and even terminal. Yet, the follower of Jesus faces illness and the consequences of the human condition aware that our Lord always shows compassion toward the infirm.

Jesus not only taught his disciples to be compassionate, but he also told them who should be the special object of their compassion. The parable of the feast with its humble guests was preceded by the instruction: "When you hold a banquet, invite the poor, the crippled, the lame, the blind" (Lk. 14:13). These were people whom Jesus healed and loved.

Catholic health care is a response to the challenge of Jesus to go and do likewise. Catholic health care services rejoice in the challenge to be Christ's healing compassion in the world and see their ministry not only as an effort to restore and preserve health, but also as a spiritual service and a sign of that final healing which will one day bring about the new creation that is the ultimate fruit of Jesus' ministry and God's love for us.

APPENDIX
THE PRINCIPLES GOVERNING COOPERATION

The principles governing cooperation differentiate the action of the wrong-doer from the action of the cooperator through two major distinctions. The first is between formal and material cooperation. If the cooperator intends the object of the wrongdoer's activity, then the cooperation is formal and, therefore, morally wrong. Since intention is not simply an explicit act of the will, formal cooperation can also be implicit. Implicit formal cooperation is attributed when, even though the cooperator denies intending the wrongdoer's object, no other explanation can distinguish the cooperator's object from the wrongdoer's object. If the cooperator does not intend the object of the wrongdoer's activity, the cooperation is material and can be morally licit.

The second distinction deals with the object of the action and is expressed by immediate and mediate material cooperation. Material cooperation is immediate when the object of the cooperator is the same as the object of the wrong-doer. Immediate material cooperation is wrong, except in some instances of duress. The matter of duress distinguishes immediate material cooperation from implicit formal cooperation. But immediate material cooperation—without duress—is equivalent to implicit formal cooperation and, therefore, is morally wrong. When the object of the cooperator's action remains distinguishable from that of the wrongdoer's, material cooperation is mediate and can be morally licit.

Moral theologians recommend two other considerations for the proper evaluation of material cooperation. First, the object of material cooperation should be as distant as possible from the wrongdoer's act. Second, any act of material cooperation requires a proportionately grave reason.

Prudence guides those involved in cooperation to estimate questions of **147** intention, duress, distance, necessity and gravity. In making a judgment about cooperation, it is essential that the possibility of scandal should be eliminated. Appropriate consideration should also be given to the church's prophetic responsibility.

21: Euthanasia

DOCUMENT 1:

SOURCE: John Paul II, "The Gospel of Life" (Mar. 25, 1995), *Origins* 24: no. 42, Apr. 6, 1995, p. 712.

64. At the other end of life's spectrum, men and women find themselves facing the mystery of death. Today as a result of advances in medicine, and in a cultural context frequently closed to the transcendent, the experience of dying is marked by new features. When the prevailing tendency is to value life only to the extent that it brings pleasure and well-being, suffering seems like an unbearable setback, something from which one must be freed at all costs. Death is considered "senseless" if it suddenly interrupts a life still open to a future of new and interesting experiences. But it becomes a "rightful liberation" once life is held to be no longer meaningful because it is filled with pain and inexorably doomed to even greater suffering.

. . . By using highly sophisticated systems and equipment, science and medical practice today are able not only to attend to cases formerly considered untreatable and to reduce or eliminate pain, but also to sustain and prolong life even in situations of extreme frailty, to resuscitate artificially patients whose basic biological functions have undergone sudden collapse and to use special procedures to make organs available for transplanting.

In this context the temptation grows to have recourse to euthanasia, that is, to take control of death and bring it about before its time, "gently" ending one's own life or the life of others. In reality what might seem logical and humane, when looked at more closely, is seen to be senseless and inhumane. Here we are faced with one of the more alarming symptoms of the "culture of death," which is advancing above all in prosperous societies, marked by an attitude of excessive preoccupation with efficiency, and which sees the growing number of elderly and disabled people as intolerable and too burdensome. . . .

65. For a correct moral judgment on euthanasia, in the first place a clear definition is required. Euthanasia in the strict sense is understood to be an action or omission which of itself and by intention causes death, with the purpose of eliminating all suffering. "Euthanasia's terms of reference, therefore, are to be found in the intention of the will and in the methods used."

Euthanasia must be distinguished from the decision to forgo so-called "aggressive medical treatment," in other words, medical procedures which no longer correspond to the real situation of the patient either because they are by now disproportionate to any expected results or because they impose an excessive burden on the patient and his family. In such situations, when death is clearly imminent and inevitable, one can in conscience "refuse forms of treatments that would only secure a precarious and burdensome prolongation of life, so long as the normal care due to the sick person in similar cases is not interrupted." Certainly there is a moral obligation to care for oneself and to allow oneself to be cared for, but this duty must take account of concrete circumstances. It needs to be determined whether the means of treatment available are objectively proportionate to the prospects for improvement. To forgo extraordinary or disproportionate means is not the equivalent of suicide or euthanasia; it rather expresses acceptance of the human condition in the face of death. . . .

DOCUMENT 2 / Euthanasia

SOURCE: Congregation for the Doctrine of the Faith, "Declaration on Euthanasia" (May 5, 1980), *Vatican Council II*, Vol. 2, pp. 510–16.

THE VALUE OF HUMAN LIFE

Human life is the basis of all goods, and is the necessary source and condition of every human activity and of all society. Most people regard life as something sacred and hold that no one may dispose of it at will, but believers see in life something greater, namely, a gift of God's love, which they are called upon to preserve and make fruitful. And it is this latter consideration that gives rise to the following consequences:

1. No one can make an attempt on the life of an innocent person without opposing God's love for that person, without violating a fundamental right, and therefore without committing a crime of the utmost gravity.

2. Everyone has the duty to lead his or her life in accordance with God's plan. That life is entrusted to the individual as a good that must bear fruit already here on earth, but that finds its full perfection only in eternal life.

3. Intentionally causing one's own death, or suicide, is therefore equally as wrong as murder; such an action on the part of a person is to be considered as a rejection of God's sovereignty and loving plan. Furthermore, suicide is also often a refusal of love for self, the denial of the natural instinct to live, a flight from the duties of justice and charity owed to one's neighbor, to various communities, or to the whole of society—although, as is generally recognized, at times there are psychological factors present that can diminish responsibility or even completely remove it.

However, one must clearly distinguish suicide from that sacrifice of one's life whereby for a higher cause, such as God's glory, the salvation of souls, or the service of one's brethren, a person offers his or her own life or puts it in danger (cf. Jn 15:14).

EUTHANASIA

In order that the question of euthanasia can be properly dealt with, it is first necessary to define the words used.

Etymologically speaking, in ancient times euthanasia meant an easy death without severe suffering. Today one no longer thinks of this original meaning of the word, but rather of some intervention of medicine whereby the sufferings of sickness or of the final agony are reduced, sometimes also with the danger of suppressing life prematurely. Ultimately, the word euthanasia is used in a more particular sense to mean "mercy killing," for the purpose of putting an end to extreme suffering or saving abnormal babies, the mentally ill, or the incurably sick from the prolongation, perhaps for many years, of a miserable life, which could impose too heavy a burden on their families or on society.

It is therefore necessary to state clearly in what sense the word is used   **151**
in the present document.

By euthanasia is understood an action or an omission which of itself or by
intention causes death, in order that all suffering may in this way be eliminated.
Euthanasia's terms of reference, therefore, are to be found in the intention of
the will and in the methods used.

It is necessary to state firmly once more that nothing and no one can in
any way permit the killing of an innocent human being, whether a fetus or an
embryo, an infant or an adult, an old person, or one suffering from an incurable
disease, or a person who is dying. Furthermore, no one is permitted to ask for
this act of killing, either for himself or herself or for another person entrusted
to his or her care, nor can he or she consent to it, either explicitly or implicitly.
Nor can any authority legitimately recommend or permit such an action. For
it is a question of the violation of the divine law, an offense against the dignity
of the human person, a crime against life, and an attack on humanity.

It may happen that, by reason of prolonged and barely tolerable pain, for
deeply personal or other reasons, people may be led to believe that they can
legitimately ask for death or obtain it for others. Although in these cases the
guilt of the individual may be reduced or completely absent, nevertheless the
error of judgment into which the conscience falls, perhaps in good faith, does
not change the nature of this act of killing, which will always be in itself
something to be rejected. The pleas of gravely ill people who sometimes ask
for death are not be to understood as implying a true desire for euthanasia; in
fact it is almost always a case of an anguished plea for help and love. What a
sick person needs, besides medical care, is love, the human and supernatural
warmth with which the sick person can and ought to be surrounded by all
those close to him or her, parents and children, doctors and nurses.

DOCUMENT 3 / Euthanasia

SOURCE: Pope John Paul II, "The Mystery of Life and Death" (Oct. 19–21, 1985), *Origins* 15: no. 25, Dec. 5, 1985, p. 416.

. . . Scientists and physicians are called to place their skill and energy at the service of life. They can never, for any reason or in any case, suppress it. For all who have a keen sense of the supreme value of the human person, believers and nonbelievers alike, euthanasia is a crime in which one must in no way cooperate or even consent to. Scientists and physicians must not regard themselves as the lords of life but as its skilled and generous servants. Only God, who created the human person with an immortal soul and saved the human body with the gift of the resurrection, is the Lord of life.

4. It is the task of doctors and medical workers to give the sick the treatment which will help to cure them and which will aid them to bear their sufferings with dignity. Even when the sick are incurable they are never untreatable; whatever their condition, appropriate care should be provided for them.

Among the useful and licit forms of treatment is the use of painkillers. Although some people may be able to accept suffering without alleviation, for the majority pain diminishes their moral strength. Nevertheless, when considering the use of these, it is necessary to observe the teaching contained in the declaration issued June 26, 1980, by the Congregation for the Doctrine of the Faith:

"Painkillers that cause unconsciousness need special consideration. For a person not only has to be able to satisfy his or her moral duties and family obligations; he or she also has to prepare himself or herself with full consciousness for meeting Christ."

DOCUMENT 4 / Euthanasia

Source: Pope John Paul II, "Opposing Euthanasia" (Sept. 6, 1984), *The Pope Speaks* 29: no. 44, 1984, pp. 353–54.

... In the light of these teachings, the believer must become ever more aware of the intangibility of every innocent human life and give proof of inflexible firmness in the face of pressures and suggestions from the dominant cultural environment by taking a stand against every attempt to legalize euthanasia and by continuing the struggle against abortion as well.

EUTHANASIA SUPPORTERS INHUMAN

But the real problem to be confronted in the growing social acceptance of euthanasia seems to be elsewhere. As has already been seen in the case of abortion, the moral condemnation of euthanasia remains unheard and incomprehensible to those who are imbued, perhaps unconsciously, with a conception of life that is irreconcilable with the Christian message and with the very dignity of the human person, correctly understood.

To find proof of this, it is sufficient to consider some of the negative characteristics in vogue in the culture that abstracts from the transcendent:

—the habit of disposing of human life at its source;

—the tendency of appreciating personal life only to the degree that it can provide riches and pleasures;

—regarding material well-being and pleasure as supreme goods, and thus viewing suffering as an absolute evil to be avoided at all costs and by every means;

—viewing death as an absurd end to a life that could have given further pleasures, or as the liberation from a life "deprived of meaning," because it was destined for further suffering.

With God out of the picture, it follows that man is responsible solely to himself and the freely established laws of society.

Paradoxically, where these attitudes have taken root among persons and social groups, it can appear logical and "humane" to "gently" put an end to one's own or another's life when that life holds only suffering or serious impairment. But, in reality, this is absurd and inhuman.

The commitment demanded of the Christian community in such a sociocultural context is more than a simple condemnation of euthanasia or the mere attempt to block the road toward its eventual spread and subsequent legalization. The basic problem is how to help the people of our time see the inhumanity of certain aspects of our culture and to rediscover the most precious values that have been obscured by it.

The emergence of euthanasia, as a further use of death in addition to abortion, must, therefore, be taken as a dramatic appeal to all believers and

154   persons of goodwill to promote, in every way possible, a true option for culture in our society's journey to the future.

Above all, therefore, the presence and decisive action of Catholics are particularly important in all those places and organizations, national and international, where the extremely important decisions for the direction of society are made.

Likewise, the same must be said about the vast field of the social communications media, for it goes without saying that they are important in forming public opinion.

But it is no less important and necessary to spread the awareness that everyone, simply by his own life-style, helps either to reinforce the Christian concept of life or to create a different one.

It is urgent, therefore, that all who can be reached by the Church be helped:

—to become aware of the dichotomy that often develops between faith and life, as a result of an uncritical, practical acceptance of hedonism, consumerism, and other concepts underlying a certain life-style;

—to discover the genuine Christian concepts concerning life, suffering, death, and the true values of a life that is seen as a vocation and a mission, for which each person is responsible before God;

—to build anew one's own individual, family, and professional existence on these concepts, without fearing to go against the time with Christian firmness. . . .

22: Family and Marriage

DOCUMENT 1:

Source: Pope Pius XI, Encyclical Letter *On Christian Marriage* (Dec. 31, 1930), *The Human Body: Papal Teachings*, pp. 5, 7–12.

I. NATURE AND DIGNITY OF CHRISTIAN MARRIAGE

. . . Let it be repeated as an immutable and inviolable fundamental doctrine that matrimony was not instituted or restored by man but by God; not by man were the laws made to strengthen and confirm and elevate it but by God, the author of nature, and by Christ our Lord, by whom nature was redeemed, and hence laws cannot be subject to any human decrees or to any contrary pact even of the spouses themselves. This is the doctrine of Holy Scripture; this is the constant tradition of the Universal Church. . . .

Therefore the sacred partnership of true marriage is constituted both by the will of God and the will of man. From God comes the very institution of marriage, the ends for which it was instituted, the laws that govern it, the blessings that flow from it; while man, through generous surrender of his own person made to another for the whole span of life, becomes, with the help and cooperation of God, the author of each particular marriage, with the duties and blessings annexed thereto from divine institution.

II. BLESSINGS AND BENEFITS OF MATRIMONY

Now when we come to explain . . . what are the blessings that God has attached to true matrimony, and how great they are, there occur to us the words of that illustrious doctor of the Church whom we commemorated recently in our encyclical *Ad Salutem* on the occasion of the fifteenth centenary of his death: "These," says St. Augustine, "are all the blessings of matrimony on account of which matrimony itself is a blessing; offspring, conjugal faith, and the sacrament." And how under these three heads is contained a splendid summary of the whole doctrine of Christian marriage, the holy doctor himself expressly declares when he said: "By conjugal faith it is provided that there should be no carnal intercourse outside the marriage bond with another man or woman; with regard to offspring, that children should be begotten of love, tenderly cared for, and educated in a religious atmosphere; finally, in its sacramental aspect that the marriage bond should not be broken and that a husband or wife, if separated, should not be joined to another even for the sake of offspring. This we regard as the law of marriage by which the fruitfulness of nature is adorned and the evil of incontinence is restrained."

. . . Christian parents must also understand that they are destined not only to propagate and preserve the human race on earth, indeed not only to

156 educate any kind of worshipers of the true God, but children who are to become members of the Church of Christ, to raise up fellow citizens of the saints, and members of God's household, that the worshipers of God and our Savior may daily increase.

For although Christian spouses even if sanctified themselves cannot transmit sanctification to their progeny, nay, although the very natural process of generating life has become the way of death by which original sin is passed on to posterity, nevertheless, they share to some extent in the blessings of that primeval marriage of paradise, since it is theirs to offer their offspring to the Church in order that by this most fruitful Mother of the children of God they may be regenerated through the lavare of Baptism unto supernatural justice and finally be made living members of Christ, partakers of immortal life, and heirs of that eternal glory to which we all aspire from our inmost heart. . . .

EDUCATION OF CHILDREN PARENTS' DUTY

The blessing of offspring, however, is not completed by the mere begetting of them, but something else must be added, namely the proper education of the offspring. For the most wise God would have failed to make sufficient provision for children that had been born, and so for the whole human race, if he had not given to those to whom he had entrusted the power and right to beget them, the power also and the right to educate them. For no one can fail to see that children are incapable of providing wholly for themselves, even in matters pertaining to their natural life, and much less in those pertaining to the supernatural, but require for many years to be helped, instructed, and educated by others. Now it is certain that both by the law of nature and of God this right and duty of educating their offspring belongs in the first place to those who began the work of nature by giving them birth, and they are indeed forbidden to leave unfinished this work and so expose it to certain ruin. But in matrimony provision has been made in the best possible way for this education of children that is so necessary, for, since the parents are bound together by an indissoluble bond, the care and mutual help of each is always at hand. . . .

CONJUGAL FIDELITY

The second blessing of matrimony, which we said we mentioned by St. Augustine, is the blessing of conjugal honor which consists in the mutual fidelity of the spouses in fulfilling the marriage contract, so that what belongs to one of the parties by reason of this contract, sanctioned by divine law, may not be denied to him or permitted to any third person; nor may there be conceded to one of the parties anything which, being contrary to the rights and laws of God and entirely opposed to matrimonial faith, can never be conceded.

DOCUMENT 2 / Family and Marriage

SOURCE: "Pastoral Constitution on the Church in the Modern World" (Dec. 7, 1965), *Vatican Council II,* Vol. 1, pp. 949–57.

THE DIGNITY OF MARRIAGE AND THE FAMILY
Marriage and the Family in the Modern World

47. The well-being of the individual person and of both human and Christian society is closely bound up with the healthy state of conjugal and family life. Hence Christians today are overjoyed, and so too are all who esteem conjugal and family life highly, to witness the various ways in which progress is being made in fostering those partnerships of love and in encouraging reverence for human life; there is progress too in services available to married people and parents for fulfilling their lofty calling: even greater benefits are to be expected and efforts are being made to bring them about.

However, this happy picture of the dignity of these partnerships is not reflected everywhere, but is overshadowed by polygamy, the plague of divorce, so-called free love, and similar blemishes; furthermore, married love is too often dishonored by selfishness, hedonism, and unlawful contraceptive practices. Besides, the economic, social, psychological, and civil climate of today has a severely disturbing effect on family life. There are also the serious and alarming problems arising in many parts of the world as a result of population expansion. On all of these counts an anguish of conscience is being generated. And yet the strength and vigor of the institution of marriage and family shines forth time and again: for despite the hardships flowing from the profoundly changing conditions of society today, the true nature of marriage and of the family is revealed in one way or another.

It is for these reasons that the Council intends to present certain key points of the Church's teaching in a clearer light; and it hopes to guide and encourage Christians and all men who are trying to preserve and to foster the dignity and supremely sacred value of the married state.

HOLINESS OF MARRIAGE AND THE FAMILY

48. The intimate partnership of life and the love which constitutes the married state has been established by the Creator and endowed by him with its own proper laws: it is rooted in the contract of its partners, that is, in their irrevocable personal consent. It is an institution confirmed by the divine law and receiving its stability, even in the eyes of society, from the human act by which the partners mutually surrender themselves to each other; for the good of the partners, of the children, and of society this sacred bond no longer depends on human decision alone. For God himself is the author of marriage and has endowed it with various benefits and with various ends in view: all of these have a very important bearing on the continuation of the human race, **157**

158 on the personal development and eternal destiny of every member of the family, on the dignity, stability, peace, and prosperity of the family and of the whole human race. By its very nature the institution of marriage and married love is ordered to the procreation and education of the offspring and it is in them that it finds its crowning glory. Thus the man and woman, who "are no longer two but one" (Mt 19:6), help and serve each other by their marriage partnership; they become conscious of their unity and experience it more deeply from day to day. The intimate union of marriage, as a mutual giving of two persons, and the good of the children demand total fidelity from the spouses and require an unbreakable unity between them.

Christ our Lord has abundantly blessed this love, which is rich in its various features, coming as it does from the spring of divine love and modeled on Christ's own union with the Church. Just as of old, God encountered his people with a covenant of love and fidelity, so our Savior, the spouse of the Church, now encounters Christian spouses through the Sacrament of Marriage. He abides with them in order that by their mutual self-giving spouses will love each other with enduring fidelity, as he loved the Church and delivered himself for it. Authentic married love is caught up into divine love and is directed and enriched by the redemptive power of Christ and the salvific action of the Church, with the result that the spouses are effectively led to God and are helped and strengthened in their lofty role as fathers and mothers. Spouses, therefore, are fortified and, as it were, consecrated for the duties and dignity of their state by a special sacrament; fulfilling their conjugal and family role by virtue of this sacrament, spouses are penetrated with the spirit of Christ and their whole life is suffused by faith, hope, and charity; thus they increasingly further their own perfection and their mutual sanctification, and together they render glory to God.

Inspired by the example and family prayer of their parents, children, and in fact everyone living under the family roof, will more easily set out upon the path of a truly human training, of salvation, and of holiness. As for the spouses, when they are given the dignity and role of fatherhood and motherhood, they will eagerly carry out their duties of education, especially religious education, which primarily devolves on them.

Children as living members of the family contribute in their own way to the sanctification of their parents. With sentiments of gratitude, affection, and trust, they will repay their parents for the benefits given to them and will come to their assistance as devoted children in times of hardship and in the loneliness of old age. Widowhood, accepted courageously as a continuation of the calling to marriage, will be honored by all. Families will generously share their spiritual treasures with other families. The Christian family springs from marriage, which is an image and a sharing in the partnership of love between Christ and the Church; it will show forth to all men Christ's living presence in the world and the authentic nature of the Church by the love and generous fruitfulness of the spouses, by their unity and fidelity, and by the loving way in which all members of the family cooperate with each other.

49. On several occasions the Word of God invites the betrothed to nourish and foster their betrothal with chaste love, and likewise spouses their marriage. Many of our contemporaries, too, have a high regard for true love between husband and wife as manifested in the worthy customs of various times and peoples. Married love is an eminently human love because it is an affection between two persons rooted in the will and it embraces the good of the whole person; it can enrich the sentiments of the spirit and their physical expression with a unique dignity and ennoble them as the special elements and signs of the friendship proper to marriage. The Lord, wishing to bestow special gifts of grace and divine love on it, has restored, perfected, and elevated it. A love like that, bringing together the human and the divine, leads the partners to a free and mutual giving of self, experienced in tenderness and action, and permeates their whole lives; besides this love is actually developed and increased by the exercise of it. This is a far cry from mere erotic attraction, which is pursued in selfishness and soon fades away in wretchedness.

Married love is uniquely expressed and perfected by the exercise of the acts proper to marriage. Hence the acts in marriage by which the intimate and chaste union of the spouses takes place are noble and honorable; the truly human performance of these acts fosters the self-giving they signify and enriches the spouses in joy and gratitude. Endorsed by mutual fidelity and, above all, consecrated by Christ's sacrament, this love abides faithfully in mind and body in prosperity and adversity and hence excludes both adultery and divorce. The unity of marriage, distinctly recognized by our Lord, is made clear in the equal personal dignity which must be accorded to man and wife in mutual and unreserved affection. Outstanding courage is required for the constant fulfillment of the duties of this Christian calling: spouses, therefore, will need grace for leading a holy life: they will eagerly practice a love that is firm, generous, and prompt to sacrifice and will ask for it in their prayers.

Authentic married love will be held in high esteem, and healthy public opinion will be quick to recognize it, if Christian spouses give outstanding witness to faithfulness and harmony in their love, if they are conspicuous in their concern for the education of their children, and if they play their part in a much needed cultural, psychological, and social renewal in matters of marriage and the family. It is imperative to give suitable and timely instruction to young people, above all in the heart of their own families, about the dignity of married love, its role and its exercise; in this way they will be able to engage in honorable courtship and enter upon marriage of their own.

THE FRUITFULNESS OF MARRIAGE

50. Marriage and married love are by nature ordered to the procreation and education of children. Indeed children are the supreme gift of marriage and greatly contribute to the good of the parents themselves. God himself said: "it is not good that man should be alone" (Gn 2:18), and "from the beginning (he) made them male and female" (Mt 19:4); wishing to associate them in a

160   special way with his own creative work, God blessed man and woman with the words: "Be fruitful and multiply" (Gn 1:28). Without intending to underestimate the other ends of marriage, it must be said that true married love and the whole structure of family life which results from it is directed to disposing the spouses to cooperate valiantly with the love of the Creator and Savior, who through them will increase and enrich his family from day to day.

Married couples should regard it as their proper mission to transmit human life and to educate their children; they should realize that they are thereby cooperating with the love of God the Creator and are, in a certain sense, its interpreters. This involves the fulfillment of their role with a sense of human and Christian responsibility and the formation of correct judgments through docile respect for God and common reflection and effort; it also involves a consideration of their own good and the good of their children already born or yet to come, an ability to read the signs of the times and of their own situation on the material and spiritual level, and, finally, an estimation of the good of the family, of society, and of the Church. It is the married couple themselves who must in the last analysis arrive at these judgments before God. Married people should realize that in their behavior they may not simply follow their own fancy but must be ruled by conscience—and conscience ought to be conformed to the law of God in the light of the teaching authority of the Church, which is the authentic interpreter of divine law. For the divine law throws light on the meaning of married love, protects it, and leads it to truly human fulfillment. Whenever Christian spouses in a spirit of sacrifice and trust in divine providence carry out their duties of procreation with generous human and Christian responsibility, they glorify the Creator and perfect themselves in Christ. Among the married couples who thus fulfill their God-given mission, special mention should be made of those who after prudent reflection and common decision courageously undertake the proper upbringing of a large number of children.

But marriage is not merely for the procreation of children: its nature as an indissoluble compact between two people and the good of the children demand that the mutual love of the partners be properly shown, that it should grow and mature. Even in cases where despite the intense desire of the spouses there are no children, marriage still retains its character of being a whole manner and communion of life and preserves its value and indissolubility.

MARRIED LOVE AND RESPECT FOR HUMAN LIFE

51. The Council realizes that married people are often hindered by certain situations in modern life from working out their married love harmoniously and that they can sometimes find themselves in a position where the number of children cannot be increased, at least for the time being: in cases like these it is quite difficult to preserve the practice of faithful love and the complete intimacy of their lives. But where the intimacy of married life is broken, it often happens that faithfulness is imperiled and the good of the children suffers: then the education of the children as well as the courage to accept more children are both endangered.

Some of the proposed solutions to these problems are shameful and some people have not hesitated to suggest the taking of life: the Church wishes to emphasize that there can be no conflict between the divine laws governing the transmission of life and the fostering of authentic married love.

God, the Lord of life, has entrusted to men the noble mission of safeguarding life, and men must carry it out in a manner worthy of themselves. Life must be protected with the utmost care from the moment of conception; abortion and infanticide are abominable crimes. Man's sexuality and the faculty of reproduction wondrously surpass the endowments of lower forms of life; therefore the acts proper to married life are to be ordered according to authentic human dignity and must be honored with the greatest reverence. When it is a question of harmonizing married love with the responsible transmission of life, it is not enough to take only the good intention and the evaluation of motives into account; the objective criteria must be used, criteria drawn from the nature of the human person and human action, criteria which respect the total meaning of mutual self-giving and human procreation in the context of true love; all this is possible only if the virtue of married chastity is seriously practiced. In questions of birth regulation the sons of the Church, faithful to these principles, are forbidden to use methods disapproved of by the teaching authority of the Church in its interpretation of the divine law.

Let all be convinced that human life and its transmission are realities whose meaning is not limited by the horizons of this life only: their true evaluation and full meaning can only be understood in reference to man's eternal destiny.

FOSTERING MARRIAGE AND THE FAMILY: A DUTY FOR ALL

52. The family is, in a sense, a school for human enrichment. But if it is to achieve the full flowering of its life and mission, the married couple must practice an affectionate sharing of thought and common deliberation as well as eager cooperation as parents in the children's upbringing. The active presence of the father is very important for their training: the mother, too, has a central role in the home, for the children, especially the younger children, depend on her considerably; this role must be safeguarded without, however, underrating woman's legitimate social advancement. The education of children should be such that when they grow up they will be able to follow their vocation, including a religious vocation, and choose their state of life with full consciousness of responsibility; and if they marry they should be capable of setting up a family in favorable moral, social, and economic circumstances. It is the duty of parents and teachers to guide young people with prudent advice in the establishment of a family; their interest should make young people listen to them eagerly; and they should beware of exercising any undue influence, directly or indirectly, to force them into marriage or compel them in their choice of partner.

The family is the place where different generations come together and help one another to grow wiser and harmonize the rights of individuals with other demands of social life; as such it constitutes the basis of society. Everyone, therefore, who exercises an influence in the community and in social groups

162 should devote himself effectively to the welfare of marriage and the family. Civil authority should consider it a sacred duty to acknowledge the true nature of marriage and the family, to protect and foster them, to safeguard public morality and promote domestic prosperity. The rights of parents to procreate and educate children in the family must be safeguarded. There should also be welfare legislation and provision of various kinds made for the protection and assistance of those who unfortunately have been deprived of the benefits of family life.

Christians, making full use of the times in which we live and carefully distinguishing the everlasting from the changeable, should actively strive to promote the values of marriage and the family; it can be done by the witness of their own lives and by concerted action along with all men of goodwill; in this way they will overcome obstacles and make provision for the requirements and the advantages of family life arising at the present day. To this end the Christian instincts of the faithful, the right moral conscience of man, and the wisdom and skill of persons versed in the sacred sciences will have much to contribute.

Experts in other sciences, particularly biology, medicine, social science, and psychology, can be of service to the welfare of marriage and the family and the peace of mind of people, if by pooling their findings they try to clarify thoroughly the different conditions favoring the proper regulation of births.

It devolves on priests to be properly trained to deal with family matters and to nurture the vocation of married people in their married and family life by different pastoral means, by the preaching of the Word of God, by liturgy, and other spiritual assistance. They should strengthen them sympathetically and patiently in their difficulties and comfort them in charity with a view to the formation of truly radiant families.

Various organizations, especially family associations, should set out by their programs of instruction and activity to strengthen young people and especially young married people, and to prepare them for family, social, and apostolic life.

Let married people themselves, who are created in the image of the living God and constituted in an authentic personal dignity, be united together in equal affection, agreement of mind, and mutual holiness. Thus, in the footsteps of Christ, the principle of life, they will bear witness by their faithful love in the joys and sacrifices of their calling, to that mystery of love which the Lord revealed to the world by his death and resurrection.

DOCUMENT 3 / Family and Marriage

SOURCE: Pope John Paul II, "The Christian Family in the Modern World" (Nov. 22, 1981), *Vatican Council II,* Vol. 2, pp. 822–26.

THE PLAN OF GOD FOR MARRIAGE AND THE FAMILY

11. God created man in his own image and likeness: calling him to existence through love, he called him at the same time for love.

God is love and in himself he lives a mystery of personal loving communion. Creating the human race in his own image and continually keeping it in being, God inscribed in the humanity of man and woman the vocation, and thus the capacity and responsibility, of love and communion. Love is therefore the fundamental and innate vocation of every human being. . . .

Christian revelation recognizes two specific ways of realizing the vocation of the human person, in its entirety, to love: marriage and virginity or celibacy. Either one is, in its own proper form, an actuation of the most profound truth of man, of his being "created in the image of God."

Consequently, sexuality, by means of which man and woman give themselves to one another through the acts which are proper and exclusive to spouses, is by no means something purely biological, but concerns the innermost being of the human person as such. It is realized in a truly human way only if it is an integral part of the love by which a man and a woman commit themselves totally to one another until death. The total physical self-giving would be a lie if it were not the sign and fruit of a total personal self-giving, in which the whole person, including the temporal dimension, is present: if the person were to withhold something or reserve the possibility of deciding otherwise in the future, by this very fact he or she would not be giving totally.

This totality, which is required by conjugal love, also corresponds to the demands of responsible fertility. This fertility is directed to the generation of a human being, and so by its nature it surpasses the purely biological order and involves a whole series of personal values. For the harmonious growth of these values a persevering and unified contribution by both parents is necessary.

The only "place" in which this self-giving in its whole truth is made possible is marriage, the covenant of conjugal love freely and consciously chosen, whereby man and woman accept the intimate community of life and love willed by God himself, which only in this light manifests its true meaning. The institution of marriage is not an undue interference by society or authority, nor the extrinsic imposition of a form. Rather it is an interior requirement of the covenant of conjugal love which is publicly affirmed as unique and exclusive, in order to live in complete fidelity to the plan of God, the Creator. A person's freedom, far from being restricted by this fidelity, is secured against every form of subjectivism or relativism and is made a sharer in creative Wisdom. . . .

164   14. According to the plan of God, marriage is the foundation of the wider community of the family, since the very institution of marriage and conjugal love are ordained to the procreation and education of children, in whom they find their crowning.

In its most profound reality, love is essentially a gift; and conjugal love, while leading the spouses to the reciprocal "knowledge" which makes them "one flesh," does not end with the couple, because it makes them capable of the greatest possible gift, the gift by which they become cooperators with God for giving life to a new human person. Thus the couple, while giving themselves to one another, give not just themselves but also the reality of children, who are a living reflection of their love, a permanent sign of conjugal unity and a living and inseparable synthesis of their being a father and a mother.

When they become parents, spouses receive from God the gift of a new responsibility. Their parental love is called to become for the children the visible sign of the very love of God, "from whom every family in heaven and on earth is named."

It must not be forgotten however that, even when procreation is not possible, conjugal life does not for this reason lose its value. Physical sterility in fact can be for spouses the occasion for other important services to the life of the human person, for example, adoption, various forms of educational work, and assistance to other families and to poor or handicapped children. . . .

23: Genetics

DOCUMENT 1:

SOURCE: National Conference of Catholic Bishops Science and Human Values Committee, "Critical Decisions; Genetic Testing and its Implications," *Origins* 25: no. 45 (May 2, 1996), pp. 770–72.

. . . Genetic testing and genetic counseling on how to deal with the results of tests will certainly grow at a rapid rate, creating a burgeoning challenge for pastors and Catholic health care providers. Obviously, the Church cannot offer a credible opinion on the quality or reliability of these tests; that is the province of the scientific and medical communities. However, genetic testing raises and will continue to raise moral issues for the individual, for the family, for racial or ethnic groups, and for society as a whole. The Church has a responsibility to offer insights based on its venerable tradition and current experience, not only to inform consciences and assist in the formation of wise public policy, but also to keep tradition vital.

Most often genetic tests show no disease, relieving anxiety. Moreover, the Catholic Church welcomes testing when it functions as an extension of sound medical practice. Catholics have served the sick for many centuries, and the Church is one of the major providers of health care in the world; naturally, it applauds every medical advance which promises healing without violating moral law. Pope John Paul II told the World Medical Association in 1983:

"A strictly therapeutic intervention whose explicit objective is the healing of various maladies such as those stemming from chromosomal defects will, in principle, be considered desirable, provided it is directed to the true promotion of the personal well-being of the individual. . . . Such an intervention would indeed fall within the logic of the Christian moral tradition."

Genetic testing can assist sound decision making in a range of situations. It is most commonly employed to detect problems with newborns. Moreover, millions of Americans are hospitalized every year because of hereditary disease and congenital defects. To the extent that genetic testing sets the stage for a cure or effective therapy, it is a blessing.

Testing has legitimate uses even in the delicate arena of human reproduction. Young couples considering marriage may want to know whether one or both partners carry a gene associated with mental retardation, cystic fibrosis, breast cancer, or some other heritable condition. While such testing carries risk, it can be considered an act of prudence, whether the couple subsequently decides to marry or not.

166   More and more frequently, expectant mothers are undergoing amniocentesis, chorionic villus sampling, and other tests to detect genetic anomalies in their unborn child. The most detailed Catholic teaching on this and related subjects appears in a 1987 statement from the Vatican Congregation for the Doctrine of the Faith called "The Gift of Life" (*Donum Vitae*). It asks: "Is prenatal diagnosis morally licit? If prenatal diagnosis respects the life and integrity of the embryo and the human fetus, and is directed toward its safeguarding or healing as an individual, then the answer is affirmative." The Holy Father builds on this declaration in his recent encyclical the "Gospel of Life" (*Evangelium Vitae*), holding that prenatal diagnostic techniques are morally permissible "when they do not involve disproportionate risks for the child and the mother, and are meant to make possible early therapy or even to favor a serene and informed acceptance of the child not yet born."

However, some prenatal testing poses significant risks to the unborn child, especially when performed on embryos before selection for implantation in the womb. Disturbing test results can also tempt individuals to make decisions not in accord with sound morality. The Holy Father goes on to note:

"But since the possibilities of prenatal therapy are today still limited, it not infrequently happens that these techniques are used with a eugenic intention which accepts selective abortion in order to prevent the birth of children affected by various types of anomalies. Such an attitude is shameful and utterly reprehensible, since it presumes to measure the value of a human life only within the parameters of 'normality' and physical well-being, thus opening the way to legitimizing infanticide and euthanasia."

The Church condemns and will never cease condemning the taking of innocent unborn life, surely the saddest aggression of our violent time.

Other uses of genetic testing, though perhaps not clearly sinful, invite serious moral reflection. Current therapies, by and large, manipulate a single gene or gene product. Science has not identified the multiple genes which may help determine high intelligence, a strong heart, immunity to cancer, a sunny personality, forcefulness of character, or other highly complex traits. Within 10 years or less, though, the Human Genome Initiative will have decoded the physical structure of all 100,000 of our genes. Decades, perhaps centuries, of research and experiment may be needed to develop sophisticated technology from this data. Even then, some traits may turn out to have no significant genetic component, while others may spring from so complex a combination of genes, environment, and experience that they remain beyond the reach of empirical analysis.

Nevertheless, the rate of discovery for genes that cause disease or influence physical and mental traits is accelerating rapidly. Within one or two generations, human beings may be able both to change significantly the individual's genetic makeup through somatic cell therapy and to affect heredity through germ-line therapy. As time passes we will learn more about our amazing diversity and our uniqueness. Unfortunately, we will also have the capacity to make finer distinctions among people and to discriminate accordingly. A predisposition to colon cancer is already detectable. If someone tests positive, should this information be available to insurance companies, whose financial success depends on minimizing risk? Potential employers? Potential marriage partners? What if the existence of a gene predisposing to homosexuality is confirmed? Who should have access to test results? These simple examples illustrate the enormous potential for abuse.

The Church's knowledge of the human heart springs from 2,000 years of moral reflection based ultimately on divine revelation. However, Catholic theology and the Catholic moral tradition mostly predate the development of genetic technologies, which offer new challenges. In an address to the Pontifical Academy for Life in November 1995, Pope John Paul II said:

"Indeed, the biomedical sciences are currently experiencing a period of rapid and marvelous growth, especially with regard to new discoveries in the areas of genetics. . . . But if scientific research is to be directed toward respect for personal dignity and support of human life, its scientific validity according to the rules of each discipline is not enough. It must also qualify positively from the ethical point of view, and this presupposes that from the outset it endeavors to promote the true good of human beings as individuals and as a community. This happens when efforts are made to eliminate the causes of disease by putting real prevention into practice, or whenever more effective therapies are sought for the treatment of serious illnesses."

Clearly, the scientific community cannot shoulder the whole burden of bringing ethics to bear. Catholic clergy and laity must become knowledgeable about emerging biotechnologies if they are to help people make the critical decisions they will inevitably face. Both the Church and the scientific community, we believe, can benefit from the effort to harmonize scientific advance with religious insight. Genetic testing is an important tool, but many will suffer if wisdom and sound morality do not guide its use.

DOCUMENT 2 / Genetics

SOURCE: Congregation for the Doctrine of the Faith, "Instruction on Respect for Human Life in Its Origin and on the Dignity of Procreation" (Feb. 22, 1987), *Origins* 16: no. 40, Mar. 19, 1987, p. 702.

I. RESPECT FOR HUMAN EMBRYOS

. . . 2. Is prenatal diagnosis morally licit?

If prenatal diagnosis respects the life and integrity of the embryo and the human fetus and is directed toward its safeguarding or healing as an individual, then the answer is affirmative.

For prenatal diagnosis makes it possible to know the condition of the embryo and of the fetus when still in the mother's womb. It permits or makes it possible to anticipate earlier and more effectively certain therapeutic, medical, or surgical procedures.

Such diagnosis is permissible, with the consent of the parents after they have been adequately informed, if the methods employed safeguard the life and integrity of the embryo and the mother, without subjecting them to disproportionate risks.* But this diagnosis is gravely opposed to the moral law when it is done with the thought of possibly inducing an abortion depending upon the results: A diagnosis which shows the existence of a malformation or a hereditary illness must not be the equivalent of a death sentence. Thus a woman would be committing a gravely illicit act if she were to request such a diagnosis with the deliberate intention of having an abortion should the results confirm the existence of a malformation or abnormality. The spouse or relatives or anyone else would similarly be acting in a manner contrary to the moral law if they were to counsel or impose such a diagnostic procedure on the expectant

---

*The obligation to avoid disproportionate risks involves an authentic respect for human beings and the uprightness of therapeutic intentions. It implies that the doctor "above all . . . must carefully evaluate the possible negative consequences which the necessary use of a particular exploratory technique may have upon the unborn child and avoid recourse to diagnostic procedures which do not offer sufficient guarantees of their honest purpose and substantial harmlessness. And if, as often happens in human choices, a degree of risk must be undertaken, he will take care to ensure that it is justified by a truly urgent need for the diagnosis and by the importance of the results that can be achieved by it for the benefit of the unborn child himself" (Pope John Paul II, Discourse to participants in the Pro-Life Movement Congress, Dec. 3, 1982, *Insegnamenti di Giovanni Paolo II*, V, 3 [1982], 1512). This clarification concerning "proportionate risk" is also to be kept in mind in the following sections of the present instruction, whenever this term appears.

mother with the same intention of possibly proceeding to an abortion. So too the specialist would be guilty of illicit collaboration if, in conducting the diagnosis and in communicating its results, he were deliberately to contribute to establishing or favoring a link between prenatal diagnosis and abortion.

In conclusion, any directive or program of the civil and health authorities or of scientific organizations which in any way were to favor a link between prenatal diagnosis and abortion, or which were to go as far as directly to induce expectant mothers to submit to prenatal diagnosis planned for the purpose of eliminating fetuses which are affected by malformations or which are carriers of hereditary illness, is to be condemned as a violation of the unborn child's right to life and as an abuse of the prior rights and duties of the spouses.

DOCUMENT 3 / Genetics

SOURCE: Pope Pius XII, "Moral Aspects of Genetics" (Sept. 7, 1953), *The Human Body: Papal Teachings*, pp. 256–58, 260.

PRACTICAL GENETICS

Genetics has not merely a theoretical interest; it is eminently practical as well. It aims at contributing towards the good of individuals and of the community—towards the common good. It proposes to accomplish this task principally in two fields: in that of genetic physiology and in that of genetic pathology.

Experience shows that natural dispositions, whether good or defective, exert a very strong influence on the education of man and on his future conduct. Undoubtedly the body, with its aptitudes and its organs, is only the instrument, while the soul is the artist that plays on that instrument. Again, the ability of the artist can compensate for many defects of the instrument; but one plays better and more easily on an instrument that is perfect; and when its quality falls below a certain level, it becomes absolutely impossible to use. (Naturally one must bear in mind the fact that, all comparison apart, the body and the soul, matter and spirit, form in man a substantial unity.)

Nevertheless, to keep to the comparison, genetics teaches us to understand the instrument better in its structure and variations and to make it play better. By observing a man's lineage, one may, on condition that one remains within certain limits, establish a diagnosis of the dispositions he has received by heredity and the prognosis of his inherited characteristics which will manifest themselves as good, and—what is more important still—also those which betray hereditary defects.

However limited the possibility of directly influencing heredity may be, practical genetics is not by any means reduced to the role of a passive spectator. Even daily life shows the extremely injurious effects of certain modes of acting of parents in the natural transmission of life. Such behavior, with the intoxications and infections to which it gives rise, must be prevented as far as possible, and genetics seeks out and points out the means to attain this end. Its conclusions bear particularly on the combinations of heredities of different lineage: it points out those that should be encouraged, those that can be tolerated, and those that should be discouraged from the point of view of genetics and eugenics.

The fundamental tendency of genetics and eugenics is to influence the transmission of hereditary factors in order to promote what is good and eliminate what is injurious. This fundamental tendency is irreproachable from the moral viewpoint. But certain methods used to attain this end, and certain protective measures, are morally questionable, as is also, in fact, a misplaced esteem for the ends to which genetics and eugenics tend. You will allow us to quote the statement of one of the most important experts in genetics at the present time. In a letter addressed to us, he expresses his regret that, notwithstanding the enormous progress it has made, genetics "from the technical and analytical point of view, has become entangled in manifold doctrinal errors, such as racialism, mutationism applied to phylogenesis, in order to explain in modern terms the evolution theory of Darwin, birth control for all persons who are really or supposedly defective either by preventive methods or by abortive practices, prenuptial certificates, etc."

In effect, there are certain defensive measures in genetics and eugenics which moral common sense, and especially Christian morals, must reject both in principle and in practice.

Amongst the methods contrary to morality, there must be included racialism, mentioned above, and eugenic sterilization. Our predecessor, Pius XI, and we ourselves were obliged to declare as contrary to the natural law, not only eugenic sterilization but every direct sterilization, whether temporary or permanent of an innocent person, either man or woman. Our opposition to sterilization has been, and still remains firm, for although racialism has come to an end, there are persons who are still desirous of, and try to suppress by sterilization, a lineage affected by hereditary diseases.

... That, gentlemen, is what we had to say to you. The practical aims being pursued by genetics are noble and worthy of recognition and encouragement. Would that your science, in weighing the means devised to achieve those ends, could remain always conscious of the fundamental difference that exists between the animal and vegetable world on the one hand, and man on the other! In the first case the means of bettering the species and race are entirely at the disposal of science. On the other hand, where man is concerned, genetics is always dealing with personal beings, with inviolable rights, with individuals who, for their part, are bound by unshakable moral laws in using their power to raise up a new life. Thus the Creator himself has established certain barriers in the moral domain, which no human power has authority to remove.

DOCUMENT 4 / Genetics

SOURCE: Pope John Paul II, "The Ethics of Genetic Manipulation" (Oct. 29, 1983), *Origins* 13: no. 23, Nov. 17, 1983, pp. 385, 388–89.

. . . Medicine is an eminent, essential form of service to mankind. It is first of all necessary to help man to live and overcome handicaps weighing upon normal functioning of all his organic functions in their psychophysical unity. Man is also at the center of the Church's concern. Her mission is, with God's grace, to save man, to restore him to his spiritual and moral integrity, to lead him toward integral development, where the body has its part. This is why the Church's ministry and the witness of Christians go hand in hand with solicitude for the sick. . . .

6. The third point is suggested to me by the very important theme which you pursued during your general assembly in Venice: the rights of the human person in view of certain new possibilities in medicine, particularly as regards "genetic manipulation," which puts a grave question to the conscience of all: how actually to reconcile such manipulation with the acknowledgment of innate dignity and untouchable autonomy in man?

A strictly therapeutic intervention, having the objective of healing various maladies—such as those stemming from chromosomic deficiencies—will be considered in principle as desirable, provided that it tends to real promotion of the personal well-being of man, without harming his integrity or worsening his life conditions. Such intervention actually falls within the logic of the Christian moral tradition, as I stated before the Pontifical Academy of Sciences Oct. 23, 1982.

But here the question rebounds. It is really of great interest to know whether an intervention upon the genetic store, exceeding the bounds of the therapeutic in the strict sense, is morally acceptable as well. For this to be so, it is necessary for several conditions to be respected and certain premises to be accepted. Let me mention some to you.

The biological nature of every human is untouchable, in the sense that it is constituent of the personal identity of the individual throughout the course of his history. Each human person—in his or her absolutely unique singularity, is not constituted only by the spirit, but also by the body.

Thus, in the body and through the body, one touches the person itself in its concrete reality. Respecting the dignity of man consequently comes down to safeguarding this identity of man *corpore et anima unus* (one in body and soul) as Vatican Council II says (*Gaudium et Spes,* 14). It is on the basis of this anthropological view that the fundamental criteria have to be found for making decisions if it is a question of interventions not strictly therapeutic, for example, interventions aimed at improving the human biological condition.

In particular, this kind of intervention must not offer harm to the origin of human life, that is procreation linked not only with the biological but also the spiritual union of the parents, united by the bond of marriage. Such an intervention must consequently respect the fundamental dignity of mankind and the common biological nature which lies at the basis of liberty; respect, consisting in avoidance of manipulations tending to modify the genetic store and to create groups of different people, at the risk of provoking fresh marginalizations in society.

For the rest, the fundamental attitudes inspiring the intervention we refer to should not derive from a racist, materialist mentality, aimed at a human happiness which is really reductive. Man's dignity transcends his biological condition.

Genetic manipulation becomes arbitrary and unjust when it reduces life to an object, when it forgets that it has to do with a human subject, capable of intelligence and liberty, and worthy of respect, whatever its limitations may be; or when genetic manipulation treats the human subject in terms of criteria not founded on the integral reality of the human person, at the risk of doing damage to his dignity. In this case it exposes man to the caprice of others, by depriving him of his autonomy.

All scientific and technical progress whatever must therefore keep the greatest respect for moral values, which constitute a safeguard of the dignity of the human person. And since, in the order of medical values, life is man's supreme and most radical good, there is need for a fundamental principle: first prevent any damage, then seek and pursue the good.

To tell the truth, the expression "genetic manipulation" remains ambiguous and ought to become the object of genuine moral discernment, for on the one hand it covers adventurous attempts aimed at promoting I know not what superman, and on the other hand salutary efforts aimed at correcting anomalies, such as certain hereditary maladies, not to mention beneficial applications in the fields of animal and vegetable biology which can be useful in food production. . . .

DOCUMENT 5 / Genetics

Source: Pontifical Academy for Life, "Reflections on Cloning," *Origins* 28: no. 1 (May 21, 1998), pp. 14–16.

Historical Background

Advances in knowledge and related developments in the procedures of molecular biology, genetics, and artificial fertilization have long made it possible to experiment with and successfully achieve the cloning of plants and animals.

Since the '30s, experiments have been made in producing identical individuals by artificial twin splitting, a procedure which can be improperly called cloning.

The practice of twin splitting in the zootechnical field has been spreading in experimental barns as an incentive to the multiple production of select exemplars. The news published in the journal *Nature,* Feb. 27, 1997, about the birth of the sheep Dolly through the efforts of the Scottish scientists Jan Vilmut and K.H.S. Campbell and their team at Edinburgh's Roslin Institute had an unusual effect on public opinion and led to statements being issued by committees and national and international authorities: this happened because it was something new and was considered troubling.

There are two new aspects of this event. The first is that it is not a question of splitting, but of a radical innovation defined as cloning, that is, an asexual and agamic reproduction meant to produce individuals biologically identical to the adult which provided the nuclear genetic inheritance. The second is that until now this type of true and proper cloning was considered impossible. It was thought that the DNA in the somatic cells of the higher forms of animal life, having already undergone the imprinting of differentiation, could no longer recover their original totipotentiality and, consequently, their ability to direct the development of a new individual. With the overcoming of this supposed impossibility, the way now seems open to human cloning, understood as the replication of one or more individuals somatically identical to the donor. The event has rightly caused concern and alarm. But after an initial phase of unanimous opposition, some have wished to call attention to the need for guaranteeing freedom of research, for not demonizing progress. The prediction has even been made that the Catholic Church herself will one day accept cloning.

Now that some time has passed, it would be useful in a more detached way to examine closely the fact that has been noted as a disturbing event.

The Biological Fact

In its biological aspects as a form of artificial reproduction, cloning is achieved without the contribution of two gametes; therefore it is an asexual and agamic reproduction. Fertilization properly so-called is replaced by the "fusion" of a nucleus taken from a somatic cell of the individual one wishes to clone, or of the somatic cell itself, with an oocyte from which the nucleus has been removed, that is, an oocyte lacking the maternal genome. Since the nucleus of the somatic cell contains the whole genetic inheritance, the individual obtained possesses—except for possible alterations—the genetic identity of the nucleus' donor. It is this essential genetic correspondence with the donor that produces in the new individual the somatic replica or copy of the donor itself. . . .

It should be stressed that the development of individuals obtained by cloning, apart from eventual possible mutations—and there could be many— should produce a body structure very similar to that of the DNA donor. This is the most disturbing result, especially when the experiment is applied to the human species.

It should be noted, however, that should the extension of cloning to the human species be desired, this duplication of body structure does not necessarily imply a perfectly identical person, understood in his ontological and psychological reality. The spiritual soul, which is the essential constituent of every subject belonging to the human species and is created directly by God, cannot be generated by the parents, prodded by artificial fertilization, or cloned. Furthermore, psychological development, culture, and environment always lead to different personalities; this is a well-known fact even among twins, whose resemblance does not mean identity. The popular image or aura of omnipotence that accompanies cloning should at least be put into perspective.

Ethical Problems

Human cloning belongs to the eugenics project and is thus subject to all the ethical and juridical observations that have amply condemned it. As Hans Jonas has already written, it is "both in method the most despotic and in aim the most slavish form of genetic manipulation; its objective is not an arbitrary modification of the hereditary material but precisely its equally arbitrary fixation in contrast to the dominant strategy of nature" (cf. Hans Jonas, *Cloniamo un Uomo: Dall'Eugenetica all'Ingegneria Genetica* in *Tecnica, Medicina ed Etica*, Einaudi, Turin 1997, pp. 122–54, p. 136).

It represents a radical manipulation of the constitutive relationality and complementarity which is at the origin of human procreation in both its biological and strictly personal aspects. It tends to make bisexuality a purely functional leftover, given that an ovum must be used without its nucleus in order to make room for the clone-embryo and requires, for now, a female womb so that its development may be brought to term. This is how all the experimental procedures in zootechny are being conducted, thus changing the specific meaning of human reproduction.

In this vision we find the logic of industrial production: market research must be explored and promoted, experimentation refined, ever newer models produced.

Women are radically exploited and reduced to a few of their purely biological functions (providing ova and womb), and research looks to the possibility of constructing artificial wombs, the last step to fabricating human beings in the laboratory.

176   In the cloning process the basic relationships of the human person are perverted: filiation, consanguinity, kinship, parenthood. A woman can be the twin sister of her mother, lack a biological father and be the daughter of her grandfather. In vitro fertilization has already led to the confusion of parentage, but cloning will mean the radical rupture of these bonds.

As in every artificial activity, what occurs in nature is "mimicked" and "imitated," but only at the price of ignoring how man surpasses his biological component, which moreover is reduced to those forms of reproduction that have characterized only the biologically simplest and least evolved organisms.

The idea is fostered that some individuals can have total dominion over the existence of others to the point of programming their biological identity—selected according to arbitrary or purely utilitarian criteria—which, although not exhausting man's personal identity, which is characterized by the spirit, is a constitutive part of it. This selective concept of man will have, among other things, a heavy cultural fallout beyond the—numerically limited—practice of cloning, since there will be a growing conviction that the value of man and woman does not depend on their personal identity but only on those biological qualities that can be appraised and therefore selected.

Human cloning must also be judged negative with regard to the dignity of the person cloned, who enters the world by virtue of being the "copy" (even if only a biological copy) of another being. This practice paves the way to the clone's radical suffering, for his psychic identity is jeopardized by the real or even by the merely virtual presence of his "other." Nor can we suppose that a conspiracy of silence will prevail, a conspiracy which, as Jonas already noted, would be impossible and equally immoral: since the "clone" was produced because he resembles someone who was "worthwhile" cloning, he will be the object of no less fateful expectations and attention, which will constitute a true and proper attack on his personal subjectivity.

If the human cloning project intends to stop "before" implantation in the womb, trying to avoid at least some of the consequences we have just indicated, it appears equally unjust from the moral standpoint.

A prohibition of cloning which would be limited to preventing the birth of a cloned child, but which would still permit the cloning of an embryo-fetus would involve experimentation on embryos and fetuses and would require their suppression before birth—a cruel, exploitative way of treating human beings.

In any case, such experimentation is immoral because it involves the arbitrary use of the human body (by now decidedly regarded as a machine composed of parts) as a mere research tool. The human body is an integral part of every individual's dignity and personal identity, and it is not permissible to use women as a source of ova for conducting cloning experiments.

It is immoral because even in the case of a clone, we are in the presence of a "man," although in the embryonic stage.

All the moral reasons which led to the condemnation of in vitro fertilization as such and to the radical censure of in vitro fertilization for merely experimental purposes must also be applied to human cloning.

The "human cloning" project represents the terrible aberration to which value-free science is driven and is a sign of the profound malaise of our civilization, which looks to science, technology and the "quality of life" as surrogates for the meaning of life and its salvation.

The proclamation of the "death of God," in the vain hope of a "superman," produces an unmistakable result: the "death of man." It cannot be forgotten that the denial of man's creaturely status, far from exalting human freedom, in fact creates new forms of slavery, discrimination, and profound suffering. Cloning risks being the tragic parody of God's omnipotence. Man, to whom God has entrusted the created world, giving him freedom and intelligence, finds no limits to his action dictated solely by practical impossibility. He himself must learn how to set these limits by discerning good and evil. Once again man is asked to choose. It is his responsibility to decide whether to transform technology into a tool of liberation or to become its slave by introducing new forms of violence and suffering.

The difference should again be pointed out between the conception of life as a gift of love and the view of the human being as an industrial product.

Halting the human cloning project is a moral duty which must also be translated into cultural, social, and legislative terms. The progress of scientific research is not the same as the rise of scientistic despotism, which today seems to be replacing the old ideologies. In a democratic, pluralistic system, the first guarantee of each individual's freedom is established by unconditionally respecting human dignity at every phase of life, regardless of the intellectual or physical abilities one possesses or is deprived. In human cloning the necessary condition for any society begins to collapse: that of treating man always and everywhere as an end, as a value and never as a mere means or simple object.

Human Rights and Freedom of Research

At the level of human rights, the possibility of human cloning represents a violation of the two fundamental principles on which all human rights are based: the principle of equality among human beings and the principle of nondiscrimination.

Contrary to what may appear at first sight, the principle of parity and equality among human beings is violated by this possible form of man's domination over man, and the discrimination comes about through the whole selective-eugenic dimension inherent in the logic of cloning. The resolution of the European Parliament (March 12, 1997) expressly states the violation of these two principles and forcefully appeals for the prohibition of human cloning and for the value of the dignity of the human person. Since 1983 the European Parliament and all the laws passed to legalize artificial procreation, even the most permissive, have always forbidden human cloning. It should be recalled that the Church's Magisterium has condemned the possibility of human cloning, twin fission, and parthenogenesis in the 1987 instruction *Donum Vitae*. The basic reasons for the inhuman nature of possible human cloning are not because it is an extreme form of artificial procreation in comparison to other legally approved forms such as in vitro fertilization, etc.

178   As we have said, the reason for its rejection is that it denies the dignity of the person subjected to cloning and the dignity of human procreation.

The most urgent need now seems to be that of re-establishing the harmony between the demands of scientific research and indispensable human values. The scientist cannot regard the moral rejection of human cloning as a humiliation; on the contrary, this prohibition eliminates the demiurgic degeneration of research by restoring its dignity. The dignity of scientific research consists in the fact that it is one of the richest resources for humanity's welfare.

Moreover, there is a place for research, including cloning, in the vegetable and animal kingdoms, wherever it answers a need or provides a significant benefit for man or for other living beings, provided that the rules for protecting the animal itself and the obligation to respect the biodiversity of species are observed.

When scientific research in man's interest aims to cure diseases, to relieve suffering, to solve problems due to malnutrition, to make better use of the earth's resources, it represents a hope for humanity, entrusted to the talent and efforts of scientists.

To enable biomedical science to maintain and strengthen its relationship with the welfare of man and society, it is necessary to foster, as the Holy Father recalls in the encyclical *Evangelium Vitae*, a "contemplative outlook" on man himself and the world, with a vision of reality as God's creation and in a context of solidarity between science, the good of the person and of society.

"It is the outlook of those who see life in its deeper meaning who grasp its utter gratuitousness, its beauty, and its invitation to freedom and responsibility. It is the outlook of those who do not presume to take possession of reality, but instead accept it as a gift, discovering in all things the reflection of the Creator and seeing in every person his living image" (*Evangelium Vitae*, 83).

24: Handicapped

DOCUMENT 1:

Source: United States Catholic Conference, "Pastoral Statement of the United States Catholic Bishops on Handicapped People" (Nov. 15, 1978), *Pastoral Letters of the United States Catholic Bishops*, Vol. IV, pp. 267–70.

1. The same Jesus who heard the cry for recognition from the handicapped of Judea and Samaria two thousand years ago calls us, his followers, to embrace our responsibility to our own handicapped brothers and sisters in the United States. . . .

2. Prejudice starts with the simple perception of difference, whether that difference is physical or psychological. Down through the ages, people have tended to interpret these differences in crude moral terms. "Our" group is not just different from "theirs"; it is better in some vague but compelling way. Few of us would admit to being prejudiced against handicapped people. We bear these people no ill will and do not knowingly seek to abrogate their rights. Yet handicapped individuals are visibly, sometimes bluntly different from the "norm," and we react to this difference. Even if we do not look down upon handicapped people, we tend all too often to think of them as somehow apart— not completely "one of us."

3. What handicapped individuals need, first of all, is acceptance in this difference that can neither be denied nor overlooked. No acts of charity or justice can be of lasting value to handicapped people unless they are informed by a sincere and understanding love that penetrates the wall of strangeness and affirms the common humanity underlying all distinction. Scripture teaches us that "any other commandment there may be [is] all summed up in this: 'You shall love your neighbor as yourself.'" In his wisdom, Jesus said, "as yourself." We must love others from the inside out, so to speak, accepting their difference from us in the same way that we accept our difference from them. . . .

THE CHURCH'S RESPONSE TO THE HANDICAPPED PERSON

7. On the most basic level, the Church responds to handicapped individuals by defending their rights. The first of these, of course, is the right to life. . . .

10. Defense of the right to life, then, implies the defense of other rights which enable the handicapped individual to achieve the fullest measure of personal development of which he or she is capable. . . .

11. It is not enough merely to affirm the rights of handicapped people. We must actively work to make them real in the fabric of modern society. Recognizing that handicapped individuals have a claim to our respect because

180   they share in the one redemption of Christ, and because they contribute to our society by their activity within it, the Church must become an advocate for and with them. It must work to increase the public's sensitivity toward the needs of handicapped people and support their rightful demand for justice. Moreover, individuals and organizations at every level within the Church should minister to handicapped persons by serving their personal and social needs. Many handicapped persons can function on their own as well as anyone in society. For others, aid would be welcome. All of us can visit the homebound, offer transportation to those who cannot drive, read to those who cannot read, speak out for those who have difficulty pleading their own case. . . .

25: Health Care Reform

DOCUMENT 1:

SOURCE: National Conference of Catholic Bishops, "Resolution on Health Care Reform" (June 18, 1993), *Origins* 23: no. 7 (July 1, 1993), pp. 99–100.

... Our approach to health care is shaped by a single, but fundamental principle: "Every person has a right to adequate health care. This right flows from the sanctity of human life and the dignity that belongs to all human persons, who are made in the image of God." Health care is more than a commodity; it is a basic human right, an essential safeguard of human life and dignity. We believe our people's health care should not depend on where they work, how much their parents earn or where they live. Our constant teaching that each human life must be protected and human dignity promoted leads us to insist that all people have a right to health care. This right is explicitly affirmed in *Pacem in Terris* and is the foundation of our advocacy for health care reform. When millions of Americans are without health coverage. When rising costs threaten the coverage of millions more, when infant mortality remains shockingly high, the right to health care is seriously undermined and our health care system is in need of fundamental reform.

... Applying our experience and principles to the choices before the nation, our bishops' conference strongly supports comprehensive reform that will ensure a decent level of health care for all without regard to their ability to pay. This will require concerted action by federal and other levels of government and by the diverse providers and consumers of health care. We believe government, an instrument of our common purpose called to pursue the common good, has an essential role to play in assuring that the rights of all people to adequate health care are respected.

We believe reform of the health care system which is truly fundamental and enduring must be rooted in values which reflect the essential dignity of each person, ensure that basic human rights are protected, and recognize the unique needs and claims of the poor. We commend to the leaders of our nation the following criteria for reform:

—*Respect for Life.* Whether it preserves and enhances the sanctity and dignity of human life from conception to natural death.

—*Priority Concern for the Poor.* Whether it gives special priority to meeting the most pressing health care needs of the poor and underserved, ensuring that they receive quality health services.

—*Universal Access.* Whether it provides ready universal access to comprehensive health care for every person living in the United States.

182   —*Comprehensive Benefits.* Whether it provides comprehensive benefits sufficient to maintain and promote good health, to provide preventive care, to treat disease, injury, and disability appropriately and to care for persons who are chronically ill or dying.

—*Pluralism.* Whether it allows and encourages the involvement of the public and private sectors, including the voluntary, religious, and non-profit sectors, in the delivery of care and services; and whether it ensures respect for religious and ethical values in the delivery of health care for consumers and for individual and institutional providers.

—*Quality.* Whether it promotes the development of processes and standards that will help to achieve quality and equity in health services, in the training of providers, and in the informed participation of consumers in decision making on health care.

—*Cost Containment and Controls.* Whether it creates effective cost containment measures that reduce waste, inefficiency, and unnecessary care; measures that control rising costs of competition, commercialism, and administration; and measures that provide incentives to individuals and providers for effective and economical use of limited resources.

—*Equitable Financing.* Whether it ensures society's obligation to finance universal access to comprehensive health care in an equitable fashion, based on ability to pay; and whether proposed cost-sharing arrangements are designed to avoid creating barriers to effective care for the poor and vulnerable.

DOCUMENT 2 / Health Care Reform

SOURCE: United States Catholic Conference, "Criteria for Evaluating Health Care Reform,"*Origins* 22: no. 2 (May 21, 1992), pp. 23–24.

Health care is not a new concern for the Catholic community. The Church has been involved in the delivery of health care services since the early days of this nation. Those early services have grown to make Catholic-sponsored health care facilities the largest network of non-profit hospitals and nursing homes in the United States, serving about 40 million Americans in a single year. In our parishes and schools, our shelters and clinics, we see the consequences of failed and confused policy—the families without insurance, the sick without options, the children without care.

Health care reform is not a new issue for the U.S. bishops' conference. In our 1981 pastoral letter "Health and Health Care," the bishops called for an adequately funded national health insurance program for all Americans:

"Following on these principles and on our belief in health care as a basic human right, we call for the development of a national health insurance program. It is the responsibility of the federal government to establish a comprehensive health care system that will ensure a basic level of health care for all Americans. The federal government should also ensure adequate funding for this basic level of care through a national health insurance program."

This public policy position is not based in some political theory, but is rooted deeply in the Judeo-Christian belief that every human person is made in the image of God (cf. Gn 1:27). As such, every person possesses an inherent dignity that must be deeply respected, and every person has the right and the responsibility to realize the fullness of that dignity.

Human life and human dignity also give rise to basic human rights, among which is the right to health care. The bishops explained in our 1981 pastoral letter:

"Every person has a basic right to adequate health care. This right flows from the sanctity of human life and the dignity that belongs to all human persons, who are made in the image of God. It implies that access to that health care which is necessary and suitable for the proper development and maintenance of life must be provided for all people, regardless of economic, social, or legal status."

In circumstances where more than 30 million Americans are without health coverage, where rising costs threaten the coverage of tens of millions more, where infant mortality remains shockingly high, and where millions of children are without basic health care, the right to health care and the responsibilities of society to ensure that care are in serious disarray.

How society is organized—in economics, politics, and health care—directly enhances or assaults human life and human dignity. When the health

184 care system leaves so many people uncared for—affecting human life itself—then this system is in need of serious and comprehensive reform.

We also bring to the question of health care reform a special concern for the poor and vulnerable, rooted in the proclamations of the Hebrew prophets, in the Gospel of Jesus of Nazareth, and in the teaching of our Church. It is the poor who suffer most acutely from the faults and failings of the health care system. It is their pain and suffering, their poor health and sickness, that sharpens our resolve to join in the call for genuine reform now.

APPLICATIONS

Applying our experience and policy to the current debate, the USCC supports national health care reform which will establish a comprehensive health care system that will ensure a decent level of health care for all Americans without regard to their ability to pay.

This will require strong steps that, in combination, address the questions of universal coverage, cost containment, and quality assurance. This will also require concerted action by federal and other levels of government and by providers and consumers of health care.

More specifically, we will use the following basic criteria in evaluating the strengths and weaknesses of proposals concerning health care reform:

1. Universal Access: whether it provides ready universal access to comprehensive health care for every person living in the United States;

2. Priority Concern for the Poor: whether it gives special priority to meeting the most pressing health care needs of the poor and underserved, ensuring that they receive quality health services;

3. Respect for Life: whether it preserves and enhances the sanctity and dignity of human life from its beginning to its end;

4. Comprehensive Benefits: whether it provides comprehensive benefits sufficient to maintain and promote good health, to treat disease, injury, and disability appropriately, and to care for persons who are chronically ill or dying; and whether it ensures government's responsibility for the public health of the population;

5. Pluralism: whether it allows and encourages the involvement of the public and private sectors, including the voluntary, religious, and non-profit sectors, in the delivery of care and services; and whether it ensures respect for religious and ethical values in the delivery of health care for consumers and for individual and institutional providers;

6. Equitable Financing: whether it ensures society's obligation to finance universal access to comprehensive health care in an equitable fashion, based on ability to pay; and whether proposed cost-sharing arrangements are designed to avoid creating barriers to effective care for the poor and vulnerable;

7. Cost Containment and Controls: whether it creates effective cost-containment measures that reduce waste, inefficiency, and unnecessary care, that control rising costs of competition, commercialism, and administration, and that provide incentives to individuals and providers for effective and economical use of limited resources;

8. Quality: whether it promotes the development of processes and standards that will help to achieve equity in the range and quality of services, in the training of providers, and in the informed participation of consumers in individual and societal decision making on health care.

On this basis, we are prepared to continue to work for reform of the U.S. health care system. In our view, the best measure of proposed health care initiatives is the extent to which they can combine universal access to quality health care with cost control, while ensuring quality care for the poor and preserving human life and dignity. In short we seek national health care reform founded on respect for human life and human dignity, that ensures quality and affordable health care for all Americans. We look forward to working with others in shaping policy which achieves these goals.

We hope our national leaders will look beyond political and ideological differences and the pleadings of the many and diverse interest groups in health care to fashion a comprehensive response which unites our nation in a new commitment to serve the common good by effectively meeting the health care needs of our people, especially the poor and vulnerable. This is a major political task, a significant policy challenge, and a moral imperative.

We look forward to working with you to achieve comprehensive national health care reform this year.

26: Health Care Administration

DOCUMENT 1:

Source: Pope John Paul II, "Health Care: Ministry in Transition" (Sept. 14, 1987), *Origins* 17: no. 17, Oct. 8, 1987, pp. 292–94.

. . . This is the high dignity to which you and your colleagues are called. This is your vocation, your commitment, and the path of your specific witness to the presence of God's kingdom in the world. Your health care ministry, pioneered and developed by congregations of women religious and by congregations of brothers, is one of the most vital apostolates of the ecclesial community and one of the most significant services which the Catholic Church offers to society in the name of Jesus Christ. . . .

2. Because of your dedication to caring for the sick and the poor, the aged and the dying, you know from your own daily experience how much illness and suffering are basic problems of human existence. When the sick flocked to Jesus during his earthly life, they recognized in him a friend whose deeply compassionate and loving heart responded to their needs. He restored physical and mental health to many. These cures, however, involved more than just healing sickness. They were also prophetic signs of his own identity and of the coming of the kingdom of God, and they very often caused a new spiritual awakening in the one who had been healed.

The power that went out from Jesus and cured people of his own time (cf. Lk 6:19) has not lost its effect in the 2,000-year history of the Church. This power remains, in the life and prayer of the Church, a source of healing and reconciliation. Ever active, this power confirms the identity of the Church today, authenticates her proclamation of the Kingdom of God, and stands as a sign of triumph over evil.

With all Catholic health care, the immediate aim is to provide for the well-being of the body and mind of the human person, especially in sickness or old age. By his example, Christ teaches the Christian "to do good by his or her suffering and to do good to those who suffer" (John Paul II, Apostolic Exhortation *On Human Suffering*, 30). This latter aspect naturally absorbs the greater part of the energy and attention of health care ministry.

Today in the United States, Catholic health care extends the mission of the Church in every state of the union, in major cities, small towns, rural areas, on the campuses of academic institutions, in remote outposts, and in inner-city neighborhoods. By providing health care in all these places, especially to the poor, the neglected, the needy, the newcomer, your apostolate penetrates and transforms the very fabric of American society. And sometimes you your-

selves, like those you serve, are called to bow, in humble and loving resignation, **187**
to the experience of sickness—or to other forms of pain and suffering.

3. All concern for the sick and suffering is part of the Church's life and
mission. The Church has always understood herself to be charged by Christ
with the care of the poor, the weak, the defenseless, the suffering, and those
who mourn. This means that as you alleviate suffering and seek to heal you
also bear witness to the Christian view of suffering and to the meaning of life
and death as taught by your Christian faith.

In the complex world of modern health care in industrialized society, this
witness must be given in a variety of ways. First, it requires continual efforts
to ensure that everyone has access to health care. I know that you have already
examined this question in the report of your task force on health care of the
poor. In seeking to treat patients equally, regardless of social and economic
status, you proclaim to your fellow citizens and to the world Christ's special
love for the neglected and powerless. This particular challenge is a consequence
of your Christian dedication and conviction, and it calls for great courage on
the part of Catholic bodies and institutions operating in the field of health care.
It is a great credit to your zeal and efficiency when, despite formidable costs,
you still succeed in preventing the economic factor from being the determinant
factor in human and Christian service.

Similarly, the love with which Catholic health care is performed and its
professional excellence have the value of a sign testifying to the Christian view
of the human person. The inalienable dignity of every human being is, of
course, fundamental to all Catholic health care. All who come to you for help
are worthy of respect and love, for all have been created in the image and
likeness of God. All have been redeemed by Christ and, in their sufferings,
bear his cross. It is fitting that our meeting is taking place on the feast of the
Triumph of the Cross. Christ took upon himself the whole of human suffering
and radically transformed it through the paschal mystery of his passion, death,
and resurrection. The triumph of the cross gives human suffering a new dimension, a redemptive value (cf. ibid., 24). It is your privilege to bear constant
witness to this profound truth in so many ways.

The structural changes which have been taking place within Catholic
health care in recent years have increased the challenge of preserving and even
strengthening the Catholic identity of the institutions and the spiritual quality
of the services given. The presence of dedicated women and men religious in
hospitals and nursing homes has ensured in the past, and continues to ensure
in the present, that spiritual dimension so characteristic of Catholic health care
centers. The reduced number of religious and new forms of ownership and
management should not lead to a loss of a spiritual atmosphere or to a loss of
a sense of vocation in caring for the sick. This is an area in which the Catholic
laity, at all levels of health care, have an opportunity to manifest the depth of
their faith and to play their own specific part in the Church's mission of
evangelization and service.

4. As I have said, Catholic health care must always be carried out within
the framework of the Church's saving mission. This mission she has received

188 from her divine founder, and she has accomplished it down through the ages with the help of the Holy Spirit, who guides her into the fullness of truth (cf. Jn 16:13; Dogmatic Constitution on the Church, 4). Your ministry therefore must also reflect the mission of the Church as the teacher of moral truth, especially in regard to the new frontiers of scientific research and technological achievement. Here too you face great challenges and opportunities.

Many times in recent years the Church has addressed issues related to the advances of biomedical technology. She does so not in order to discourage scientific progress or to judge harshly those who seek to extend the frontiers of human knowledge and skill, but in order to affirm the moral truths which must guide the application of this knowledge and skill. Ultimately, the purpose of the Church's teaching in this field is to defend the innate dignity and fundamental rights of the human person. In this regard the Church cannot fail to emphasize the need to safeguard the life and integrity of the human embryo and fetus.

5. The human person is a unique composite—a unity of spirit and matter, soul and body, fashioned in the image of God and destined to live forever. Every human life is sacred, because every human person is sacred. It is in the light of this fundamental truth that the Church constantly proclaims and defends the dignity of human life from the moment of conception to the moment of natural death. It is also in the light of this fundamental truth that we see the great evil of abortion and euthanasia. . . .

6. In the exercise of your professional activities you have a magnificent opportunity, by your constant witness to moral truth, to contribute to the formation of society's moral vision. As you give the best of yourselves in fulfilling your Christian responsibilities, you will also be aware of the important contribution you must make to building a society based on truth and justice. Your service to the sick enables you with great credibility to proclaim to the world the demands and values of the Gospel of Jesus Christ, and to foster hope and renewal of heart. In this respect, your concern with the Catholic identity of your work and your institutions is not only timely and commendable, it is essential for the success of your ecclesial mission.

You must always see yourselves and your work as part of the Church's life and mission. You are indeed a very special part of the people of God. You and your institutions have precise responsibilities toward the ecclesial community, just as that community has responsibilities toward you. It is important at every level—national, state, and local—that there be close and harmonious links between you and the bishops, who "preside in place of God over the flock whose shepherds they are, as teachers of doctrine, priests of sacred worship, and officers of good order" (Dogmatic Constitution on the Church, 20). They, for their part, wish to support you in your witness and service.

. . . Today you are faced with new challenges, new needs. One of these is the present crisis of immense proportions which is that of AIDS and AIDS-related complex. Besides your professional contribution and your human sensitivities toward all affected by this disease, you are called to show the love and compassion of Christ and his Church. As you courageously affirm and

implement your moral obligation and social responsibility to help those who   **189**
suffer, you are individually and collectively living out the parable of the good
Samaritan (cf. Lk 10:30–32).

The good Samaritan of the parable showed compassion to the injured
man. By taking him to the inn and giving of his own material means, he truly
gave of himself. This action, a universal symbol of human concern, has become
one of the essential elements of moral culture and civilization. How beautifully
the Lord speaks of the Samaritan! He "was neighbor to the man who fell in
with the robbers" (Lk 10:36). To be "neighbor" is to express love, solidarity, and
service, and to exclude selfishness, discrimination, and neglect. The message of
the parable of the good Samaritan echoes a reality connected with today's feast
of the Triumph of the Cross: "The kindness and love of God our Savior appeared
. . . that we might be justified by his grace and become heirs, in hope, of eternal
life" (Ti 3:4–7). In the changing world of health care, it is up to you to ensure
that this "kindness and love of God our Savior" remains the heart and soul of
Catholic health services. . . .

27: Homosexuality

DOCUMENT 1:

SOURCE: Congregation for the Doctrine of the Faith, "The Pastoral Care of Homosexual Persons" (Oct. 30, 1986), *Origins* 16: no. 22, Nov. 13, 1986, pp. 377, 379–81.

. . . The Catholic moral viewpoint is founded on human reason illumined by faith and is consciously motivated by the desire to do the will of God, our Father. The Church is thus in a position to learn from scientific discovery but also to transcend the horizons of science and to be confident that her more global vision does greater justice to the rich reality of the human person in his spiritual and physical dimensions created by God and heir, by grace, to eternal life. . . .

4. An essential dimension of authentic pastoral care is the identification of causes of confusion regarding the Church's teaching. One is a new exegesis of Sacred Scripture which claims variously that Scripture has nothing to say on the subject of homosexuality or that it somehow tacitly approves of it or that all of its moral injunctions are so culture-bound that they are no longer applicable to contemporary life. These views are gravely erroneous and call for particular attention here.

5. It is quite true that the biblical literature owes to the different epochs in which it was written a good deal of its varied patterns of thought and expression (*Dei Verbum*, 12). The Church today addresses the Gospel to a world which differs in many ways from ancient days. But the world in which the New Testament was written was already quite diverse from the situation in which the Sacred Scriptures of the Hebrew people had been written or compiled, for example.

What should be noticed is that in the presence of such remarkable diversity there is nevertheless a clear consistency within the Scriptures themselves on the moral issue of homosexual behavior. The Church's doctrine regarding this issue is thus based not on isolated phrases for facile theological argument, but on the solid foundation of a constant biblical testimony. The community of faith today, in unbroken continuity with the Jewish and Christian communities within which the ancient Scriptures were written, continues to be nourished by those same Scriptures and by the Spirit of truth whose word they are. It is likewise essential to recognize that the Scriptures are not properly understood when they are interpreted in a way which contradicts the Church's living tradition. To be correct, the interpretation of Scripture must be in substantial accord with that tradition.

Vatican Council II in *Dei Verbum*, no. 10, put it this way: "It is clear, **191** therefore, that in the supremely wise arrangement of God, sacred tradition, Sacred Scripture, and the Magisterium of the Church are so connected and associated that one of them cannot stand without the others. Working together, each in its own way under the action of the one Holy Spirit, they all contribute effectively to the salvation of souls." In that spirit we wish to outline briefly the biblical teaching here.

6. Providing a basic plan for understanding this entire discussion of homosexuality is the theology of creation we find in Genesis. God, by his infinite wisdom and love, brings into existence all of reality as a reflection of his goodness. He fashions mankind, male and female, in his own image and likeness. Human beings, therefore, are nothing less than the work of God himself, and in the complementarity of the sexes they are called to reflect the inner unity of the Creator. They do this in a striking way in their cooperation with him in the transmission of life by a mutual donation of the self to the other.

In Genesis 3, we find that this truth about persons being an image of God has been obscured by original sin. There inevitably follows a loss of awareness of the convenantal character of the union these persons had with God and with each other. The human body retains "spousal significance," but this is now clouded by sin. Thus, in Genesis 19:1–11, the deterioration due to sin continued in the story of the men of Sodom. There can be no doubt of the moral judgment made there against homosexual relations. In Leviticus 18:22 and 20:13, in the course of describing the conditions necessary for belonging to the chosen people, the author excludes from the people of God those who behave in a homosexual fashion.

Against the background of this exposition of theocratic law, an eschatological perspective is developed by St. Paul when, in 1 Corinthians 6:9, he proposes the same doctrine and lists those who behave in a homosexual fashion among those who shall not enter the kingdom of God.

In Romans 1:18–32, still building on the moral traditions of his forebears but in the new context of the confrontation between Christianity and the pagan society of his day, Paul uses homosexual behavior as an example of the blindness which has overcome humankind. Instead of the original harmony between Creator and creatures, the acute distortion of idolatry has led to all kinds of moral excess. Paul is at a loss to find a clearer example of this disharmony than homosexual relations. Finally, 1 Timothy 1, in full continuity with the biblical position, singles out those who spread wrong doctrine and in verse 10 explicitly names as sinners those who engage in homosexual acts.

7. The Church, obedient to the Lord who founded her and gave to her the sacramental life, celebrates the divine plan of the loving and life-giving union of men and women in the sacrament of marriage. It is only in the marital relationship that the use of the sexual faculty can be morally good. A person engaging in homosexual behavior therefore acts immorally.

To choose someone of the same sex for one's sexual activity is to annul the rich symbolism and meaning, not to mention the goals, of the Creator's sexual design. Homosexual activity is not a complementary union able to

192   transmit life; and so it thwarts the call to a life of that form of self-giving which the Gospel says is the essence of Christian living. This does not mean that homosexual persons are not often generous and giving of themselves; but when they engage in homosexual activity they confirm within themselves a disordered sexual inclination which is essentially self-indulgent.

As in every moral disorder, homosexual activity prevents one's own fulfillment and happiness by acting contrary to the creative wisdom of God. The Church, in rejecting erroneous opinions regarding homosexuality, does not limit but rather defends personal freedom and dignity realistically and authentically understood.

8. Thus, the Church's teaching today is in organic continuity with the scriptural perspective and with her own constant tradition. Though today's world is in many ways quite new, the Christian community senses the profound and lasting bonds which join us to those generations who have gone before us, "marked with the sign of faith."

Nevertheless, increasing numbers of people today, even within the Church, are bringing enormous pressure to bear on the Church to accept the homosexual condition as though it were not disordered and to condone homosexual activity. Those within the Church who argue in this fashion often have close ties with those with similar views outside it. These latter groups are guided by a vision opposed to the truth about the human person, which is fully disclosed in the mystery of Christ. They reflect, even if not entirely consciously, a materialistic ideology which denies the transcendent nature of the human person as well as the supernatural vocation of every individual. . . .

10. It is deplorable that homosexual persons have been and are the object of violent malice in speech or in action. Such treatment deserves condemnation from the Church's pastors wherever it occurs. It reveals a kind of disregard for others which endangers the most fundamental principles of a healthy society. The intrinsic dignity of each person must always be respected in word, in action, and in law. . . .

11. It has been argued that the homosexual orientation in certain cases is not the result of deliberate choice; and so the homosexual person would then have no choice but to behave in a homosexual fashion. Lacking freedom, such a person, even if engaged in homosexual activity, would not be culpable.

Here, the Church's wise moral tradition is necessary since it warns against generalizations in judging individual cases. In fact, circumstances may exist or may have existed in the past which would reduce or remove the culpability of the individual in a given instance; or other circumstances may increase it. What is at all costs to be avoided is the unfounded and demeaning assumption that the sexual behavior of homosexual persons is always and totally compulsive and therefore inculpable. What is essential is that the fundamental liberty which characterizes the human person and gives him his dignity be recognized as belonging to the homosexual person as well. As in every conversion from evil, the abandonment of homosexual activity will require a profound collaboration of the individual with God's liberating grace. . . .

DOCUMENT 2 / Homosexuality

SOURCE: Congregation for the Doctrine of the Faith, "Declaration on Certain Problems of Sexual Ethics" (Dec. 29, 1975), *Vatican Council II*, Vol. 2, 1982, pp. 490–91.

8. In our day there are those who, relying on the findings of psychology, have begun to judge homosexual relationships indulgently and even to excuse them completely. This goes against the constant teaching of the Magisterium and the moral sense of the Christian people.

They draw a distinction, not without reason, between two kinds of homosexuals. The first kind consists of homosexuals whose condition is temporary or at least is not incurable. It can be due to a faulty education, a lack of normal sexual development, to habit or bad example, or other similar causes. The second type consists of homosexuals whose condition is permanent and who are such because of some kind of innate impulse or because of a constitutional defect presumed to be incurable.

Many argue that the condition of the second type of homosexual is so natural that it justifies homosexual relations for them, in the context of a genuine partnership in life and love analogous to marriage, and granted that they feel quite incapable of leading solitary lives.

Certainly, pastoral care of such homosexuals should be considerate and kind. The hope should be instilled in them of one day overcoming their difficulties and their alienation from society. Their culpability will be judged prudently. However, it is not permissible to employ any pastoral method or theory to provide moral justification for their actions, on the grounds that they are in keeping with their condition. Sexual relations between persons of the same sex are necessarily and essentially disordered according to the objective moral order. Sacred Scripture condemns them as gravely depraved and even portrays them as the tragic consequence of rejecting God. Of course, the judgment of Sacred Scripture does not imply that all who suffer from this deformity are by that very fact guilty of personal fault. But it does show that homosexual acts are intrinsically disordered and may never be approved in any way whatever.

DOCUMENT 3 / Homosexuality

SOURCE: Congregation for the Doctrine of the Faith, "Responding to Legislative Proposals on Discrimination Against Homosexuals" (July 23, 1992), *Origins* 22: no. 10 (Aug. 6, 1992), pp. 174–177.

Recently, legislation has been proposed in various places which would make discrimination on the basis of sexual orientation illegal. In some cities, municipal authorities have made public housing, otherwise reserved for families, available to homosexual (and unmarried heterosexual) couples. Such initiatives, even where they seem more directed toward support of basic civil rights than condonement of homosexual activity or a homosexual lifestyle, may in fact have a negative impact on the family and society. Such things as the adoption of children, the employment of teachers, the housing needs of genuine families, landlords' legitimate concerns in screening potential tenants, for example, are often implicated.

While it would be impossible to anticipate every eventuality in respect to legislative proposals in this area, these observations will try to identify some principles and distinctions of a general nature which should be taken into consideration by the conscientious legislator, voter, or Church authority who is confronted with such issues.

The first section will recall relevant passages from the Congregation for the Doctrine of the Faith's "Letter to the Bishops of the Catholic Church on the Pastoral Care of Homosexual Persons" of 1986. The second section will deal with their application.

I. Relevant Passages from the CDF's "Letter"

1. The letter recalls that the CDF's "Declaration on Certain Questions Concerning Sexual Ethics" of 1975 "took note of the distinction commonly drawn between the homosexual condition or tendency and individual homosexual actions"; the latter are "intrinsically disordered" and "in no case to be approved of" (no. 3).

2. Since "in the discussion which followed the publication of the (aforementioned) declaration . . . an overly benign interpretation was given to the homosexual condition itself, some going so far as to call it neutral or even good," the letter goes on to clarify:

"Although the particular inclination of the homosexual person is not a sin, it is a more or less strong tendency ordered toward an intrinsic moral evil; and thus the inclination itself must be seen as an objective disorder. Therefore special concern and pastoral attention should be directed toward those who have this condition, lest they be led to believe that the living out of this orientation in homosexual activity is a morally acceptable option. It is not" (no. 3).

3. "As in every moral disorder, homosexual activity prevents one's own fulfillment and happiness by acting contrary to the creative wisdom of God. The Church, in rejecting erroneous opinions regarding homosexuality, does not limit but rather defends personal freedom and dignity realistically and authentically understood" (no. 7).

4. In reference to the homosexual movement, the letter states: "One tactic used is to protest that any and all criticism of or reservations about homosexual people, their activity and lifestyle are simply diverse forms of unjust discrimination" (no. 9).

5. "There is an effort in some countries to manipulate the Church by gaining the often well-intentioned support of her pastors with a view to changing civil statutes and laws. This is done in order to conform to these pressure groups' concept that homosexuality is at least a completely harmless, if not an entirely good, thing. Even when the practice of homosexuality may seriously threaten the lives and well-being of a large number of people, its advocates remain undeterred and refuse to consider the magnitude of the risks involved" (no. 9).

6. "She (the Church) is also aware that the view that homosexual activity is equivalent to or as acceptable as the sexual expression of conjugal love has a direct impact on society's understanding of the nature and rights of the family and puts them in jeopardy" (no. 9).

7. "It is deplorable that homosexual persons have been and are the object of violent malice in speech or in action. Such treatment deserves condemnation from the Church's pastors wherever it occurs. It reveals a kind of disregard for others which endangers the most fundamental principles of a healthy society. The intrinsic dignity of each person must always be respected in word, in action, and in law.

"But the proper reaction to crimes committed against homosexual persons should not be to claim that the homosexual condition is not disordered. When such a claim is made and when sexual activity is consequently condoned, or when civil legislation is introduced to protect behavior to which no one has any conceivable right, neither the Church nor society at large should be surprised when other distorted notions and practices gain ground, and irrational and violent reactions increase" (no. 10).

8. "What is at all costs to be avoided is the unfounded and demeaning assumption that the sexual behavior of homosexual persons is always totally compulsive and therefore inculpable. What is essential is that the fundamental liberty which characterizes the human person and gives him his dignity be recognized as belonging to the homosexual person as well" (no. 11).

9. "In assessing proposed legislation, the bishops should keep as their uppermost concern the responsibility to defend and promote family life" (no. 17).

Applications

10. "Sexual orientation" does not constitute a quality comparable to race, ethnic background, etc., in respect to non-discrimination. Unlike these,

196 homosexual orientation is an objective disorder (cf. "Letter," no. 3) and evokes moral concern.

11. There are areas in which it is not unjust discrimination to take sexual orientation into account, for example, in the placement of children for adoption or foster care, in employment of teachers or athletic coaches, and in military recruitment.

12. Homosexual persons, as human persons, have the same rights as all persons, including the right of not being treated in a manner that offends their personal dignity (cf. no. 10). Among other rights, all persons have the right to work, to housing, etc. Nevertheless, these rights are not absolute. They can be legitimately limited for objectively disordered external conduct. This is sometimes not only licit but obligatory. This would obtain moreover not only in the case of culpable behavior but even in the case of actions of the physically or mentally ill. Thus it is accepted that the state may restrict the exercise of rights, for example, in the case of contagious or mentally ill persons, in order to protect the common good.

13. Including "homosexual orientation" among the considerations on the basis of which it is illegal to discriminate can easily lead to regarding homosexuality as a positive source of human rights, for example, in respect to so-called affirmative action or preferential treatment in hiring practices. This is all the more deleterious since there is no right to homosexuality (cf. no. 10), which therefore should not form the basis for judicial claims. The passage from the recognition of homosexuality as a factor on which basis it is illegal to discriminate can easily lead, if not automatically, to the legislative protection and promotion of homosexuality. A person's homosexuality would be invoked in opposition to alleged discrimination, and thus the exercise of rights would be defended precisely via the affirmation of the homosexual condition instead of in terms of a violation of basic human rights.

14. The "sexual orientation" of a person is not comparable to race, sex, age, etc. also for another reason than that given above which warrants attention. An individual's sexual orientation is generally not known to others unless he publicly identifies himself as having this orientation or unless some overt behavior manifests it. As a rule, the majority of homosexually oriented persons who seek to lead chaste lives do not publicize their sexual orientation. Hence the problem of discrimination in terms of employment, housing, etc. does not usually arise.

Homosexual persons who assert their homosexuality tend to be precisely those who judge homosexual behavior or lifestyle to be "either completely harmless, if not an entirely good thing" (no. 3), and hence worthy of public approval. It is from this quarter that one is more likely to find those who seek to "manipulate the Church by gaining the often well-intentioned support of her pastors with a view to changing civil statutes and laws" (no. 5), those who use the tactic of protesting that "any and all criticism of or reservations about homosexual people . . . are simply diverse forms of unjust discrimination" (no. 9).

In addition, there is a danger that legislation which would make homosex- **197** uality a basis for entitlement could actually encourage a person with a homosexual orientation to declare his homosexuality or even to seek a partner in order to exploit the provisions of the law.

15. Since in the assessment of proposed legislation uppermost concern should be given to the responsibility to defend and promote family life (cf. no. 17), strict attention should be paid to the single provisions of proposed measures. How would they affect adoption or foster care? Would they protect homosexual acts, public or private? Do they confer equivalent family status on homosexual unions, for example, in respect to public housing or by entitling the homosexual partner to the privileges of employments, which could include such things as 'family" participation in the health benefits given to employees.

Finally, where a matter of the common good is concerned, it is inappropriate for Church authorities to endorse or remain neutral toward adverse legislation even if it grants exceptions to Church organizations and institutions. The Church has the responsibility to promote family life and the public morality of the entire civil society on the basis of fundamental moral values, not simply to protect herself from the application of harmful laws.

DOCUMENT 4 / Homosexuality

SOURCE: Cardinal George Basil Hume, "Note on Church Teaching Concerning Homosexual People," *Origins* 24: no. 45 (Apr. 27, 1995), pp. 767–68.

PRINCIPLES

Dignity of the Human Person

The Church recognizes the dignity of all people and does not define or label them in terms of their sexual orientation. "The pastor and counselor must see all people, irrespective of their sexuality, as children of God and destined for eternal life" (Catholic Social Welfare Commission of the Bishops' Conference of England and Wales, "An Introduction to the Pastoral Care of Homosexual People," p. 10). The Congregation states this even more fully:

"The human person, made in the image and likeness of God, can hardly be adequately described by a reductional reference to his or her sexual orientation. Everyone living on the face of the earth has personal problems and difficulties, but has challenges to growth, strengths, talents and gifts as well. Today the Church provides a badly needed context for the care of the human person when she refuses to consider the person as heterosexual or homosexual and insists that every person has a fundamental identity: a creature of God, and by grace, his child and heir to eternal life" (Congregation for the Doctrine of the Faith, "Letter on the Pastoral Care of Homosexual Persons," 16).

Sexuality and Marriage

In upholding the dignity of people who are homosexual, the Church is being consistent to its teaching. There are two fundamental principles which determine the Catholic Church's teaching on sexual matters. First, the Church has always taught that the sexual (genital) expression of love is intended by God's plan of creation to find its place exclusively within marriage between a man and a woman. The Church therefore cannot in any way equate a homosexual partnership with a heterosexual marriage. Second, the sexual (genital) expression of love must be open to the possible transmission of new life. For these two reasons the Church does not approve of homosexual genital acts. When the Church describes such acts as "intrinsically disordered" (CDF, "Pastoral Care," 3), it means that these acts are not consistent with the two fundamental principles mentioned above. It is in this sense that the Church teaches that there can be no moral right to homosexual acts, even though they are no longer held to be criminal in any secular legal systems. No individual, bishop, priest, or layperson is in a position to change the teaching of the Church, which she considers to be God-given.

FURTHER CONSIDERATIONS

Homosexual Orientation

It is necessary to distinguish between sexual orientation or inclination, and engaging in sexual (genital) activity, heterosexual or homosexual. Neither a homosexual nor a heterosexual orientation leads inevitably to sexual activity. **199** Furthermore, an individual's sexual orientation can be unclear, even complex. Also, it may vary over the years.

Meaning of "Objectively Disordered"

The particular orientation or inclination of the homosexual person is not a moral failing. An inclination is not a sin. An inclination toward acts which are contrary to the teaching of the Church has, however, been described as "objectively disordered." The word disordered is a harsh one in our English language. It immediately suggests a sinful situation or at least implies a demeaning of the person or even a sickness. It should not be so interpreted.

First, the word is a term belonging to the vocabulary of traditional Catholic moral theology and philosophy. It is used to describe an inclination which is a departure from what is generally regarded to be the norm. The norm consists of an inclination toward a sexual relationship with a person of the opposite sex and not between persons of the same sex. Being a homosexual person is, then, neither morally good nor morally bad; it is homosexual genital acts that are morally wrong.

Second, when the Church speaks of the inclination to homosexuality as being "an objective disorder" (PC, 3), the Church can be thinking only of an inclination toward homosexual genital acts. The Church does not consider the whole personality and character of the individual to be thereby disordered. Homosexual people, as well as heterosexual people, can and often do give a fine example of friendship and the art of chaste loving.

Friendship

Friendship is a gift from God. Friendship is a way of loving. Friendship is necessary for every person. To equate friendship and full sexual involvement with another is to distort the very concept of friendship. Sexual loving presupposes friendship, but friendship does not require full sexual involvement. It is a mistake to say or think or presume that if two persons of the same or different sexes enjoy a deep and lasting friendship then they must be sexually involved.

To love another, whether of the same sex or of a different sex, is to have entered the area of the richest human experience. But that experience of love is spoiled, whether it is in marriage or in friendship, when we do not think and act as God wills us to think and act. Human loving is precarious, for human nature is wounded and frail. Thus marriage and friendship will never be easy to handle. We shall often fail, but the ideal remains.

28: Human Life

DOCUMENT 1:

Source: Congregation for the Doctrine of the Faith, "Instruction on Respect for Human Life in Its Origin and on the Dignity of Procreation" (Feb. 22, 1987), *Origins* 16: no. 40, Mar. 19, 1987, pp. 699–701.

2. SCIENCE AND TECHNOLOGY AT THE SERVICE OF THE HUMAN PERSON

God created man in his own image and likeness: "Male and female he created them" (Gn 1:27), entrusting to them the task of "having dominion over the earth" (Gn 1:28). Basic scientific research and applied research constitute a significant expression of this dominion of man over creation. Science and technology are valuable resources for man when placed at his service and when they promote his integral development for the benefit of all; but they cannot of themselves show the meaning of existence and of human progress. Being ordered to man, who initiates and develops them, they draw from the person and his moral values the indication of their purpose and the awareness of their limits.

It would, on the one hand, be illusory to claim that scientific research and its applications are morally neutral; on the other hand one cannot derive criteria for guidance from mere technical efficiency, from research's possible usefulness to some at the expense of others or, worse still, from prevailing ideologies. Thus science and technology require for their own intrinsic meaning an unconditional respect for the fundamental criteria of the moral law. That is to say, they must be at the service of the human person, of his inalienable rights and his true and integral good according to the design and will of God.

The rapid development of technological discoveries gives greater urgency to this need to respect the criteria just mentioned: Science without conscience can only lead to man's ruin. "Our era needs such wisdom more than bygone ages if the discoveries made by man are to be further humanized. For the future of the world stands in peril unless wiser people are forthcoming."

3. ANTHROPOLOGY AND PROCEDURES IN THE BIOMEDICAL FIELD

Which moral criteria must be applied in order to clarify the problems posed today in the field of biomedicine? The answer to this question presupposes a proper idea of the nature of the human person in his bodily dimension.

For it is only in keeping with his true nature that the human person can achieve self-realization as a "unified totality," and this nature is at the same time corporal and spiritual. By virtue of its substantial union with a spiritual soul, the human body cannot be considered as a mere complex of tissues, organs, and functions, nor can it be evaluated in the same way as the body of animals; rather it is a constitutive part of the person who manifests and expresses himself through it.

The natural moral law expresses and lays down the purposes, rights and duties which are based upon the bodily and spiritual nature of the human person. Therefore this law cannot be thought of as simply a set of norms on the biological level; rather it must be defined as the rational order whereby man is called by the Creator to direct and regulate his life and actions and in particular to make use of his own body.

A first consequence can be deduced from these principles: an intervention on the human body affects not only the tissues, the organs, and their functions, but also involves the person himself on different levels. It involves, therefore, perhaps in an implicit but nonetheless real way, a moral significance and responsibility. Pope John Paul II forcefully reaffirmed this to the World Medical Association when he said:

"Each human person, in his absolutely unique singularity, is constituted not only by his spirit, but by his body as well. Thus, in the body and through the body, one touches the person himself in his concrete reality. To respect the dignity of man consequently amounts to safeguarding this identity of the man *corpore et anima unus*, as the Second Vatican Council says (*Gaudium et Spes*, 14.1). It is on the basis of this anthropological vision that one is to find the fundamental criteria for decision making in the case of procedures which are not strictly therapeutic, as, for example, those aimed at the improvement of the human biological condition."

Applied biology and medicine work together for the integral good of human life when they come to the aid of a person stricken by illness and infirmity and when they respect his or her dignity as a creature of God. No biologist or doctor can reasonably claim, by virtue of his scientific competence, to be able to decide on people's origin and destiny. This norm must be applied in a particular way in the field of sexuality and procreation, in which man and woman actualize the fundamental values of love and life.

God, who is love and life, has inscribed in man and woman the vocation to share in a special way in his mystery of personal communion and in his work as Creator and Father. For this reason marriage possesses specific goods and values in its union and in procreation which cannot be likened to those existing in lower forms of life. Such values and meanings are of the personal order and determine from the moral point of view the meaning and limits of artificial interventions on procreation and on the origin of human life. These interventions are not to be rejected on the grounds that they are artificial. As such, they bear witness to the possibilities of the art of medicine. But they must be given a moral evaluation in reference to the dignity of the human person, who is called to realize his vocation from God to the gift of love and the gift of life.

4. FUNDAMENTAL CRITERIA FOR A MORAL JUDGMENT

The fundamental values connected with the techniques of artificial human procreation are two: the life of the human being called into existence and the

202   special nature of the transmission of human life in marriage. The moral judgment on such methods of artificial procreation must therefore be formulated in reference to these values.

Physical life, with which the course of human life in the world begins, certainly does not itself contain the whole of a person's value nor does it represent the supreme good of man, who is called to eternal life. However it does constitute in a certain way the "fundamental" value of life precisely because upon this physical life all the other values of the person are based and developed. The inviolability of the innocent human being's right to life "from the moment of conception until death" is a sign and requirement of the very inviolability of the person to whom the Creator has given the gift of life.

By comparison with the transmission of other forms of life in the universe, the transmission of human life has a special character of its own, which derives from the special nature of the human person. "The transmission of human life is entrusted by nature to a personal and conscious act and as such is subject to the all-holy laws of God: immutable and inviolable laws which must be recognized and observed. For this reason one cannot use means and follow methods which could be licit in the transmission of the life of plants and animals."

Advances in technology have now made it possible to procreate apart from sexual relations through the meeting in vitro of the germ cells previously taken from the man and the woman. But what is technically possible is not for that very reason morally admissible. Rational reflection on the fundamental values of life and of human procreation is therefore indispensable for formulating a moral evaluation of such technological interventions on a human being from the first stage of his development.

5. TEACHINGS OF THE MAGISTERIUM

On its part, the Magisterium of the Church offers to human reason in this field too the light of revelation. The doctrine concerning man taught by the Magisterium contains many elements which throw light on the problems being faced here.

From the moment of conception, the life of every human being is to be respected in an absolute way because man is the only creature on earth that God has "wished for himself" and the spiritual soul of each man is "immediately created" by God; his whole being bears the image of the Creator. Human life is sacred because from its beginning it involves "the creative action of God," and it remains forever in a special relationship with the Creator, who is its sole end. God alone is the Lord of life from its beginning until its end: no one can in any circumstance claim for himself the right to destroy directly an innocent human being. . . .

DOCUMENT 2 / Human Life

SOURCE: Pope John Paul II, "The Gospel of Life" (Mar. 25, 1995), *Origins* 24: no. 42, Apr. 6, 1995, pp. 701–02.

34. Life is always a good. This is an instinctive perception and a fact of experience, and man is called to grasp the profound reason why this is so.

Why is life a good? This question is found everywhere in the Bible, and from the very first pages it receives a powerful and amazing answer. The life which God gives man is quite different from the life of all other living creatures inasmuch as man, although formed from the dust of the earth (cf. Gn 2:7, 3:19; Jb 34:15; Ps 103:14; 104:29), is a manifestation of God in the world, a sign of his presence, a trace of his glory (cf. Gn 1: 26–27; Ps 8:6). This is what St. Irenaeus of Lyons wanted to emphasize in his celebrated definition: "Man, living man, is the glory of God." Man has been given a sublime dignity based on the intimate bond which unites him to his Creator: in man there shines forth a reflection of God himself.

The Book of Genesis affirms this when in the first account of creation it places man at the summit of God's creative activity as its crown, at the culmination of a process which leads from indistinct chaos to the most perfect of creatures. Everything in creation is ordered to man, and everything is made subject to him: "Fill the earth and subdue it; and have dominion over . . . every living thing" (1:28); this is God's command to the man and the woman. A similar message is found also in the other account of creation: "The Lord God took the man and put him in the garden of Eden to till it and keep it" (Gn 2:15). We see here a clear affirmation of the primacy of man over things; these are made subject to him and entrusted to his responsible care, whereas for no reason can he be made subject to other men and almost reduced to the level of a thing.

In the biblical narrative, the difference between man and other creatures is shown above all by the fact that only the creation of man is presented as the result of a special decision on the part of God. . . .

DOCUMENT 3 / Human Life

SOURCE: Pope John Paul II, "Biological Experimentation" (Oct. 23, 1982), *The Pope Speaks* 28: no. 1, 1983, pp. 74–75.

The work which you have accomplished during these days, besides having a high scientific value, is also of great interest for religion. My predecessor, Paul VI, in his discourse to the United Nations Organization Oct. 4, 1963, spoke from the viewpoint of being an "expert in humanity." This expertise is judged linked with the Church's own wisdom, but it likewise comes from culture, of which the natural sciences are an ever more important expression.

In my talk to UNESCO June 2, 1980, I mentioned, and now I wish to repeat it to you scientists, that there exists "an organic and constitutive link between culture and religion." I must also confirm before this illustrious assembly what I said in my address of Oct. 3, 1981, to the Pontifical Academy of Sciences, on the occasion of the annual study week: "I have firm confidence in the world scientific community, and in a very particular way in the Pontifical Academy of Sciences, being certain that, thanks to them, biological progress and research, as also all other scientific research and its technological application, will be accomplished in full respect for the norms of morality, safeguarding the dignity of people and their freedom and equality."

And I added: "It is necessary that science should always be accompanied and guided by the wisdom that belongs to the permanent spiritual heritage of humanity, and which is inspired by the design of God inscribed in creation before being subsequently proclaimed by his Word."

FOR MAN'S SERVICE

Science and wisdom, which in their truest and most varied expressions constitute a most precious heritage of humanity, are at the service of man. The Church is called, in its essential vocation, to foster the progress of man, since, as I wrote in my first encyclical, ". . . man is the primary route which the Church must travel in fulfilling its mission: he is the primary and fundamental way for the Church, the way traced out by Christ himself."

Man also is for you the ultimate term of scientific research, the whole man, spirit and body, even if the immediate object of the sciences which you profess is the body with all its organs and tissues. The human body is not independent of the spirit, just as the spirit is not independent of the body, because of the deep unity and mutual connection which exists between one and the other.

The substantial unity between spirit and body, and indirectly with the cosmos, is so essential that every human activity, even the most spiritual one, is in some way permeated and colored by the bodily condition; at the same time the body must in turn be directed and guided to its final end by the spirit.

There is no doubt that the spiritual activities of the human person proceed   **205**
from the personal center of the individual, who is predisposed by the body to
which the spirit is substantially united.

Hence the great importance, for the life of the spirit, of the sciences which
promote the knowledge of corporeal reality and activity. . . .

DOCUMENT 4 / Human Life

Source: Pope John Paul II, "A Patient is a Person" (Oct. 27, 1980), *The Pope Speaks* 26: no. 1, 1981, pp. 1–3.

. . . In recent years the medical arts have made significant advances, thus notably increasing the possibilities of therapeutic intervention. This has led to a gradual modification of the very concept of medicine, extending its role beyond the ancient function of fighting disease to that of promoting the overall health of human beings. A consequence of this new outlook is that the relation between physician and patient has gradually taken on increasingly organized and complex forms that are meant to safeguard the citizen's health from birth to old age.

The safeguarding of children and the elderly; medical care in schools and factories; prevention of occupational diseases and work-related accidents; mental hygiene; care of the handicapped, addicts and the mentally ill; prevention of contagious diseases; environmental control; and so on; all these are facets of the contemporary way of conceiving the "service to human beings" to which you are called in the practice of your art.

There is no reason why you should not rejoice since it can now be said that, from the point of view just indicated, the right of the human person to life has never been so fully recognized. This is one of the characteristic traits of the extraordinary acceleration of history that marks our age.

By reason of this remarkable development, medicine is playing a role of the first order in shaping contemporary society.

A calm and attentive examination of the contemporary situation in its entirety, however, must lead us to recognize that insidious ways of violating the right all human beings have to a life worthy of them have, in fact, not disappeared. It can even be said that from certain points of view there has been the emergence of negative trends as I pointed out in my encyclical *Redemptor Homines*:

"If, then, our age . . . seems a time of splendid progress, it shows itself simultaneously to be full of imminent dangers to the human race. . . . Every phase of contemporary progress must, therefore, be subjected to examination, that is, we must, as it were, X-ray every aspect of this progress. . . . The danger already exists, and is now being seen, that while human beings are increasing their economic mastery, they may lose sight of the basic reasons for this mastery, let their humanity take second place to material things, and—even though they may not immediately see that this is happening—allow themselves to be manipulated in many ways."

NORMS GOVERNING MEDICINE

The truth is that the technological progress so characteristic of our age suffers from a radical ambivalence. On the one hand, it allows human beings to take control of their own destiny but, on the other, it exposes them to the temptation of going beyond the limits of a reasonable mastery of nature, thus endangering the integrity and even the very survival of the human person.

Limiting ourselves to the realm of biology and medicine, we may consider the implicit dangers to which the human right to life is exposed by discoveries in the field of artificial insemination, birth control and fertility control, hibernation and "delayed death," genetic engineering, mind-altering drugs, organic transplants, and so on. Scientific knowledge does, of course, have its own laws and must observe these, but it also must recognize, especially in the area of medicine, the inviolable limits created by respect for the person and by the protection of the person's right to live a life worthy of a human being.

If a new research technique, for example, injures or risks injuring this right, the technique is not to be considered permissible simply because it increases our store of knowledge. Science is not the highest value, to which all others are to be subordinated. Higher in the scale of values is the personal right of each individual to physical and spiritual life and to psychic and functional integrity. The person is the measure and criterion of goodness or fault in every human manifestation. Scientific progress cannot, therefore, claim to stand on neutral ground. Ethical norms, which are based on respect for the human person, must light the way for, and control, the stages of research and the application of the results obtained by research.

For some time now, voices have been raised in alarm to call attention to the harmful consequences of medical practice that is more concerned with itself than with the human beings it is meant to serve. . . .

29: Human Rights

DOCUMENT 1:

Source: Pope John Paul II, "The Gospel of Life" (Mar. 25, 1995), *Origins* 24: no. 42, Apr. 6, 1995, pp. 696–697.

19. . . . The theory of human rights is based precisely on the affirmation that the human person, unlike animals and things, cannot be subjected to domination by others. We must also mention the mentality which tends to equate personal dignity with the capacity for verbal and explicit, or at least perceptible, communication. It is clear that on the basis of these presuppositions there is no place in the world for anyone who, like the unborn or the dying, is a weak element in the social structure, or for anyone who appears completely at the mercy of others and radically dependent on them, and can only communicate through the silent language of a profound sharing of affection. In this case it is force which becomes the criterion for choice and action in interpersonal relations and in social life. But this is the exact opposite of what a state ruled by law, as a community in which the "reasons of force" are replaced by the "force of reason," historically intended to affirm.

At another level, the roots of the contradiction between the solemn affirmation of human rights and their tragic denial in practice lie in a notion of freedom which exalts the isolated individual in an absolute way and gives no place to solidarity, to openness to others and service of them. While it is true that the taking of life not yet born or in its final stages is sometimes marked by a mistaken sense of altruism and human compassion, it cannot be denied that such a culture of death, taken as a whole, betrays a completely individualistic concept of freedom, which ends up by becoming the freedom of "the strong" against the weak who have no choice but to submit.

It is precisely in this sense that Cain's answer to the Lord's question "where is Abel your brother?" can be interpreted: "I do not know; am I my brother's keeper?" (Gn 4:9). Yes, every man is his "brother's keeper," because God entrusts us to one another. And it is also in view of this entrusting that God gives everyone freedom, a freedom which possesses an inherently relational dimension. This is a great gift of the Creator, placed as it is at the service of the person and of his fulfillment through the gift of self and openness to others; but when freedom is made absolute in an individualistic way, it is emptied of its original content, and its very meaning and dignity are contradicted.

There is an even more profound aspect which needs to be emphasized: freedom negates and destroys itself and becomes a factor leading to the destruction of others when it no longer recognizes and respects its essential link with

the truth. When freedom, out of a desire to emancipate itself from all forms of   **209**
tradition and authority, shuts out even the most obvious evidence of an objective
and universal truth, which is the foundation of personal and social life, then
the person ends up by no longer taking as the sole and indisputable point of
reference for his own choices the truth about good and evil, but only his
subjective and changeable opinion or, indeed, his selfish interest and whim.

20. This view of freedom leads to a serious distortion of life in society. If
the promotion of the self is understood in terms of absolute autonomy, people
inevitably reach the point of rejecting one another. Everyone else is considered
an enemy from whom one has to defend oneself. Thus society becomes a mass
of individuals placed side by side, but without any mutual bonds. Each one
wishes to assert himself independently of the other and in fact intends to make
his own interests prevail. Still, in the face of other people's analogous interests,
some kind of compromise must be found if one wants a society in which the
maximum possible freedom is guaranteed to each individual. In this way, any
reference to common values and to a truth absolutely binding on everyone is
lost, and social life ventures on to the shifting sands of complete relativism.
At that point, everything is negotiable, everything is open to bargaining, even
the first of the fundamental rights, the right to life. . . .

DOCUMENT 2 / Human Rights

Source: Pope John XXIII, *Pacem in Terris* (Apr. 1963), *The Pope Speaks* 9: no. 1, 1963, pp. 15–17.

THE RIGHT TO LIFE AND TO A WORTHY STANDARD OF LIVING

11. But first we must speak of man's rights. Man has the right to live. He has the right to bodily integrity and to the means necessary for the proper development of life, particularly food, clothing, shelter, medical care, rest, and finally, the necessary social services. In consequence, he has the right to be looked after in the event of ill-health, disability stemming from his work, widowhood, old age, enforced unemployment, or whenever through no fault of his own he is deprived of the means of livelihood. . . .

THE RIGHT TO CHOOSE FREELY ONE'S STATE IN LIFE

15. Human beings have also the right to choose for themselves the kind of life which appeals to them: whether it is to found a family—in the founding of which both the man and the woman enjoy equal rights and duties—or to embrace the priesthood or the religious life.

16. The family, founded upon marriage freely contracted, one and dissoluble, must be regarded as the natural, primary cell of human society. The interests of the family must be taken very specially into consideration in social and economic affairs, as well as in the spheres of faith and morals. For all of these have to do with strengthening the family and assisting it in the fulfillment of its mission.

17. Of course, the support and education of children is a right which belongs primarily to the parents.

ECONOMIC RIGHTS

18. In the economic sphere, it is evident that a man has the inherent right not only to be given the opportunity to work, but also to be allowed the exercise of personal initiative in the work he does.

19. The conditions in which a man works form a necessary corollary to these rights. They must not be such as to weaken his physical or moral fiber, or militate against the proper development of adolescents to manhood. Women must be accorded such conditions of work as are consistent with their needs and responsibilities as wives and mothers.

20. A further consequence of man's personal dignity is his right to engage in economic activities suited to his degree of responsibility. The worker is likewise entitled to a wage that is determined in accordance with the precepts of justice. This needs stressing. The amount a worker receives must be sufficient, in proportion to available funds, to allow him and his family a standard of living consistent with human dignity. . . .

DOCUMENT 3 / Human Rights

SOURCE: United States Catholic Conference, "USCC Platform Testimony" (June 12, 1984), *Origins* 14: no. 8, July 12, 1984, pp. 116–19.

In presenting this testimony on behalf of the U.S. Catholic Conference, I wish not only to state our positions on issues, but to indicate their ethical and moral basis. As much as the positions themselves, the system of norms and principles which shapes our view of issues speaks to the requirements of sound political and social policy in our times.

Although the system to which I refer is the social doctrine of the Catholic Church, it is no narrowly sectarian body of thought and teaching. For its fundamental insight is the dignity of the human person, and its applications in specific cases flow directly from that insight. . . .

. . . Catholic social doctrine embodies and elaborates two fundamental truths about the human person: human life is uniquely sacred, and human life is essentially social. Because life is sacred, it must be protected and fostered at all stages and in all circumstances. Because it is social, society itself must be formed as an environment congenial to the development and flourishing of all lives.

. . . Hence our view of the role of the state and of other key social institutions. The state exists for people, not people for the state. And because human life requires a social environment for its development and flourishing, the state has a positive role to play in relation to the needs and rights of persons: it must protect life from attack and foster political, economic, and cultural conditions in keeping with human dignity. It follows that the state should adopt and put into effect sound policies with regard to such matters as nutrition, housing, education, health care, and employment.

Although the state has unique responsibilities in society, it does not have sole responsibility. Other institutions—churches, unions, professional organizations, corporations and business enterprises, cultural agencies—are part of the social fabric which sustains and fosters human dignity. From the societal perspective, each should be evaluated in terms of its contribution to the common good. Each too should be left free by the others and by the state to perform its particular functions in relation to the good of persons.

The common good can be understood as the mix of temporal and spiritual conditions which must pertain in a society if all its members are to have opportunity to develop their potential in relation to all the aspects of their personhood. Thus the common good is, in a sense, the good of all. In considering its concrete implications, however, Catholic social teaching emphasizes concern for the poor, the oppressed, and the least powerful. . . .

212 **ABORTION AND THE RIGHT TO LIFE**

Abortion directly destroys an unborn human being and thus violates the right to life. A legal system which permits abortion contradicts the principle that human rights are inherent and inalienable. Thus the 1973 Supreme Court decisions on abortion and subsequent decisions which rely on them should be reversed, while society's resources should be redirected to solving the problems for which abortion is mistakenly proposed as a solution. . . .

We support legal equity for women and reject efforts to link abortion "rights" to this objective. Women have been at the forefront of the drive to secure legal protection for the unborn and are generally more opposed to abortion than men are. Women's equity measures should be scrutinized and, where necessary, amended so that their legitimate and important goals are not exploited as vehicles for abortion and abortion funding. . . .

CIVIL RIGHTS

Discrimination on the basis of race, ethnicity, sex, age, or handicapping condition continues to haunt our land. Such discrimination is present not only in the hearts of many persons, but in the fabric of our nation's institutions. . . .

CRIME AND CRIMINAL JUSTICE

Crime and violence are major and legitimate concerns for many. We support strong and effective action to control handguns, leading to their eventual elimination from our society. We advocate greater utilization of community-based correctional facilities, effective programs of education, rehabilitation and job training for offenders, and the compensation of victims of crime.

We oppose the use of capital punishment. A return to the use of the death penalty can only lead to further erosion of respect for life. . . .

EDUCATION

We support public policy which guarantees the rights of all persons to an adequate education regardless of race, sex, national origin, economic status, or personal disability. In particular, we advocate policies to improve the educational opportunities available to economically disadvantaged persons and minorities, including bilingual education, as well as compliance in schools with the legal requirements of all civil-rights statutes regarding race, sex, age, and handicapping conditions.

We also support—and urge the platform committee to support—constitutionally acceptable means of providing tax assistance for the education of children in non-public schools, in order to guarantee the free exercise of parental rights in choosing educational opportunities for their children. . . .

EMPLOYMENT AND INCOME

Our nation should provide jobs for those who can work and a decent income for those who cannot. . . .

Present levels of unemployment, although down from the extreme levels of two years ago, are still far too high. . . .

We reaffirm our support for the right of workers to join together to **213** bargain collectively with their employers and ask that protection of this right be extended to those whose rights are currently unprotected, especially farm laborers.

We urge a guarantee of a decent income for those who cannot work and adequate assistance for those in need. To achieve these goals, we support a comprehensive reform of the welfare system which will provide an adequate income base for all Americans and replace the present system of fragmented programs. . . .

FOOD AND AGRICULTURAL POLICY

The right to eat follows from the right to life. We support a national policy aimed at securing this right, including nutrition programs which help meet the needs of hungry and malnourished Americans, especially children, the poor, the unemployed, and the elderly. The food-stamp program and child-nutrition programs should be funded at adequate levels. . . .

HEALTH CARE

Adequate health care is a basic human need to which society must respond according to its best ability. Yet our society appears in recent years to have retreated from this goal. Budget cuts, rising health care costs, and high unemployment have deprived millions of adequate preventive and acute care. . . .

HUMAN RIGHTS

The dignity of the human person requires the defense and promotion of human rights in global and domestic affairs. With respect to human rights internationally, there is a pressing need for the United States to pursue a double task: to strengthen and expand international mechanisms by which human rights can be protected and promoted and to take seriously the human rights dimensions of U.S. foreign policy. . . .

30: Hydration and Nutrition

DOCUMENT 1:

SOURCE: John Paul II, *Ad Limina* address to Bishops from California, Nevada, and Hawaii. "Building a Culture of Life," (October 2, 1998), *Origins* 28, no. 18, Oct. 15, 1998, p. 316.

. . . As ecumenical witness in defense of life develops, a great teaching effort is needed to clarify the substantive moral difference between discontinuing medical procedures that may be burdensome, dangerous or disproportionate to the expected outcome—what the Catechism of the Catholic Church calls the refusal of "overzealous treatment" (n. 2278; cf *Evangelium Vitae*, 65)—and taking away the ordinary means of preserving life such as feeding, hydration and normal medical care. The statement of the U.S. bishops' pro-life committee "Nutrition and Hydration: Moral and Pastoral Considerations," rightly emphasizes that the omission of nutrition and hydration intended to cause a patient's death must be rejected and that, while giving careful consideration to all the factors involved, the presumption should be in favor of providing medically assisted nutrition and hydration to all patients who need them. To blur this distinction is to introduce a source of countless injustices and much additional anguish, affecting both those already suffering from ill health or the deterioration which comes with age, and their loved ones.

DOCUMENT 2 / Hydration and Nutrition

SOURCE: National Conference of Catholic Bishops Committee for Pro-Life Activities, "Nutrition and Hydration: Moral and Pastoral Reflections," *Origins* 21: no. 44 (Apr. 9, 1992), pp. 705–12.

Introduction

Modern medical technology seems to confront us with many questions not faced even a decade ago. Corresponding changes in medical practice have benefited many, but have also prompted fears by some that they will be aggressively treated against their will or denied the kind of care that is their due as human persons with inherent dignity. Current debates about life-sustaining treatment suggest that our society's moral reflection is having difficulty keeping pace with its technological progress.

A religious view of life has an important contribution to make to these modern debates. Our Catholic tradition has developed a rich body of thought on these questions, which affirms a duty to preserve human life but recognizes limits to that duty.

Our first goal in making this statement is to reaffirm some basic principles of our moral tradition, to assist Catholics and others in making treatment decisions in accord with respect for God's gift of life.

These principles do not provide clear and final answers to all moral questions that arise as individuals make difficult decisions. Catholic theologians may differ on how best to apply moral principles to some questions not explicitly resolved by the Church's teaching authority. Likewise, we understand that those who must make serious health care decisions for themselves or for others face a complexity of issues, circumstances, thoughts and emotions in each unique case.

This is the case with some questions involving the medically assisted provision of nutrition and hydration to helpless patients—those who are seriously ill, disabled, or persistently unconscious. These questions have been made more urgent by widely publicized court cases and the public debate to which they have given rise.

Our second purpose in issuing this statement, then, is to provide some clarification of the moral issues involved in decisions about medically assisted nutrition and hydration. We are fully aware that such guidance is not necessarily final, because there are many unresolved medical and ethical questions related to these issues and the continuing development of medical technology will necessitate ongoing reflection . . .

Questions About Medically Assisted Nutrition and Hydration

1. Is the withholding or withdrawing of medically assisted nutrition and hydration always a direct killing?

215

216   In answering this question one should avoid two extremes.

First, it is wrong to say that this could not be a matter of killing simply because it involves an omission rather than a positive action. In fact a deliberate omission may be an effective and certain way to kill, especially to kill someone weakened by illness. Catholic teaching condemns as euthanasia "an action or an omission which of itself or by intention causes death, in order that all suffering may in this way be eliminated." Thus "euthanasia includes not only active mercy killing but also the omission of treatment when the purpose of the omission is to kill the patient."

Second, we should not assume that all or most decisions to withhold or withdraw medically assisted nutrition and hydration are attempts to cause death. To be sure, any patient will die if all nutrition and hydration are withheld. But sometimes other causes are at work—for example, the patient may be imminently dying, whether feeding takes place or not, from an already existing terminal condition. At other times, although the shortening of the patient's life is one foreseeable result of an omission, the real purpose of the omission was to relieve the patient of a particular procedure that was of limited usefulness to the patient or unreasonably burdensome for the patient and the patient's family or caregivers. This kind of decision should not be equated with a decision to kill or with suicide.

The harsh reality is that some who propose withdrawal of nutrition and hydration from certain patients do directly intend to bring about a patient's death and would even prefer a change in the law to allow for what they see as more "quick and painless" means to cause death. In other words, nutrition and hydration (whether orally administered or medically assisted) are sometimes withdrawn not because a patient is dying, but precisely because a patient is not dying (or not dying quickly) and someone believes it would be better if he or she did, generally because the patient is perceived as having an unacceptably low "quality of life" or as imposing burdens on others.

When deciding whether to withhold or withdraw medically assisted nutrition and hydration, or other forms of life support, we are called by our moral tradition to ask ourselves: What will my decision do for this patient? And what am I trying to achieve by doing it? We must be sure that it is not our intent to cause the patient's death—either for its own sake or as a means to achieving some other goal such as the relief of suffering.

3. What are the benefits of medically assisted nutrition and hydration?

According to international codes of medical ethics, a physician will see a medical procedure as appropriate "if in his or her judgment it offers hope of saving life, re-establishing health or alleviating suffering."

Nutrition and hydration, whether provided in the usual way or with medical assistance, do not by themselves remedy pathological conditions, except those caused by dietary deficiencies. But patients benefit from them in several ways. First, for all patients who can assimilate them, suitable food and fluids sustain life, and providing them normally expresses loving concern and solidarity with the helpless. Second, for patients being treated with the hope

of a cure, appropriate food and fluids are an important element of sound health   **217**
care. Third, even for patients who are imminently dying and incurable, food
and fluids can prevent the suffering that may arise from dehydration, hunger,
and thirst.

The benefit of sustaining and fostering life is fundamental, because life
is our first gift from a loving God and the condition for receiving his other
gifts. But sometimes even food and fluids are no longer effective in providing
this benefit because a patient has entered the final stage of a terminal condition.
At such times we should make the dying person as comfortable as possible
and provide nursing care and proper hygiene as well as companionship and
appropriate spiritual aid. Such a person may lose all desire for food and drink
and even be unable to ingest them. Initiating medically assisted feeding or
intravenous fluids in this case may increase the patient's discomfort while
providing no real benefit; ice chips or sips of water may instead be appropriate
to provide comfort and counteract the adverse effects of dehydration." Even
in the case of the imminently dying patient, of course, any action or omission
that of itself or by intention causes death is to be absolutely rejected.

As Christians who trust in the promise of eternal life we recognize that
death does not have the final word. Accordingly we need not always prevent
death until the last possible moment; but we should never intentionally cause
death or abandon the dying person as though he or she were unworthy of care
and respect.

6. Do persistently unconscious patients represent a special case?

Even Catholics who accept the same basic moral principles may strongly
disagree on how to apply them to patients who appear to be persistently
unconscious—that is, those who are in a permanent coma or a "persistent
vegetative state" (PVS). Some moral questions in this area have not been explicitly resolved by the Church's teaching authority.

On some points there is wide agreement among Catholic theologians:

(1) An unconscious patient must be treated as a living human person
with inherent dignity and value. Direct killing of such a patient is as morally
reprehensible as the direct killing of anyone else. Even the medical terminology
used to describe these patients as "vegetative" unfortunately tends to obscure
this vitally important point, inviting speculation that a patient in this state is
a "vegetable" or a subhuman animal.

(2) The area of legitimate controversy does not concern patients with
conditions like mental retardation, senility, dementia, or even temporary unconsciousness. Where serious disagreement begins is with the patient who has
been diagnosed as completely and permanently unconscious after careful testing over a period of weeks or months.

Some moral theologians argue that a particular form of care or treatment
is morally obligatory only when its benefits outweigh its burdens to a patient
or the care providers. In weighing burdens, they say, the total burden of a
procedure and the consequent requirements of care must be taken into account.
If no benefit can be demonstrated, the procedure, whatever its burdens, cannot

218   be obligatory. These moralists also hold that the chief criterion to determine the benefit of a procedure cannot be merely that it prolongs physical life, since physical life is not an absolute good but is relative to the spiritual good of the person. They assert that the spiritual good of the person is union with God, which can be advanced only by human acts, i.e., conscious, free acts. Since the best current medical opinion holds that persons in the persistent vegetative state (PVS) are incapable now or in the future of conscious, free human acts, these moralists conclude that, when careful diagnosis verifies this condition, it is not obligatory to prolong life by such interventions as a respirator, antibiotics, or medically assisted hydration and nutrition. To decide to omit non-obligatory care, therefore, is not to intend the patient's death, but only to avoid the burden of the procedure. Hence, though foreseen, the patient's death is to be attributed to the patient's pathological condition and not to the omission of care. Therefore, these theologians conclude, while it is always wrong directly to intend or cause the death of such patients, the natural dying process which would have occurred without these interventions may be permitted to proceed.

While this rationale is convincing to some, it is not theologically conclusive and we are not persuaded by it. In fact, other theologians argue cogently that theological inquiry could lead one to a more carefully limited conclusion.

These moral theologians argue that while particular treatments can be judged useless or burdensome, it is morally questionable and would create a dangerous precedent to imply that any human life is not a positive good or "benefit." They emphasize that while life is not the highest good, it is always and everywhere a basic good of the human person and not merely a means to other goods. They further assert that if the "burden" one is trying to relieve by discontinuing medically assisted nutrition and hydration is the burden of remaining alive in the allegedly undignified condition of PVS, such a decision is unacceptable because one's intent is only achieved by deliberately ensuring the patient's death from malnutrition or dehydration. Finally, these moralists suggest that PVS is best seen as an extreme form of mental and physical disability—one whose causes, nature and prognosis are as yet imperfectly understood—and not as a terminal illness or fatal pathology from which patients should generally be allowed to die. Because the patient's life can often be sustained indefinitely by medically assisted nutrition and hydration that is not unreasonably risky or burdensome for that patient, they say, we are not dealing here with a case where "inevitable death is imminent in spite of the means used." Rather, because the patient will die in a few days if medically assisted nutrition and hydration are discontinued, but can often live a long time if they are provided, the inherent dignity and worth of the human person obligates us to provide patient with care and support.

. . . In the face of the uncertainties and unresolved medical and theological issues, it is important to defend and preserve important values. On the one hand, there is a concern that patients and families should not be subjected to unnecessary burdens, ineffective treatments, and indignities when death is approaching. On the other hand, it is important to ensure that the inherent dignity of human persons, even those who are persistently unconscious, is

respected and that no one is deprived of nutrition and hydration with the   **219**
intent of bringing on his or her death.

    . . . In light of these concerns, it is our considered judgment that while
legitimate Catholic moral debate continues, decisions about these patients
should be guided by a presumption in favor of medically assisted nutrition
and hydration. A decision to discontinue such measures should be made in
light of a careful assessment of the burdens and benefits of nutrition and
hydration for the individual patient and his or her family and community.
Such measures must not be withdrawn in order to cause death, but they may
be withdrawn if they offer no reasonable hope of sustaining life or pose excessive risks or burdens. We also believe that social and health care policies should
be carefully framed so that these patients are not routinely classified as "terminal" or as prime candidates for the discontinuance of even minimal means of
life support. . . .

DOCUMENT 3 / Hydration and Nutrition

SOURCE: Pontifical Council Cor Unum, *Questions of Ethics Regarding the Fatally Ill and the Dying*, Vatican Press, 1981, pp. 8–9.

2.4.3 THE CRITERION OF THE QUALITY OF LIFE: ITS IMPORTANCE

Among all the criteria for decision, particular importance must be given to the quality of the life to be saved or kept living by the therapy. The letter of Cardinal Villot to the Congress of the International Federation of Catholic Medical Associations is very clear on this subject: "It must be emphasized that it is the sacred character of life which forbids a physician to kill and makes it a duty for him at the same time to use every resource of his art to fight against death. This does not, however, mean that a physician is under obligation to use all and every one of the life-maintaining techniques offered him by the indefatigable creativity of science. Would it not be a useless torture, in many cases, to impose vegetative reanimation during the last phase of an incurable disease?" (*Documentation Catholique*, 1970, p. 963.)

But the criterion of the quality of life is not the only one to be taken into account, since, as we have said above, subjective considerations must enter into a properly cautious judgment as to what therapy to undertake and what therapy not. The fundamental point is that the decision should be made according to rational arguments that have taken well into account the many and various aspects of the situation, including what effect will be had upon the family. The principle to follow is, therefore, that no moral obligation to have recourse to extraordinary measures exists; and that, incidentally, a doctor must follow the wishes of a sick person who refuses such measures.

2.4.4 OBLIGATORY MINIMAL MEASURES

On the contrary, there remains the strict obligation to apply under all circumstances those therapeutic measures which are called "minimal": that is, those which are normally and customarily used for the maintenance of life (alimentation, blood transfusions, injections, etc.). To interrupt these minimal measures would, in practice, be equivalent to wishing to put an end to the patient's life.

DOCUMENT 4 / Hydration and Nutrition

SOURCE: Joint Statement by 16 of the 18 Texas Catholic Bishops and the Texas Conference of Catholic Health Facilities, "On Withdrawing Artificial Nutrition and Hydration," *Origins* 20: no. 4 (June 7, 1990), p. 53.

. . . Catholic health facilities have a special duty to reflect Roman Catholic teaching while carrying out the compassionate healing ministry of Jesus Christ.

. . . The Texas Conference of Catholic Health Facilities, to ensure consonance with the teachings of the Catholic Church in all of its activities, consulted the bishops of Texas on the subject of forgoing and withdrawing of artificial nutrition and hydration. This consultation contributed to this statement, which addresses the moral aspects of this issue.

BASIC MORAL PRINCIPLES

. . . Although life always is a good, there are conditions which, if present, lessen or remove one's obligation to sustain life.

. . . If the reasonable foreseen benefits to the patient in the use of any means outweigh the burdens to the patient or others, then those means are morally obligatory. . . . There is no moral distinction to be made between the forgoing and withdrawing of life-sustaining procedures.

. . . If the means used to prolong life are disproportionately burdensome compared with the benefits to the patient, then those means need not be used, they are morally optional.

. . . The Declaration on Euthanasia, as well as the teaching of Pius XII, explicitly states that such forgoing or withdrawing are not suicide, rather they should be considered as the acceptance of the human condition and simply letting nature take its course. The omission of life-sustaining means (whether it be a mechanical respirator, a cardiac pacemaker, a renal dialysis machine, or artificial nutrition and hydration) can be acceptable under conditions which render those means morally non-obligatory. In those appropriate cases the decision maker is not guilty of murder, suicide, or assisted suicide, since there is no moral obligation under these circumstances to impede the normal consequences of the underlying pathology. The physical cause of death is ultimately the pathology which required the use of those means in the first place.

APPLICATION TO PERSISTENT VEGETATIVE STATE

. . . Patients, competently diagnosed to be in a persistent vegetative state or in an irreversible coma, remain human persons. Nonetheless, those individuals are stricken with a lethal pathology which, without artificial nutrition and hydration, will lead to death.

. . . The morally appropriate forgoing or withdrawing of artificial nutrition and hydration from a permanently unconscious person is not abandoning that **221**

222   person. Rather, it is accepting the fact that the person has come to the end of his or her pilgrimage and should not be impeded from taking the final step. The forgoing or withdrawing of artificial nutrition and hydration should only occur after there has been sufficient deliberation based upon the best medical and personal information available.

31: Informed Consent

DOCUMENT 1:

SOURCE: Pope Pius XII, "The Intangibility of the Human Person" (Sept. 13, 1952), *The Human Body: Papal Teachings*, pp. 198–201.

THE INTERESTS OF THE PATIENT

... First of all, one must suppose that the doctor, as a private person, cannot take any measure or try an intervention without the consent of the patient. The doctor has only that power over the patient which the latter gives him, be it explicitly, or implicitly and tacitly. The patient, for his part, cannot confer rights which he does not possess. The decisive point, in this problem, is the moral legitimacy of the right which the patient has at his own disposal. This is where is marked out the moral frontier for the doctor who acts with the consent of the patient.

... The patient has not the right to involve his physical and psychic integrity in medical experiments or researches, when these interventions entail, either immediately or subsequently, acts of destruction, or of mutilation and wounds, or grave dangers.

Furthermore, in exercising his right to dispose of himself, of his faculties and organs, the individual must observe the hierarchy of the scale of values, and within an identical order of values, the hierarchy of individual goods, to the extent demanded by the laws of morality. So, for example, man cannot perform upon himself or allow medical operations, either physical or somatic, which beyond doubt do remove serious defects or physical or psychic weaknesses, but which entail at the same time permanent destruction of, or a considerable and lasting lessening of freedom, that is to say, of the human personality in its particular and characteristic function. Thus is man degraded to the level of a being purely sensitive to acquired reflexes, or of an automaton. Such a reversal of values the moral law does not support; therefore here it establishes the limits and frontiers of the "medical interests of the patient."

... So far, we have spoken directly of the patient, not of the doctor, and we have explained at what point the personal rights of the patient to dispose of himself, of his mind, of his body, of his faculties, organs, and functions, come face to face with a moral limit. At the same time, we have found an answer to the question: Where does the moral frontier exist for the doctor in research and the use of new methods and processes in the "interests of the patient"? The frontier is the same as for the patient: It is the one fixed by the judgment of right reason, and it is traced by the demands of the moral law, which is derived from the natural finality or purpose stamped on beings, and

224   from the scale of values expressed by the very nature of things. The boundaries are the same for the doctor as for the patient, because, as we have already said, the doctor, as does the private individual, disposes of rights and those rights alone, which are granted by the patient, and because the patient cannot give more than he possesses himself.

32: In Vitro Fertilization

DOCUMENT 1:

SOURCE: Congregation for the Doctrine of the Faith, "Instruction on Respect for Human Life in Its Origin and on the Dignity of Procreation" (Feb. 22, 1987), *Origins* 16: no. 40, Mar. 19, 1987, pp. 704–07.

PART II—INTERVENTIONS UPON HUMAN PROCREATION

By artificial procreation or artificial fertilization are understood here the different technical procedures directed toward obtaining a human conception in a manner other than the sexual union of man and woman. This Instruction deals with fertilization of an ovum in a test tube (in vitro fertilization) and artificial insemination through transfer into the woman's genital tracts of previously collected sperm.

A preliminary point for the moral evaluation of such technical procedures is constituted by the consideration of the circumstances and consequences which those procedures involve in relation to the respect due the human embryo. Development of the practice of in vitro fertilization has required innumerable fertilizations and destructions of human embryos. Even today, the usual practice presupposes a hyper ovulation on the part of the woman: a number of ova are withdrawn, fertilized, and then cultivated in vitro for some days. Usually not all are transferred into the genital tracts of the woman; some embryos, generally called "spare," are destroyed or frozen. On occasion, some of the implanted embryos are sacrificed for various eugenic, economic, or psychological reasons. Such deliberate destruction of human beings, or their utilization for different purposes to the detriment of their integrity and life, is contrary to the doctrine on procured abortion already recalled.

The connection between in vitro fertilization and the voluntary destruction of human embryos occurs too often. This is significant: through these procedures, with apparently contrary purposes, life and death are subjected to the decision of man, who thus sets himself up as the giver of life and death by decree. This dynamic of violence and domination may remain unnoticed by those very individuals who, in wishing to utilize this procedure, become subject to it themselves. The facts recorded and the cold logic which links them must be taken into consideration for a moral judgment on IVF and ET (in vitro fertilization and embryo transfer): the abortion mentality which has made this procedure possible thus leads, whether one wants it or not, to man's domination over the life and death of his fellow human beings and can lead to a system of radical eugenics.

225

226   Nevertheless, such abuses do not exempt one from a further and thorough ethical study of the techniques of artificial procreation considered in themselves, abstracting as far as possible from the destruction of embryos produced in vitro.

The present instruction will therefore take into consideration in the first place the problems posed by heterologous artificial fertilization (II, 1–3)* and, subsequently, those linked with homologous artificial fertilization (II, 4–6).**

Before formulating an ethical judgment on each of these procedures, the principles and values which determine the moral evaluation of each of them will be considered.

B. HOMOLOGOUS ARTIFICIAL FERTILIZATION

Since heterologous artificial fertilization has been declared unacceptable, the question arises of how to evaluate morally the process of homologous artificial fertilization: IVF and ET and artificial insemination between husband and wife. First a question of principle must be clarified.

4. What connection is required from the moral point of view between procreation and the conjugal act?

a) The Church's teaching on marriage and human procreation affirms the "inseparable connection, willed by God and unable to be broken by man on his own initiative, between the two meanings of the conjugal act: the unitive meaning and the procreative meaning. Indeed, by its intimate structure the conjugal act, while most closely uniting husband and wife, capacitates them for the generation of new lives according to laws inscribed in the very being

---

*By the term *heterologous artificial fertilization or procreation*, the Instruction means techniques used to obtain a human conception artificially by the use of gametes coming from at least one donor other than the spouses who are joined in marriage. Such techniques can be of two types:

a) *Heterologous "in vitro" fertilization* and *embryo transfer*—the technique used to obtain a human conception through the meeting in vitro of gametes taken from at least one donor other than the two spouses joined in marriage.

b) *Heterologous artificial insemination*—the technique used to obtain a human conception through the transfer into the genital tracts of the woman of the sperm previously collected from a donor other than the husband.

**By *artificial homologous fertilization* or *procreation*, the Instruction means the technique used to obtain a human conception using the gametes of the two spouses joined in marriage. Homologous artificial fertilization can be carried out by two different methods:

a) *Homologous "in vitro" fertilization* and *embryo transfer*—the technique used to obtain a human conception through the meeting in vitro of the gametes of the spouses joined in marriage.

b) *Homologous artificial insemination*—the technique used to obtain a human conception through the transfer into the genital tracts of a married woman of the sperm previously collected from her husband.

of man and of woman." This principle, which is based upon the nature of marriage and the intimate connection of the goods of marriage, has well-known consequences on the level of responsible fatherhood and motherhood. "By safeguarding both these essential aspects, the unitive and the procreative, the conjugal act preserves in its fullness the sense of true mutual love and its ordination toward man's exalted vocation to parenthood."

The same doctrine concerning the link between the meanings of the conjugal act and between the goods of marriage throws light on the moral problem of homologous artificial fertilization, since "it is never permitted to separate these different aspects to such a degree as positively to exclude either the procreative intention or the conjugal relation."

Contraception deliberately deprives the conjugal act of its openness to procreation and in this way brings about a voluntary dissociation of the ends of marriage. Homologous artificial fertilization, in seeking a procreation which is not the fruit of a specific act of conjugal union, objectively effects an analogous separation between the goods and the meanings of marriage.

Thus fertilization is licitly sought when it is the result of a "conjugal act which is per se suitable for the generation of children, to which marriage is ordered by its nature and by which the spouses become one flesh." But from the moral point of view procreation is deprived of its proper perfection when it is not desired as the fruit of the conjugal act, that is to say, of the specific act of the spouses' union.

b) The moral value of the intimate link between the goods of marriage and between the meanings of the conjugal act is based upon the unity of the human being, a unity involving body and spiritual soul. Spouses mutually express their personal love in the "language of the body," which clearly involves both "spousal meanings" and parental ones. The conjugal act by which the couples mutually express their self-gift at the same time expresses openness to the gift of life. It is an act that is inseparably corporal and spiritual. It is in their bodies and through their bodies that the spouses consummate their marriage and are able to become father and mother. In order to respect the language of their bodies and their natural generosity, the conjugal union must take place with respect for its openness to procreation; and the procreation of a person must be the fruit and the result of married love. The origin of the human being thus follows from a procreation that is "linked to the union, not only biological but also spiritual, of the parents, made one by the bond of marriage." Fertilization achieved outside the bodies of the couple remains by this very fact deprived of the meanings and the values which are expressed in the language of the body and in the union of human persons.

c) Only respect for the link between the meanings of the conjugal act and respect for the unity of the human being make possible procreation in conformity with the dignity of the person. In his unique and irrepeatable origin, the child must be respected and recognized as equal in personal dignity to those who give him life. The human person must be accepted in his parents' act of union and love; the generation of a child must therefore be the fruit of that

228   mutual giving which is realized in the conjugal act wherein the spouses cooperate as servants and not as masters in the work of the Creator, who is love.

In reality, the origin of a human person is the result of an act of giving. The one conceived must be the fruit of his parents' love. He cannot be desired or conceived as the product of an intervention of medical or biological techniques; that would be equivalent to reducing him to an object of scientific technology. No one may subject the coming of a child into the world to conditions of technical efficiency which are to be evaluated according to standards of control and dominion.

The moral relevance of the link between the meanings of the conjugal act and between the goods of marriage, as well as the unity of the human being and the dignity of his origin, demand that the procreation of a human person be brought about as the fruit of the conjugal act specific to the love between spouses. The link between procreation and the conjugal act is thus shown to be of great importance on the anthropological and moral planes, and it throws light on the positions of the Magisterium with regard to homologous artificial fertilization.

5. Is homologous "in vitro" fertilization morally licit?

The answer to this question is strictly dependent on the principles just mentioned. Certainly one cannot ignore the legitimate aspirations of sterile couples. For some, recourse to homologous in vitro fertilization and embryo transfer appears to be the only way of fulfilling their sincere desire for a child. The question is asked whether the totality of conjugal life in such situations is not sufficient to ensure the dignity proper to human procreation. It is acknowledged that in vitro fertilization and embryo transfer certainly cannot supply for the absence of sexual relations and cannot be preferred to the specific acts of conjugal union, given the risks involved for the child and the difficulties of the procedure. But it is asked whether, when there is no other way of overcoming the sterility which is a source of suffering, homologous in vitro fertilization may not constitute an aid, if not a form of therapy, whereby its moral licitness could be admitted.

The desire for a child—or at the very least an openness to the transmission of life—is a necessary prerequisite from the moral point of view for responsible human procreation. But this good intention is not sufficient for making a positive moral evaluation of in vitro fertilization between spouses. The process of in vitro fertilization and embryo transfer must be judged in itself and cannot borrow its definitive moral quality from the totality of conjugal life of which it becomes part nor from the conjugal acts which may precede or follow it.

It has already been recalled that in the circumstances in which it is regularly practiced in vitro fertilization and embryo transfer involve the destruction of human beings, which is something contrary to the doctrine on the illicitness of abortion previously mentioned. But even in a situation in which every precaution was taken to avoid the death of human embryos, homologous in vitro fertilization and embryo transfer dissociates from the conjugal act the actions which are directed to human fertilization. For this reason the very

nature of homologous in vitro fertilization and embryo transfer also must be   **229**
taken into account, even abstracting from the link with procured abortion.

Homologous in vitro fertilization and embryo transfer is brought about outside the bodies of the couple through actions of third parties whose competence and technical activity determine the success of the procedure. Such fertilization entrusts the life and identity of the embryo into the power of doctors and biologists and establishes the domination of technology over the origin and destiny of the human person. Such a relationship of domination is in itself contrary to the dignity and equality that must be common to parents and children.

Conception in vitro is the result of the technical action which presides over fertilization. Such fertilization is neither in fact achieved nor positively willed as the expression and fruit of a specific act of the conjugal union. In homologous "in vitro" fertilization and embryo transfer, therefore, even if it is considered in the context of de facto existing sexual relations, the generation of the human person is objectively deprived of its proper perfection: namely, that of being the result and fruit of a conjugal act in which the spouses can become "cooperators with God for giving life to a new person."

These reasons enable us to understand why the act of conjugal love is considered in the teaching of the Church as the only setting worthy of human procreation. For the same reasons the so-called "simple case," i.e., a homologous in vitro fertilization and embryo transfer procedure that is free of any compromise with the abortive practice of destroying embryos and with masturbation, remains a technique which is morally illicit because it deprives human procreation of the dignity which is proper and connatural to it.

Certainly, homologous in vitro fertilization and embryo transfer fertilization is not marked by all that ethical negativity found in extraconjugal procreation; the family and marriage continue to constitute the setting for the birth and upbringing of the children. Nevertheless, in conformity with the traditional doctrine relating to the goods of marriage and the dignity of the person, the Church remains opposed from the moral point of view to homologous "in vitro" fertilization. Such fertilization is in itself illicit and in opposition to the dignity of procreation and of the conjugal union, even when everything is done to avoid the death of the human embryo.

Although the manner in which human conception is achieved with in vitro fertilization and embryo transfer cannot be approved, every child who comes into the world must in any case be accepted as a living gift of the divine goodness and must be brought up with love.

DOCUMENT 2 / In Vitro Fertilization

Source: Pope Pius XII, "Fertility and Sterility" (May 19, 1956), *The Human Body: Papal Teachings,* pp. 387–90.

But the Church has likewise rejected the opposite attitude which would pretend to separate, in generation, the biological activity from the personal relation of the married couple. The child is the fruit of the conjugal union when that union finds full expression by bringing into play the organic functions, the associated sensible emotions, and the spiritual and disinterested love which animates the union. It is in the unity of this human act that we should consider the biological conditions of generation. Never is it permitted to separate these various aspects to the positive exclusion either of the procreative intention or of the conjugal relationship. The relationship which unites the father and the mother to their child finds its root in the organic fact and still more in the deliberate conduct of the spouses, who give themselves to each other and whose will to give themselves blossoms forth and finds its true attainment in the being which they bring into the world.

Furthermore, only this consecration of self, begun in generosity and brought to realization in hardship, by the conscious acceptance of the responsibilities which it involves, can guarantee that the task of educating children will be pursued with all the care and courage and patience which it demands. It can therefore be affirmed that human fecundity, beyond the physical factors, takes on essential moral aspects which must necessarily be considered, even when the subject is treated from the medical point of view.

It is quite evident that when the scholar and the physician approach a problem in their specialized field, they have the right to concentrate their attention on its strictly scientific elements and to solve the problem on the basis of these data alone. But when one is confronted with practical applications to man, it is impossible not to take into account the repercussions which the proposed methods will have on the person and his destiny. The greatness of a human act consists precisely in its going beyond the moment itself at which the act is posited to consider the entire orientation of a life, and to bring it into relation with the absolute. This is already true of everyday activity; how much more is it true of an act which involves, with the reciprocal love of the spouses, their future and that of their posterity.

We also believe that it is of capital importance for you, Gentlemen, not to neglect this perspective when you consider the methods of artificial fecundation. The means by which one tends toward the production of a new life take on an essential human significance inseparable from the desired end and susceptible of causing grave harm to this very end if these means are not conformable to reality and to the laws inscribed in the nature of beings.

We have been asked to give some directives on this point also. On the subject of the experiments in artificial human fecundation "in vitro," let it suffice for us to observe that they must be rejected as immoral and absolutely illicit. With regard to the various moral problems which are posed by artificial fecundation, in the ordinary meaning of the expression, or "artificial insemination," we have already expressed our thought in a discourse addressed to physicians on Sept. 29, 1949. (a) For the details we refer you to what we said then and we confine ourself here to repeating the concluding judgment given there: "With regard to artificial fecundation, not only is there reason to be extremely reserved, but it must be absolutely rejected. In speaking thus, one is not necessarily forbidding the use of certain artificial means destined solely to facilitate the natural act or to achieve the attainment of the natural act normally performed." (b) But since artificial fecundation is being more and more widely used, and in order to correct some erroneous opinions which are being spread concerning what we have taught, we have the following to add:

Artificial fecundation exceeds the limits of the right which spouses have acquired by the matrimonial contract, namely, that of fully exercising their natural sexual capacity in the natural accomplishment of the marital act. The contract in question does not confer on them a right to artificial fecundation, for such a right is not in any way expressed in the right to the natural conjugal act and cannot be deduced from it. Still less can one derive it from the right to the "child," the primary "end" of marriage. The matrimonial contract does not give this right, because it has for its object not the "child," but the "natural acts" which are capable of engendering new life and are destined to this end. It must likewise be said that artificial fecundation violates the natural law and is contrary to justice and morality. . . .

33: Labor Relations

DOCUMENT 1:

SOURCE: Pope John Paul II, "On Human Work" (Sept. 15, 1981), *Origins* 11: no. 15, Sept. 24, 1981, p. 232.

9. WORK AND PERSONAL DIGNITY

Remaining within the context of man as the subject of work, it is now appropriate to touch upon, at least in a summary way, certain problems that more closely define the dignity of human work in that they make it possible to characterize more fully its specific moral value. In doing this we must always keep in mind the biblical calling to "subdue the earth," in which is expressed the will of the Creator that work should enable man to achieve that "dominion" in the visible world that is proper to him.

God's fundamental and original intention with regard to man, whom he created in his image and after his likeness, was not withdrawn or canceled out even when man, having broken the original covenant with God, heard the words: "In the sweat of your face you shall eat bread." These words refer to the sometimes heavy toil that from then onward has accompanied human work; but they do not alter the fact that work is the means whereby man achieves that "dominion" which is proper to him over the visible world, by "subjecting" the earth. Toil is something that is universally known, for it is universally experienced. It is familiar to those doing physical work under sometimes exceptionally laborious conditions. It is familiar not only to agricultural workers, who spend long days working the land, which sometimes "bears thorns and thistles," but also to those who work in mines and quarries, to steelworkers at their blast furnaces, to those who work in builders' yards and in construction work, often in danger of injury or death. It is also familiar to those at an intellectual workbench; to scientists; to those who bear the burden of grave responsibility for decisions that will have a vast impact on society. It is familiar to doctors and nurses, who spend days and nights at their patients' bedside. It is familiar to women, who sometimes without proper recognition on the part of society and even of their own families bear the daily burden and responsibility for their homes and the upbringing of their children. It is familiar to all workers and, since work is a universal calling, it is familiar to everyone.

And yet in spite of all this toil—perhaps, in a sense, because of it—work is a good thing for man. Even though it bears the mark of a *bonum arduum*, in the terminology of St. Thomas, this does not take away the fact that, as such, it is a good thing for man. It is not only good in the sense that it is useful or

something to enjoy; it is also good as being something worthy, that is to say,   **233**
something that corresponds to man's dignity, that expresses this dignity and
increases it. If one wishes to define more clearly the ethical meaning of work,
it is this truth that one must particularly keep in mind. Work is a good thing
for man—a good thing for his humanity—because through work man not only
transforms nature, adapting it to his own needs, but he also achieves fulfillment
as a human being and indeed in a sense becomes "more a human being."

Without this consideration it is impossible to understand the meaning of
the virtue of industriousness, and more particularly it is impossible to understand why industriousness should be a virtue: for virtue, as a moral habit, is
something whereby man becomes good as man. This fact in no way alters our
justifiable anxiety that in work, whereby matter gains in nobility, man himself
should not experience a lowering of his own dignity. Again, it is well known
that it is possible to use work in various ways against man, that it is possible
to punish man with the system of forced labor in concentration camps, that
work can be made into a means for oppressing man, and that in various ways
it is possible to exploit human labor, that is to say, the worker. All this pleads
in favor of the moral obligation to link industriousness as a virtue with the
social order of work, which will enable man to become in work "more a human
being" and not be degraded by it not only because of the wearing out of his
physical strength (which, at least up to a certain point, is inevitable), but
especially through damage to the dignity and subjectivity that are proper to him.

20. IMPORTANCE OF UNIONS

All these rights, together with the need for the workers themselves to
secure them, give rise to yet another right: the right of association, that is, to
form associations for the purpose of defending the vital interests of those
employed in the various professions. These associations are called labor or
trade unions. The vital interests of the workers are to a certain extent common
for all of them; at the same time, however, each type of work, each profession,
has its own specific character which should find a particular reflection in these
organizations.

In a sense, unions go back to the medieval guilds of artisans, insofar as
those organizations brought together people belonging to the same craft and
thus on the basis of their work. However, unions differ from the guilds on this
essential point: the modern unions grew up from the struggle of the workers—
workers in general but especially the industrial workers—to protect their just
rights vis-à-vis the entrepreneurs and the owners of the means of production.
Their task is to defend the existential interests of workers in all sectors in which
their rights are concerned. The experience of history teaches that organizations
of this type are an indispensable element of social life, especially in modern
industrialized societies. Obviously this does not mean that only industrial
workers can set up associations of this type. Representatives of every profession
can use them to ensure their own rights. . . .

Just efforts to secure the rights of workers who are united by the same
profession should always take into account the limitations imposed by the

234 general economic situation of the country. Union demands cannot be turned into a kind of group or class "egoism," although they can and should also aim at correcting—with a view to the common good of the whole of society—everything defective in the system of ownership of the means of production or in the way these are managed. Social and socioeconomic life is certainly like a system of "connected vessels," and every social activity directed toward safeguarding the rights of particular groups should adapt itself to this system. . . .

One method used by unions in pursuing the just rights of their members is the strike or work stoppage, as a kind of ultimatum to the competent bodies, especially the employers. This method is recognized by Catholic social teaching as legitimate in the proper conditions and within just limits. In this connection workers should be assured the right to strike, without being subjected to personal penal sanctions for taking part in a strike. While admitting that it is a legitimate means, we must at the same time emphasize that a strike remains, in a sense, an extreme means. It must not be abused; it must not be abused especially for "political" purposes. Furthermore, it must never be forgotten that when essential community services are in question, they must in every case be ensured, if necessary, by means of appropriate legislation. Abuse of the strike weapon can lead to the paralysis of the whole of socioeconomic life, and this is contrary to the requirements of the common good of society, which also corresponds to the properly understood nature of work itself.

DOCUMENT 2 / Labor Relations

SOURCE: Bishops of Texas and the Texas Conference of Catholic Health Facilities, "Labor Relations in Catholic Hospitals" (April 1983), *Origins* 13: no. 3 (June 2, 1983), pp. 53–54.

Catholic health care facilities have the important role of carrying forward a ministry of the Church in promoting health and caring for the sick and elderly. Although independent of diocesan structures in their routine operations, nonetheless they reflect the teachings of the Church in their private and public posture. Applying these teachings in a health care setting can be at once challenging and complex. To meet one such challenge—that of service to patients while at the same time safeguarding the rights of employees—the Texas Conference of Catholic Health Facilities and the bishops of Texas have formulated the following joint statement on labor relations.

Catholic health care facilities in Texas have a long-standing tradition of serving the aged, the sick, and the dying—the poor as well as the rich. Their commitment is not simply to the well-being of the patients, but to their spiritual, psychological, and emotional needs as well, a commitment that is both a sign and an instrument of the healing ministry of the Church.

Catholic employers are well aware of the dedication of their employees in the health care ministry. They are also keenly aware of the greatly changing socioeconomic conditions affecting both institutions and workers. Rising costs and reduced third-party reimbursement are threatening the very existence of many health care facilities. The problems generated by these conditions can tear at the very fabric of cooperation between employer and employee in their attempts to maintain a spirit of trust and collaboration.

As an employer desiring to uphold the dignity of the worker and as an authentic witness to the Church's teachings, each Catholic health care facility recognizes and supports the rights of its employees, including:

—a just, living wage;

—benefits intended to promote the life and health of both workers and their families;

—a reasonable degree of job satisfaction, good working conditions, and continuing dialogue with management;

—personnel policies that provide a formal grievance procedure, permitting arbitration as a final step in the process;

—the seeking of union representation and collective bargaining without fear of reprisal.

The Catholic Church has a deep interest in issues related to the obligations and rights of the worker. In his encyclical letter "On Human Work," Pope John Paul II stated:

236 "All these rights, together with the need for the workers themselves to secure them, give rise to yet another right: the right of association, that is, to form associations for the purpose of defending the vital interests of those employed in the various professions" (no. 20).

Recognition must therefore be given to the worker's right to seek union representation and to bargain collectively without fear of threat, coercion, or intimidation, however subtle. The choice of the worker to select or reject union representation must be a free one. However, any discussion concerning unionization in a Catholic health care facility must take into special account the unique services that such institutions provide. Since their primary concern is the care of the sick and the preservation of life and dignity, both labor and management must hold the welfare of the patient as their first priority. Indeed, the principles of social justice apply equally to employee, employer, and patient.

Employees must always remember that if their services are collectively withdrawn, the welfare of the patient can be seriously jeopardized. Therefore, no action should be taken by workers that would endanger the life or quality of care of the patients entrusted to them. For, as Pope John Paul II has said relative to the abuse of the right to strike, "It must never be forgotten that when essential community services are in question, they must in every case be ensured, if necessary, by means of appropriate legislation" (no. 20).

In any union organizing drive both labor organizers and management should be cautioned against becoming overly zealous in their efforts to influence the votes of employees. Any communication in these matters on the part of organizers or management in Catholic health care facilities should be open, honest, and nonoppressive, and always with a view toward the common good.

The decision of a Catholic health care facility to recruit a consultant during any union organizing effort is also reasonable and should not be seen as a threat to the worker. Before hiring a consultant, however, the institutions should ensure that his or her approach will be consistent with the rights of both employee and employer, as reflected in Church teachings. The methods espoused must not violate the worker's freedom or generate a spirit of mistrust.

Resolution of all matters of controversy between labor and management must be focused on the common responsibility—namely, the patient's welfare. For their part, the employees will work to capacity and will respect the right of patients to quality care and will contribute to the achievement of the goals set by the facility. Management, on the other hand, will continually seek ways to promote justice, seeking to integrate employees more fully into the life of the facility through open communication and participatory decision making.

34: Living Will

DOCUMENT 1:

Source: National Conference of Catholic Bishops Committee on Pro-Life Activities, "The Rights of the Terminally Ill" (July 2, 1986), *Origins* 16: no. 12, Sept. 4, 1986, pp. 222–24.

In proposing a Uniform Rights of the Terminally Ill Act for enactment by state legislatures, the National Conference of Commissioners on Uniform State Laws has presented legislators with a new and complex challenge. The Uniform Act is designed to eliminate disparities among state laws on withholding and withdrawing life-sustaining treatment; such laws have been enacted in most of the fifty states over the past decade. Yet some of the provisions of the Uniform Act raise new and significant moral problems, highlighting the need for serious debate on the purpose and risks of legislation on this subject.

As Catholic bishops in the United States we feel a responsibility to contribute to this debate. We are concerned that legislation which is ethically unsound will further compromise the right to life and respect for life in American society. Moreover, we are confident that our Church's moral tradition can be of great assistance in determining the extent to which legislative proposals in this area are consistent with sound moral principles.

In keeping with this tradition we uphold the duty to preserve life while recognizing certain limits to that duty. We absolutely reject euthanasia, by which we mean "an act or an omission which of itself or by intention causes death, in order that all suffering may in this way be eliminated" (Vatican Declaration on Euthanasia, 1980). We maintain that one is obliged to use "ordinary" means of preserving life—that is, means which can effectively preserve life without imposing grave burdens on the patient—and we see the failure to supply such means as "equivalent to euthanasia" (U.S. Catholic Conference, "Ethical and Religious Directives for Catholic Health Facilities," 1975, no.28). But we also recognize and defend a patient's right to refuse "extraordinary" means, that is, means which provide no benefit or which involve too grave a burden. In cases where patients cannot speak for themselves, we urge family members, others qualified to interpret the patient's intentions, and physicians to be guided by these fundamental moral principles.

The task of judging how these principles can best be incorporated into social policy is complex and difficult. For example, various proposals giving legal force to an advance declaration or "living will" have been offered as ways of clarifying a terminally ill patient's legitimate right to refuse extraordinary medical treatment. From one perspective, clarification of this right seems

238 increasingly necessary as physicians, concerned about legal liability, seek guidance concerning their legal rights and responsibilities. Indeed, public support for such legislation is due in large part to a concern that some physicians are resisting even morally appropriate requests for withdrawal of treatment when these requests have no explicit statutory recognition.

Yet the operative provisions of such legislation, and their degree of conformity with Catholic moral teaching, vary widely from state to state. Some "living will" proposals have been formulated and promoted by right-to-die groups which see them as stepping stones to the eventual legalization of euthanasia. In fact, some existing laws and proposals could be read not merely as stepping stones but as actually authorizing euthanasia in certain circumstances. Many "living will" statutes reflect a bias toward facilitating only the right to refuse means for sustaining life, instead of facilitating morally responsible decisions either to provide or to withhold treatment in accord with the wishes and best interests of the patient.

Due to concerns such as these, the Bishops' Committee for Pro-Life Activities has neither endorsed nor encouraged the trend toward enactment of "living will" legislation. Indeed, many people dedicated to the protection of human life have judged these concerns serious enough to warrant outright opposition to some legislative proposals of this kind, and have sought to amend other proposals to reduce their potential for abuse. As more states have debated and enacted a variety of legislative standards on this subject, we have sought to provide guidance by pointing out serious problems which deserve the special attention of legislators.

Our most comprehensive set of criteria for assessing these problems can be found in the "Guidelines for Legislation on Life-Sustaining Treatment" issued by the bishops' committee in November 1984. Such criteria should not be taken as implying support for legislation of this kind; but if incorporated into law they can help safeguard the rights of the terminally ill and uphold the value of human life in this complex area.

THE UNIFORM ACT: AN ANALYSIS

The Uniform Rights of the Terminally Ill Act merits special consideration because it is designed for nationwide enactment and will undoubtedly be considered in many state legislatures. Assessing the proposed Act in the light of Catholic moral principles, we find that it poses at least three serious problems not always encountered in laws of this kind.

1. The Scope of the Uniform Act. Like most "living will" laws, the Uniform Act is intended to authorize withdrawal of life-sustaining treatment from patients in the final stage of a terminal condition, that is, patients who will inevitably die soon. But the ambiguity of key terms in the Uniform Act's "definitions" section creates the potential for a much broader application. For example, the Act could be read as authorizing withdrawal of life-sustaining treatment in cases where the patient could live a long time with treatment but will die quickly without it. Patients who have an incurable or irreversible disabling condition might be seen as falling within this broader scope. In such

cases, even treatment that is not unduly burdensome and could effectively **239** prolong life may be dismissed as merely "prolonging the process of dying" and hence removed. Such an interpretation would allow withholding of customary and beneficial medical procedures in order to hasten the patient's death. Thus the potential for abuse is greater here than in laws whose scope is clearly limited to patients in the final stage of a terminal condition.

2. Nutrition and Hydration. Because human life has inherent value and dignity regardless of its condition, every patient should be provided with measures which can effectively preserve life without involving too grave a burden. Since food and water are necessities of life for all human beings, and can generally be provided without the risks and burdens of more aggressive means for sustaining life, the law should establish a strong presumption in favor of their use.

The Uniform Act states that it will not affect any existing responsibility to provide measures such as nutrition and hydration to promote comfort. But it does not adequately recognize a distant and more fundamental benefit of such measures—that of sustaining life itself. This is a serious lapse in light of the ambiguous scope of the Uniform Act, which may include cases in which a patient will live a long time with treatment but die quickly without it. For most patients, measures for providing nourishment are morally obligatory even when other treatment can be withdrawn due to its burdensomeness or ineffectiveness.

Negative judgments about the "quality of life" of unconscious or otherwise disabled patients have led some in our society to propose withholding nourishment precisely in order to end these patients' lives. Society must take special care to protect against such discrimination. Laws dealing with medical treatment may have to take account of exceptional circumstances, when even means for providing nourishment may become too ineffective or burdensome to be obligatory. But such laws must establish clear safeguards against intentionally hastening the deaths of vulnerable patients by starvation or dehydration.

3. Treatment of Pregnant Women. The Uniform Act explicitly allows a pregnant woman to refuse treatment that could save the life of her unborn child whenever she herself fulfills the conditions of the Uniform Act. The State is thus placed in the position of ratifying and facilitating a decision to end the life of the child. This provision goes beyond even the U.S. Supreme Court's decisions which removed most legal restrictions on abortion. Instead of ignoring the unborn child's independent interest in life, the law should provide for continued treatment if it could benefit the child.

OTHER PROBLEM AREAS

Although the above are the most serious flaws in the proposed Uniform Act, it also contains other problem areas which deserve comment:

—The absence of a preamble stating the exact purpose of the Act is a notable deficiency, because such a preamble could assert a presumption in favor of life and thereby help to eliminate ambiguities in the judicial interpretation of the Uniform Act. For example, a preamble could clearly recognize that a

240 patient's right to refuse treatment is limited by certain legitimate state interests, such as interests in preserving life, preventing suicide and homicide, protecting dependent third parties, and maintaining sound ethics in the medical profession.

—The Act fails to define euthanasia, or to explain whether this word is meant to include euthanasia by omission, thus reducing the effectiveness of its disclaimer that it does not authorize euthanasia.

—The broad immunities given for withdrawing life-sustaining treatment, and the penalties imposed upon physicians who do not obey a patient's directive, reinforce the Act's bias toward withdrawing treatment and even encourage such withdrawal in doubtful cases.

—The Act does not encourage communication among patient, family, and physician, but tends to exclude family members from the decision-making process.

—The vaguely worded directive intended for a patient's signature provides very little information to help the patient appreciate the scope of the power being granted to a physician. For example, the patient is given no warning that his or her directive may authorize withdrawal of food and water, or that it may apply to situations where he or she could live a long time with continued treatment.

CONCLUSION

The NCCB Committee for Pro-Life Activities has provided this analysis in order to indicate some serious problems raised by much current "living will" legislation and by the proposed Uniform Rights of the Terminally Ill Act. We believe that legislators considering such proposals must appreciate the importance of examining them in the light of sound moral principles, precisely because these are matters of life and death for some of the most helpless members of our society. Above all, public policy in this area must be based on a positive attitude toward disabled and terminally ill patients, who have a right to live with dignity and with reasonable care until the moment of death.

DOCUMENT 2 / Living Will

SOURCE: National Conference of Catholic Bishops Committee for Pro-Life Activities, "Guidelines for Legislation on Life-Sustaining Treatment" (Nov. 10, 1984), *Origins* 14: no. 32, Jan. 24, 1985, pp. 526–28.

MORAL PRINCIPLES

Our Judeo-Christian heritage celebrates life as the gift of a loving God, and respects the life of each human being because each is made in the image and likeness of God. As Christians we also celebrate the fact that we are redeemed by Christ and called to share eternal life with him. From these roots the Roman Catholic tradition has developed a distinctive approach to fostering and sustaining human life. Our tradition not only condemns direct attacks on innocent life, but also promotes a general view of life as a sacred trust over which we can claim stewardship but not absolute dominion. As conscientious stewards, we see a duty to preserve life while recognizing certain limits to that duty, as was reiterated most recently in the Vatican Declaration on Euthanasia. This and other documents have set forth the following moral principles defining a "stewardship of life" ethic:

1. The Second Vatican Council condemned crimes against life, including "euthanasia or willful suicide" (*Gaudium et Spes*, 27). Grounded as it is in respect for the dignity and fundamental rights of the human person, this teaching cannot be rejected on grounds of political pluralism or religious freedom.

2. As human life is the basis and necessary condition for all other human goods, it has a special value and significance; both murder and suicide are violations of human life.

3. "Euthanasia" is "an action or an omission which of itself or by intention causes death, in order that all suffering may in this way be eliminated" (Declaration on Euthanasia). It is an attack on human life which no one has a right to make or request. Although individual guilt may be reduced or absent because of suffering or emotional factors which cloud the conscience, this does not change the objective wrong of the act. It should also be recognized that an apparent plea for death may really be a plea for help and love.

4. Suffering is a fact of human life and has special significance for the Christian as an opportunity to share in Christ's redemptive suffering. Nevertheless there is nothing wrong in trying to relieve someone's suffering as long as this does not interfere with other moral and religious duties. For example, it is permissible in the case of terminal illness to use painkillers which carry the risk of shortening life, so long as the intent is to relieve pain effectively rather than to cause death.

5. Everyone has the duty to care for his or her own health and to seek necessary medical care from others, but this does not mean that all possible

242 remedies must be used in all circumstances. One is not obliged to use "extraordinary" means, that is, means which offer no reasonable hope of benefit or which involve excessive hardship. Such decisions are complex and should be made by the patient in consultation with his or her family and physician whenever possible.

Although these principles have grown out of a specific religious tradition, they appeal to a common respect for the dignity of the human person rather than to any specific denomination stance. We offer them without hesitation to the consideration of men and women of goodwill, and commend them to the attention of legislators and other policy makers. We see them as especially appropriate to a society which, whatever its moral and political pluralism, was founded on the belief that all human beings are created equal as bearers of the inalienable right to life.

LEGISLATIVE GUIDELINES

Today the application of these principles to the legislative debate regarding treatment of the terminally ill is both difficult and necessary. The medical treatment of terminally ill patients, including the withdrawal of extraordinary means, has always been subject to legal constraints. Since 1975, however, an increasing number of court decisions and legislative enactments have interpreted and changed these constraints. Some decisions and enactments have been constructive, but others have not. Technological changes in medicine occur so rapidly that it is difficult to keep pace with them. These changes have had a drastic effect on the physician-patient relationship and make much more difficult the decision process by which a patient determines treatment with the counsel and support of physician and family.

As problems and confusions surrounding the treatment of terminally ill patients continue to multiply, new legislation dealing with this subject is being enacted in some states and proposed in many others. Yet the law relating to the treatment of terminally ill patients still differs from state to state and does not always adequately reflect the moral principles which we endorse. The Church therefore feels an obligation to provide its guidance through participation in the current debate.

In light of these considerations, we suggest the following as ways of respecting the moral principles listed above as well as related concerns of the Church, whenever there is a debate on whether existing or proposed legislation adequately addresses this subject. Such legislation should:

(a) Presuppose the fundamental right to life of every human being, including the disabled, the elderly, and the terminally ill. In general, phrases which seem to romanticize death, such as "right to die" or "death with dignity," should be avoided.

(b) Recognize that the right to refuse medical treatment is not an independent right, but is a corollary to the patient's right and moral responsibility to request reasonable treatment. The law should demonstrate no preference for protecting only the right to refuse treatment, particularly when life-sustaining treatment is under consideration.

(c) Place the patient's right to determine medical care within the context   **243**
of other factors which limit the exercise of that right—e.g., the state's interest
in protecting innocent third parties, preventing homicide and suicide, and
maintaining good ethical standards in the health care profession. Policy statements which define the right to refuse treatment in terms of the patient's
constitutional rights (e.g., a "right of privacy") tend to inhibit the careful balancing of all the interests that should be considered in such cases.

(d) Promote communication among patient, family, and physician. Current "living will" laws tend to have the opposite effect—that of excluding
family members and other loved ones from the decision-making process. As a
general rule, documents and legal proceedings are no substitute for a physician's personal consultation with the patient and/or family at the time a decision must be made on a particular course of treatment.

(e) Avoid granting unlimited power to a document or proxy decision
maker to make health care decisions on a patient's behalf. The right to make
such decisions on one's own behalf is itself not absolute and in any event
cannot be fully exercised when a patient has had no opportunity to assess the
burdens and benefits of treatment in a specific situation. Laws which allow a
decision to be made on behalf of a mentally incompetent patient must include
safeguards to ensure that the decision adequately represents the patient's wishes
or best interests and is in accord with responsible medical practice.

(f) Clarify the rights and responsibilities of physicians without granting
blanket immunity from all legal liability. No physician should be protected from
liability for acting homicidally or negligently. Nor should new legal penalties be
imposed on a physician for failing to obey a patient's or proxy's wishes when
such obedience would violate the physician's ethical convictions or professional standards.

(g) Reaffirm public policies against homicide and assisted suicide. Medical
treatment legislation may clarify procedures for discontinuing treatment which
only secures a precarious and burdensome prolongation of life for the terminally
ill patient, but should not condone or authorize any deliberate act or omission
designed to cause a patient's death.

(h) Recognize the presumption that certain basic measures such as nursing
care, hydration, nourishment, and the like must be maintained out of respect
for the human dignity of every patient.

(i) Protect the interests of innocent parties who are not competent to make
treatment decisions on their own behalf. Life-sustaining treatment should not
be discriminatorily withheld or withdrawn from mentally incompetent or retarded patients.

(j) Provide that life-sustaining treatment should not be withdrawn from
a pregnant woman if continued treatment may benefit her unborn child.

These guidelines are not intended to provide an exhaustive description of
good legislation or to endorse the viewpoint that every state requires new legislation on treatment of the terminally ill. They outline a general approach which, we
believe, will help clarify rights and responsibilities with regard to such treatment
without sacrificing a firm commitment to the sacredness of human life.

DOCUMENT 3 / Living Will

Source: Pennsylvania Bishops, "Living Will and Proxy for Health Care Decisions," *Origins* 23: no. 10 (Aug. 12, 1993), p. 162.

Preamble

Our Judeo-Christian heritage holds that life is the gift of a loving God. I understand also as a Catholic that I may never choose to cause my death. Therefore, I believe that euthanasia and suicide constitute an unwarranted destruction of human life and are not morally permissible.

I understand that I have the right to make decisions about my health care. There may come a time when I am unable, due to physical or mental incapacity, to express my own health care decisions. In these circumstances, those caring for me will need direction concerning my care and will turn to someone who knows my values and health care wishes. I am, therefore, signing the attached living will, which is my advance directive for health care, to provide the guidance and authority needed to implement my decisions.

35: Medical Profession

DOCUMENT 1:

SOURCE: Pope Pius XII, "The Exalted Character of the Medical Profession" (Feb. 13, 1945), *The Human Body: Papal Teachings*, pp. 67–70.

We are delighted to extend a welcome to you, distinguished members of the Army Medical Corps; and to express to you in person the satisfaction we held on hearing of your congress here in Rome. Despite the demands of a violent and unabating war, you have found it possible, shall we not say necessary, to meet together for a few days to discuss the problems of your profession, and to perfect through mutual help the means of confronting and solving them. It shows that you are keenly alive to the first duty of every physician, to be constantly increasing his fund of knowledge, and to keep quite abreast of the scientific progress being made in his particular field.

This duty arises at once from the doctor's responsibility to the individual and the community. God is not the author of death. That monster gained entrance into the world through sin—that original sin which, while it snuffed out the supernatural life in man's soul, laid heavy hand also on his body, robbing it of that gift of immortality which God had willed to grant it despite the exigencies of its nature. And man began that struggle, more or less constant, more or less acute, against physical weakness, pain and suffering, and decomposition that increasingly mark the stages of his path, until the point is reached when the inexorable sentence hanging over all flesh brings blessed relief. But in that struggle God has not abandoned the creature of his omnipotent love. "The most High hath created medicines out of the earth; and a wise man will not abhor them. . . . The virtue of these things is come to the knowledge of men; the Most High hath given knowledge to men, that he may be honored in his wonders." So you read in the Book of Ecclesiasticus; and the inspired writer continues: "My son, in the sickness neglect not thyself . . . give place to the physician, for the Lord hath created him; and let him not depart from thee, for his works are necessary" (verses 9–12).

Yes, necessary; and man's need will be the measure of the doctor's responsibility. How exalted, how worthy of all honor is the character of your profession! The doctor has been appointed by God himself to minister to the needs of suffering humanity. He who created that fever-consumed or mangled frame, now in your hands, who loves it with an eternal love, confides to you the ennobling charge of restoring it to health. You will bring to the sickroom and to the operating table something of the charity of God, of the love and tenderness of Christ, the Master Physician of soul and body. That charity is not a superficial,

246   irresolute sentiment; it does not write a diagnosis to please or curry favor; it is blind as well to the alluring trappings of wealth as to the unpleasant wretchedness of poverty or destitution; it is deaf to the appeals of base passion that would seek cooperation in evil-doing. For it is a love that embraces the whole man, a fellow human being, whose sickly body is still vivified by an immortal soul bonded by every right of creation and redemption to the will of its divine Master. That will is clearly written for those who wish to read, first in the essential scope that nature has manifestly attributed to the human organs, and then positively in the Ten Commandments. That genuine love will exclude any reason, however grave, that may be adduced as a warrant for a patient or doctor to do or counsel aught that would contravene that supreme will.

That is why a doctor, worthy of his profession, rising to the full height of unselfish, fearless devotion to his noble mission of healing and saving life, will scorn any suggestion made to destroy life, however frail or humanly useless it may appear, knowing that unless a man is guilty of some crime deserving the death penalty, God alone, no power on earth, may dispose of his life. As a special minister of the God of nature he will never countenance the deliberate frustration of nature's priceless power to generate life. Uncompromisingly loyal to these and to other fundamental principles of ethics and Christian morality the medical profession will be the truest friend of the individual and the community, the firmest bulwark against the enemies from without and within, a veritable channel of earthly and heavenly blessings to the nation which it honors. The skill of the physician shall raise him to eminence among men, and in the sight of great men he shall be praised; the gifts of the king shall be reserved for him. That the blessing of the King of Kings may descend upon you and all your dear ones and your loved countries and remain forever, is the wish and prayer that rise from our affectionate paternal heart.

DOCUMENT 2 / Medical Profession
(Cf. also Confidentiality)

SOURCE: Pope Pius XII, "The Foundation of Medical Morality" (Oct. 19, 1953), *The Human Body: Papal Teachings,* pp. 281–83.

As your reports show, the problem of moral limits became clear in your own discussions, and various opinions were then expressed. We said last year that the doctor justifies his decisions by the interests of science, of the patient, and of the common good. The interest of science has already been discussed. As for the interests of the patient, the doctor has no more right to intervene than the patient gives him. The patient, on his part, the individual himself, has no right to dispose of his own existence, of the integrity of his organism, of his particular organs, and of their functional capacity, except in the measure demanded by the good of the whole organism.

This provides the key for the answer to the question which has interested you. May the doctor apply a dangerous remedy, undertake interventions which will probably or certainly be fatal, solely because the patient wishes it and consents? Likewise to the question, in itself understandable by the doctor working just behind the front lines or at a military hospital; could he, in a case of insupportable or incurable suffering, or horrible wounds, administer, at the express demand of the patient, injections which are equivalent to euthanasia?

Now with regard to the interest of the community, public authority has, in general, no direct right to dispose of the existence and the integrity of the organs of its innocent subjects. As to the question of corporal punishment and the death penalty, we do not discuss it here, since we are speaking of the doctor, not of the executioner. Since the state does not possess this direct right of disposition, it cannot then communicate it to the doctor for any motive or end whatsoever. The political community is not a physical being as is an organic body, but a whole which possesses only a unity of purpose and action. Man does not exist for the state but the state for man. When there is a question of irrational beings, plants or animals, man is free to dispose of their existence and life (not forgetting the obligation which he has before God and his own dignity to avoid unjustified brutality and cruelty), but not of other men or of subordinates.

The military doctor derives from this a sure directive, which, without taking away from him the responsibility of his decision, is capable of saving him from errors of judgment, by furnishing him with a clear, objective standard.

A word remains to be said about the control and the sanctions of the medical conscience.

The final and highest control is the Creator himself, God. We would not do justice to the fundamental principles of your program and to the consequences derived therefrom, were we to describe them merely as requirements of

248 mankind, as humanitarian ends and aims. They are also that, but they are essentially more. The ultimate source whence they derive force and dignity is the Creator of human nature. If it were simply a matter of principles elaborated by the will of men only, then their obligation would have no more binding force than men have; they could be applicable today and be passed over tomorrow; one country could accept them and another refuse them. The case is just the opposite if the authority of the Creator intervenes. Now, the basic principles of medical ethics are a part of the Divine Law. This, then, is the motive which authorizes the doctor to place unconditional confidence in these principles of medical ethics.

DOCUMENT 3 / Medical Profession

Source: Pope John Paul II, "Catholic Doctors: Higher Witnesses" (Oct. 3, 1982), *The Pope Speaks* 28: no. 1, 1983, pp. 30–35.

. . . The subject of your congress takes up and synthesizes the problem of basic human rights, which is of great concern to me. During every age, man's right to life has been recognized as the first and fundamental right, and as the root and source of every other right.

Life, therefore, is one of the highest values, since it comes directly from God, the origin of every life. Man, as a living being created in the image of the Creator, is, by his nature, immortal.

I see that the concept of the totality of life is appropriately emphasized in the various parts of the congress, in the reports, papers, subjects of discussion. This pleases me since I hold such a basis to be of fundamental importance.

If, in fact, service to life defines the final aim of medicine, the limits of such service can be set only by the true and integral concepts of life. In other words; the service to which you are called must include and at the same time transcend corporality precisely because this is not all there is to life. . . .

. . . For good reason, therefore, you distinguished doctors, convened here to study the many problems which relate to health, have placed emphasis upon the defense of life, inasmuch as in that supreme value are found the ultimate reasons which justify your commitment in the various areas of the respective specializations. Yours is the task of safeguarding life, of taking care that it evolves and develops throughout the span of existence, with respect for the plan mapped out by the Creator.

The increased knowledge of the phenomena which control life has greatly broadened the limits of medical science, whose service takes place in the areas of preventive, curative, rehabilitative medicine, with an inexhaustible effort to prepare, to defend, to correct, to recover vital functions, accompanying the human individual from the earliest stages of life up to the inevitable end.

In addition, today medicine is more than ever at the center of community life, as a determining factor in educational tendencies, in assessment of the whole man, in the organization of related lifestyles, in the recovery of compromised or lost values, in offering to mankind an always new reason for hope.

The Church, since its origin, has always looked upon medicine as an important support of its redemptive mission with regard to mankind. From the ancient xenodochia (houses for the care of the sick) to the first hospital complexes and up to the present, the ministry of Christian witness has progressed at the same pace as that of concern for the sick. And how can we not emphasize the fact that the very presence of the Church in missionary lands is distinguished by careful attention to health problems?

250   This happens not in order to replace or substitute for the function of public institutions, but because services to the spirit of man cannot be fully effective if not presented as a service to his psycho-physical unit. The Church well knows that physical illness imprisons the spirit, just as illness of the spirit enslaves the body.

On the other hand, it is not without significance that saints canonized by the Church—such as John of God and Camillus de Lellis, not to mention many others—have introduced important innovations in the field of an ever more alert and compassionate care for the sick.

On the other hand, a careful study of Christian ascetical norms would reveal no minor contributions to the education of man for the total care of his physical and psychic health. And was it not a colleague of yours, Alexis Carrel, who maintained, for example, that prayer reconciles man with God and with himself, confirming it as a medicine of the spirit with documentable effects upon the total health of the person? (A. Carrel, *La Priere*, Paris 1935).

In consideration of this, the Fathers of the Second Vatican Council, in their appeal to men of knowledge and science, affirmed with moving pride: "Your journey is ours. Your paths are never unrelated to those which are properly ours. We are the friends of your vocation as researchers, the allies of your toils, the leading spirits of your conquests and, if necessary, the comforters of your discouragements and failures. Therefore, we have a message for you too: Continue to search without ever giving up, without ever despairing of the truth. . . ."

In the recent encyclical *Laborem Exercens*, I myself paid tribute to the importance of your role, insisting on the primary right of every individual to what is necessary for the care of his health and, therefore, to adequate health service.

I would like to return to this subject in order to reiterate the duty that is incumbent upon medical science to make progress in order to improve the conditions and the environment in which work, that basic human activity, is carried out. If we want work to become always more personalizing, it is primarily necessary that its wholesomeness be guaranteed.

SPIRIT OF SERVICE

Your commitment, distinguished gentlemen, cannot be limited to only professional correctness but must be sustained by that interior attitude which is fittingly called "spirit of service." In fact, the patient to whom you dedicate your care and your studies is not a nameless individual to whom the fruit of your knowledge is applied, but a responsible person who must be called upon to participate in the improvement of his health and the achievement of his cure. He must be put in the position of being able to make personal choices and not have to submit to the decisions and choices of others.

The appeal to "humanize" the doctor's work and the places where it is practiced is placed in these terms. Such humanization means the proclamation of the dignity of the human person, respect for his corporality, for his spirit, for his culture. It is your task to seek to discover ever more deeply the biological

mechanisms which control life so as to be able to intervene in them, on the   **251**
strength of a power over things, which the Lord has willed to give man.

In so doing, it is also your commitment constantly to keep within the perspective of the human person and of the requirements which spring from his dignity. In more concrete terms, no one of you can limit yourself to being a doctor of an organ or apparatus, but must treat the whole person and, what is more, the interpersonal relationships which contribute to his well-being.

In this regard, the presence of scientists, clinicians, physicians, and health workers from every part of the world inspires me to recall a grave and urgent problem: that of providing for the safeguarding, the defense, and the promotion of human life through the filter of the various cultures.

Inasmuch as he is the image of God, man is the reflection of the infinite countenances which the Creator assumes in his creatures: countenances sketched by the environment, by social conditions, by tradition, in a word, by culture. It is essential that in the various cultural contexts the brilliance of that reflection be not dimmed, nor the features of that image disfigured. It is the task of every citizen, but especially of those who, as you, have direct social responsibilities, to work for the recognition and effective prevention of possible forms of intervention upon man which appear to be in contrast with his dignity as a creature of God.

In order to do this, individual action is not sufficient. Collective, intelligent, well-planned, constant and generous work is required, and not only within the individual countries, but also on an international scale. Coordination on a worldwide level would, in fact, allow a better proclamation and a more effective defense of your faith, of your culture, of your Christian commitment in scientific research and in your profession.

There is a message which I sense in your congress and which must be made ever more explicit through your individual and collective action. It is the appeal to the social community and to those responsible for it that the limitless resources consumed in the technologies of death be transformed into the support and the development of the technologies of life.

Because of a mystery rooted in the complexity and the frailty of the human heart, the option for good and for evil often makes use of identical instruments. Technologies which could work for good are at the same time capable of working immense evil, and only man is the arbiter of their application and their use.

In addition, there are numerous projects in the field of scientific research which have long been awaiting better support in order to be carried on, but instead have been set aside because of lack of funds. Laboratories, from which a word of hope is awaited to combat illnesses particularly widespread in our age, seem to be languishing, certainly not through the fault of well-prepared men, but because the necessary financing is diverted to ways of destruction, war and death.

Nor is the problem different with regard to some other very grave phenomena of our age. Allow me to point out in particular the problem of malnutrition and underdevelopment. Vast areas and entire populations suffering from poverty and hunger emerge today on the demographic map. While rich nations

252   suffer from metabolic illnesses due to overfeeding, hunger still cuts down its victims, especially among the weak, children, and the aged.

It is not admissible to remain silent and passive in the face of this tragedy, especially when the possible solution can be seen in a wiser utilization of available resources. May our voices join those of all persons of good will in calling upon those responsible in the public area for a more determined commitment to place in the forefront the immediate and concrete resolution of this tremendous and dramatic problem.

DOCUMENT 4 / Medical Profession

Source: Pope John Paul II, "The Ethics of Genetic Manipulation" (Oct. 29, 1983), *Origins* 13: no. 23, Nov. 17, 1983, pp. 385–89.

Medicine is an eminent, essential form of service to mankind. It is first of all necessary to help man to live and overcome handicaps weighing upon the normal functioning of all his organic functions in their psychophysical unity. Man is also at the center of the Church's concern. Her mission is, with God's grace, to save man, to restore him to his spiritual and moral integrity, to lead him toward integral development, where the body has its part. This is why the Church's ministry and the witness of Christians go hand in hand with solicitude for the sick.

I therefore express best wishes, together with you, for medical science and the art of healing to make further progress. The struggle against acquired acute and chronic maladies has already become very effective. What has been organized against inherited illnesses is also called upon to make progress.

How not wish, then, that you will find sufficient attention and aid in contemporary society—which already does so much for the comfort of the healthy—to bring to the sick of today and of tomorrow the care which they require?

DOCUMENT 5 / Medical Profession

SOURCE: Pope John Paul II, "Physicians, Health Care Educators Must Assert Christian Identity," *Health Progress* (Oct. 1984), pp. 20–22.

... The medical profession today is suffering fundamentally from an identity crisis: the grave danger exists that this profession, born and developed as a commitment of service to suffering persons, can become deviated by ideologies and can be used to the detriment of human life. Where the medical profession is called upon to suppress conceived life; where it is used to eliminate the dying; where it allows itself to be led to intervene against the plan of the Creator in the life of the family or to be taken by the temptation to manipulate human life, and when it loses sight of its authentic direction of purpose toward the person who is most unfortunate and most sick, it loses its ethos, it becomes sick in its turn, it loses and obscures its own dignity and moral autonomy.

It was necessary at that time, and is even more necessary today, to have a school where all the components work harmoniously toward the achievement of the educational purpose, which is to maintain and enrich in the medical profession the ethical dimension and the Christian view of human beings. Research, teaching, witness, and the education environment converge in a university institution in order to foster a tradition and a "school" that can offer to eager young people an educational wealth that is not otherwise attainable. Students who are believers and teachers who are aware of their faith and their educational responsibilities can be found in every other similar civil institution, but it is precisely these persons, who live out the experience and the Christian witness in the diaspora of the secularized world, who expect from a providential institution such as this a line, a thought, and a point of reference.

DOCUMENT 6 / Medical Profession

SOURCE: Pope John Paul II, "Care Providers: Neither Lords Of Life nor Conquerors of Death," *Health Progress* (Dec. 1985), pp. 31, 72.

On October 21 Pope John Paul II addressed scientists assembled at the Vatican by invitation of the Pontifical Academy of Sciences. Following are excerpts from his message.

Since life is a treasure, it is appropriate that scientists promote research which can enhance and prolong human life and that physicians be well informed of the most advanced scientific means available to them in the field of medicine.

Scientists and physicians are called to place their skill and energy at the service of life. They can never, for any reason or in any case, suppress it. For all who have a keen sense of the supreme value of the human person, believers and nonbelievers alike, euthanasia is a crime in which one must in no way cooperate or even consent. Scientists and physicians must not regard themselves as the lords of life, but as its skilled and generous servants. Only God, who created the human person with an immortal soul and saved the human body with the gift of the resurrection, is the Lord of life.

It is the task of doctors and medical workers to give the sick the treatment which will help to cure them and which will aid them to bear their sufferings with dignity. Even when the sick are incurable they are never untreatable: whatever their condition, appropriate care should be provided for the. . . .

The physician is not the lord of life, but neither is he the conqueror of death. Death is an inevitable fact of human life, and the use of means for avoiding it must take into account the human condition. With regard to the use of ordinary and extraordinary means the Church expressed herself in the following terms in the Sacred Congregation for the Doctrine of the Faith's "Declaration on Euthanasia":

"If there are no other sufficient remedies, it is permitted, with the patient's consent, to have recourse to the means provided by the most advanced medical techniques, even if these means are still at the experimental stage and are not without a certain risk. . . . It is also permitted, with the patient's consent, to interrupt these means, where the results fall short of expectations. But for such a decision to be made, account will have to be taken of the reasonable wishes of the patient and the patient's family, as also of the advice of the doctors who are specially competent in the matter. . . . When inevitable death is imminent in spite of the means used, it is permitted in conscience to take the decision to refuse forms of treatments that would only secure a precarious and burdensome prolongation of life, so long as the normal care due to the sick person in similar cases is not interrupted."

DOCUMENT 7 / Medical Profession

SOURCE: Joseph Cardinal Bernardin, "AMA Address: Medicine's Moral Crisis," *Origins* 25: no. 27 (Dec. 21, 1995), pp. 454–56.

Your profession and mine have much in common—the universal human need for healing and wholeness. What special qualities do ministry and medicine share?

First, we both are engaged in something more than a profession—a vocation. In its truest sense, it means a life to which we are called. In my own case I was called to both professions. As an undergraduate I had decided to become a doctor and followed a pre-med curriculum. But long before I graduated, I heard a stronger call to the priesthood.

Second, we both are centered on promoting and restoring wholeness of life. The key words in our professions—*heal, health, holy* and *whole*—share common roots in Old English.

Third, and most fundamentally, we both are engaged in a moral enterprise. We both respond to those who are in need, who ask us for help, who expose to us their vulnerabilities and who place their trust in us.

As someone who has cared for others and who has been cared for by you and your colleagues, I hope you will allow me to speak frankly about the moral crisis that I believe currently grips the medical profession generally and physicians individually.

In speaking of a "moral crisis" I realize that I am assuming a position with which some within your profession would disagree. They would assert that the marketplace is the only valid reference point for evaluating medical practice. I respectfully, though forcefully, disagree with such an assertion. I believe that medicine, like other professions such as teaching, law, and ministry, does have a moral center, even though this center is under attack. And I think you believe deep down as I do that such a moral center exists and that it must not be lost. Dr. Bristow's priority on medical standards as a hallmark of his administration reflects this concern.

What do I mean when I speak of a "moral crisis" in medicine? I mean that more and more members of the community of medicine no longer agree on the universal moral principles of medicine or on the appropriate means to realize those principles. Conscientious practitioners are often perplexed as to how they should act when they are caught up in a web of economics, politics, business practice, and social responsibility. The result is that the practice of medicine no longer has the surety of an accurate compass to guide it through these challenging and difficult times. In other words, medicine, along with other professions, including my own, is in need of a moral renewal.

My purpose today is not to dictate the details of medicine's moral renewal. Rather, it is to invite you to join me in a conversation that will lead to a restoration of medicine's first principles. I am convinced that with good will and persistence this process will benefit society, reinvigorate the medical profession, preserve its independence, and infuse your lives with a quality of meaning that has too often been missing.

How did we arrive at this situation? Medicine, like other professions, does not exist in a vacuum. The upheavals in our society, especially those of the past 30 years, have left their imprint on the practice and organization of medicine. Each of us has his or her own list of such upheavals. My list includes the shift from family and community to the individual as the primary unit of society, an overemphasis on individual self-interest to the neglect of the common good, the loss of a sense of personal responsibility and the unseemly flight to the refuge of "victimhood," the loss of confidence in established institutions, the decline in religious faith, the commercialization of our national existence, the growing reliance on the legal system to redress personal conflicts.

In addition to societal changes there are causes specific to the medical enterprise that contribute to medicine's disconnection from its underlying moral foundation. For example, advances in medical science and technology have improved the prospect of cure but have de-emphasized medicine's traditional caring function. Other contributors include the commercialization of medical practice, the growing preoccupation of some physicians with monetary concerns, and the loss of a sense of humility and humanity by certain practitioners.

None of this, I am sure, is news to you. In surveys, newspaper articles, and personal conversations, many physicians report that they are increasingly concerned with the condition and directions of medical practice.

What may surprise you, however, is my contention that, to reverse these trends, you, as individuals and as a profession, must accept a major share of the responsibility for where you are today. Physicians have too often succumbed to the siren songs of scientific triumph, financial success, and political power. In the process medicine has grown increasingly mechanistic, commercial, and soulless. The age-old covenants between doctors and patient, between the profession and society have been ignored or violated.

This dire view is tempered by hope. If the present predicament is the product of choices—explicit and implicit—made by members of your profession, then it is possible that you can choose to change it.

The change I have in mind is "renewing the covenant with patients and society." That covenant is grounded in the moral obligations that arise from the nature of the doctor-patient relationship. They are moral obligations— as opposed to legal or contractual obligations—because they are based on fundamental human concepts of right and wrong. While, as I noted earlier, it is not currently fashionable to think of medicine in terms of morality, morality is, in fact, the core of the doctor-patient relationship and the foundation of the medical profession. Why do I insist on a moral model as opposed to the economic and contractual models now in vogue?

258   Allow me to describe four key aspects of medicine that give it a moral status and establish a covenantal relationship:

—First, the reliance of the patient on the doctor. Illness compels a patient to place his or her fate in the hands of a doctor. A patient relies not only on the technical competence of a doctor, but also on his or her moral compass, on the doctor's commitment to put the interests of the patient first.

—Second, the holistic character of medical decisions. A physician is a scientist and a clinician, but as a doctor is and must be more. A doctor is and must be a caretaker of the patient's person, integrating medical realities into the whole of the patient's life. A patient looks to his or her doctor as a professional adviser, a guide through some of life's most difficult journeys.

—Third, the social investment in medicine. The power of modern medicine—of each and every doctor—is the result of centuries of science, clinical trials, and public and private investments.

Above all, medical science has succeeded because of the faith of people in medicine and in doctors. This faith creates a social debt and is the basis of medicine's call—its vocation—to serve the common good.

—Fourth, the personal commitments of doctors. Relationship with a patient creates an immediate, personal, nontransferable fiduciary responsibility to protect that patient's best interests. Regardless of markets, government programs, or network managers, patients depend on doctors for a personal commitment and for advocacy through an increasingly complex and impersonal system.

This moral center of the doctor-patient relationship is the very essence of being a doctor. It also defines the outlines of the covenant that exists between physicians and their patients, their profession, and their society. The covenant is a promise that the profession makes a solemn promise, that it is and will remain true to its moral center. In individual terms the covenant is the basis on which patients trust their doctors. In social terms, the covenant is the grounds for the public's continued respect and reliance on the profession of medicine.

36: Murder

DOCUMENT 1:

SOURCE: Pope John Paul II, "The Gospel of Life" (Mar. 25, 1995), *Origins* 24: no. 42 (Apr. 6, 1995), p. 709.

57. If such great care must be taken to respect every life, even that of criminals and unjust aggressors, the commandment "you shall not kill" has absolute value when it refers to the innocent person. And all the more so in the case of weak and defenseless human beings, who find their ultimate defense against the arrogance and caprice of others only in the absolute binding force of God's commandment.

In effect, the absolute inviolability of innocent human life is a moral truth clearly taught by Sacred Scripture, constantly upheld in the Church's tradition and consistently proposed by her Magisterium. This consistent teaching is the evident result of that "supernatural sense of the faith" which, inspired and sustained by the Holy Spirit, safeguards the people of God from error when "it shows universal agreement in matters of faith and morals."

Faced with the progressive weakening in individual consciences and in society of the sense of the absolute and grave moral illicitness of the direct taking of all innocent human life, especially at its beginning and at its end, the Church's Magisterium, particularly insistent in this regard, has always been seconded by that of the bishops, with numerous and comprehensive doctrinal and pastoral documents issued either by episcopal conferences or by individual bishops. The Second Vatican Council also addressed the matter forcefully in a brief but incisive passage.

Therefore, by the authority which Christ conferred upon Peter and his successors, and in communion with the bishops of the Catholic Church, I confirm that the direct and voluntary killing of an innocent human being is always gravely immoral. This doctrine, based upon that unwritten law which man, in the light of reason, finds in his own heart (cf. Rom 2:14–15), is reaffirmed by Sacred Scripture, transmitted by the tradition of the Church, and taught by the ordinary and universal Magisterium.

The deliberate decision to deprive an innocent human being of his life is always morally evil and can never be licit either as an end in itself or as a means to a good end. It is in fact a grave act of disobedience to the moral law, and indeed to God himself, the author and guarantor of that law; it contradicts the fundamental virtues of justice and charity. "Nothing and no one can in any way permit the killing of an innocent human being, whether a fetus or an embryo, an infant or an adult, an old person or one suffering from an incurable

260   disease, or a person who is dying. Furthermore, no one is permitted to ask for this act of killing, either for himself or herself or for another person entrusted to his or her care, nor can he or she consent to it, either explicitly or implicitly. Nor can any authority legitimately recommend or permit such an action.

As far as the right to life is concerned, every innocent human being is absolutely equal to all others. This equality is the basis of all authentic social relationships which, to be truly such, can only be founded on truth and justice, recognizing and protecting every man and woman as a person and not as an object to be used. Before the moral norm which prohibits the direct taking of the life of an innocent human being, "there are no privileges or exceptions for anyone. It makes no difference whether one is the master of the world or the 'poorest of the poor' on the face of the earth. Before the demands of morality we are all absolutely equal."

37: National Health Insurance

DOCUMENT 1:

Source: United States Catholic Conference, Catholic Hospital Association, and National Conference of Catholic Charities, "Statement on National Health Insurance" (July 2, 1974), United States Catholic Conference, Washington, DC, 1974, pp. 2–8, 11–12, 14.

... As representatives of the Catholic Church's concern for adequate health care in America, our basic approach to the issue of national health insurance is rooted in the fundamental tenet that every person has the right to life, to bodily integrity, and the means which are necessary and suitable for the development of life. The right to life clearly implies the right to health care; indeed, the two are philosophically and practically inseparable. The right of persons to health care further implies that such health care will be available, and that the route of access to necessary and comprehensive care will not be strewn with impediments.

In spite of the enormous dimension of the national commitment to health, we recognize the inadequacies of the health system. There exist presently widespread disparities throughout the country in the availability of treatment, facilities, and personnel. And in a significant number of rural areas, inner cities, ghettos, and barrios, there are few medical facilities and, in some cases, no physicians or nurses, contributing to haphazard and generally poor standards of health for millions of people. Health care costs have risen to the point where many will not or cannot seek necessary treatment because of severe or ruinous financial demands.

... With such facts and statistics in mind, we strongly endorse the prospect of a national health care insurance program. We believe it is only through a well-planned national approach that the United States can begin to strike a balance between the actual delivery of health care to all persons living within our borders and our undisputed excellence in the areas of health research and technology. We believe that there can be no further delay in recognizing the moral necessity of developing a national health care insurance program within which all participate. The question, in other words, is not whether we should have a national program; it is how such a program should be developed and implemented.

Our testimony today reflects the principles we would wish to see included in any national health care program which will finally emerge and seeks to address specifically those elements within several of the pending bills which we likewise feel should be included in the legislation. No one bill, in our view, **261**

262   provides a total and practical solution to the inadequacies in the present health care system, nor does any one bill speak adequately of the preservation of the better aspects of our present delivery system. . . .

COVERAGE

We believe that by attaching restrictions on who may be covered under a national health insurance program, or by attempting to define eligibility, many thousands, and possibly millions, of persons will either never be covered or will lose protection for a variety of economic reasons, including, in some cases, nonenrollment in the social security system. Distinctions among people, classes of people, or places of national origin are, in terms of the right to health care, an affront to the dignity of man. Therefore, coverage should be universal, including all U.S. citizens, resident aliens, and aliens admitted for employment. Any other approach would compromise too severely a truly national approach. . . .

BENEFITS

We believe that the legislative enactment of a mandated package of benefits should include the following: preventive services, all physician services, and all inpatient, outpatient, and medical services. This is intended to include coverage for all catastrophic illnesses, all prescription drugs, post-hospital extended care, nursing home care, medical home health services, rehabilitation services, care for the developmentally disabled, dental care including orthodontia, therapeutic devices, prosthetic devices including hearing aids and eyeglasses, health-oriented social services, mental health services, and necessary medical transportation. . . .

HEALTH EDUCATION

Our conviction about the right to all health care prompts us to speak within the context of preventive health care for an equally strong program of health education. . . .

PREVENTIVE MEDICINE

We believe there should be substantially more emphasis on preventive medicine and services than is reflected in most of the pending bills. We recognize that there may be present financial limitations in respect to immediate creation of a far-ranging effort to institutionalize, in effect, the practice of preventive medicine. Legislation should include authorities for the development of preventive health services and strong encouragement for the conversion of our present inclination to treatment of episodic illnesses to an approach which places more emphasis on comprehensive prevention of sickness. . . .

FINANCING

. . . We endorse the establishment of a national trust fund within the Social Security Administration to handle the collection and disbursement of funds— in terms of purchasing and reimbursing services. . . .

THE ROLE OF THE CONSUMER IN NATIONAL HEALTH INSURANCE 263

. . . We believe that consumer initiatives in respect to bringing health services into a community must actively be encouraged. Accordingly, we feel that the legislation should provide clearly for federal override of any state regulations or legislation which curtails or discourages consumer initiatives in relation to federal health funds and programs. Without such protection, consumer participation will vary widely and significantly among the states, to the detriment of a national health insurance program. We urge also appropriate procedures for appeals. . . .

FAMILY PLANNING

. . . In summary, we believe that participation by persons and institutions in any system of national health insurance must not be contingent upon nor result in the violation of deeply held beliefs by persons of many faiths. Catholic people and Catholic health care institutions could not participate in any plan which would require the violation of such beliefs, most emphatically in the areas of abortion services.

DOCUMENT 2 / National Health Insurance

SOURCE: United States Catholic Conference, "Pastoral Letter on Health and Health Care," (Nov. 16–19, 1981) *Origins* 11: no. 25, Dec. 3, 1981, pp. 401–02.

... It is appropriate in this context to call attention to the significant impact that public policy has on health care in our society. The government, working for the common good, has an essential role to play in ensuring that the right of all people to adequate health care is protected. The function of government reaches beyond the limited resources of individuals and private groups. Private agencies and institutions alone are unable to develop a comprehensive national health policy or to ensure that all Americans have adequate health insurance or to command the vast resources necessary to implement an effective national health policy. These functions are in large part the responsibility of government. However, in accord with the traditional Catholic principle of subsidiarity, we believe voluntary institutions must continue to play an essential role in our society.

Christian people have a responsibility to participate actively in the shaping and executing of public policy that relates to health care. On this issue, as on all issues of basic human rights, the Church has an important role to play in bringing gospel values to the social and political order. ...

1. Every person has a basic right to adequate health care. This right flows from the sanctity of human life and the dignity that belongs to all human persons, who are made in the image of God. It implies that access to that health care which is necessary and suitable for the proper development and maintenance of life must be provided for all people, regardless of economic, social or legal status. Special attention should be given to meeting the basic health needs of the poor. With increasingly limited resources in the economy, it is the basic rights of the poor that are frequently threatened first. The Church should work with government to avoid this danger.

2. Pluralism is an essential characteristic of the health care delivery system of the United States. Any comprehensive health system that is developed, therefore, should use the cooperative resources of both the public and private sectors, the voluntary, religious, and nonprofit sectors. In any national health system, provision should be made for the protection of conscience in the delivery of care. This applies not only to individual and institutional providers, but also to consumers.

3. The benefits provided in a national health care policy should be sufficient to maintain and promote good health as well as to treat disease and disability. Emphasis should be placed on the promotion of health, the prevention of disease, and the protection against environmental and other hazards to physical and mental health. If health is viewed in an integrated and comprehensive manner, the social and economic context of illness and health care must

become an important focus of concern and action. Toward this end, public policy should provide incentives for preventive care, early intervention, and alternative delivery systems. All of these actions should be carried out in the context of our fundamental commitment to the sanctity and dignity of human life.

4. Consumers should be allowed a reasonable choice of providers whether they be individual providers, groups, clinics, or institutions. Likewise, to enhance personal and family responsibility in health care, public policy should ensure broad consumer participation in the planning and decision making that affects health maintenance and health care delivery both in the community and in institutions.

5. Health care planning is an essential element in the development of an efficient and coordinated health care system. Public policy should ensure that uniform standards are part of the health care delivery system. This is the joint responsibility of the private and public sectors. They should work cooperatively to ensure the provision of standards that will help to achieve equity in the range and quality of services and in the training of providers.

6. Methods of containing and controlling costs are an essential element of national health policy. Incentives should be developed at every level for administering health care efficiently, effectively, and economically.

Following on these principles and on our belief in health care as a basic human right, we call for the development of a national health insurance program. It is the responsibility of the federal government to establish a comprehensive health care system that will ensure a basic level of health care for all Americans. The federal government should also ensure adequate funding for this basic level of care through a national health insurance program. Such a program should reflect sound human values and should, in our view, be based on the principles which we have set forth in this statement.

38: Natural Family Planning

DOCUMENT 1:

Source: John Paul II, "Why Natural Family Planning Differs From Contraception," *Origins* 27: no. 40 (Mar. 27, 1998), p. 680.

. . . I hope that everyone will benefit from a closer study of the Church's teaching on the "truth" of the act of love in which spouses become sharers in God's creative action.

The truth of this act stems from its being an expression of the spouses reciprocal personal giving, a giving that can only be total since the person is one and indivisible. In the act that expresses their love, spouses are called to make a reciprocal gift of themselves to each other in the totality of their person: nothing that is part of their being can be excluded from this gift. This is the reason for the intrinsic unlawfulness of contraception. It introduces a substantial limitation into this reciprocal giving, breaking that "inseparable connection" between the two meanings of the conjugal act, the unitive and the procreative, which, as Pope Paul VI pointed out, are written by God himself into the nature of the human being (no. 12).

Continuing in this vein, the great pontiff rightly emphasized the "essential difference" between contraception and the use of natural methods in exercising "responsible procreation." It is an anthropologic difference because in the final analysis it involves two irreconcilable concepts of human sexuality (cf. *Familiaris Consortio*, 32).

It is not uncommon in current thinking for the natural methods of fertility regulation to be separated from their proper ethical dimension and to be considered in their merely functional aspect. It is not surprising then that people no longer perceive the profound difference between these and the artificial methods. As a result, they go so far as to speak of them as if they were another form of contraception. But this is certainly not the way they should be viewed or applied.

On the contrary, it is only in the logic of the reciprocal gift between man and woman that the natural relation of fertility can be correctly understood and authentically lived as the proper expression of a real and mutual communion of love and life. It is worth repeating here that "the person can never be considered as a means to an end, above all never a means of 'pleasure.' The person is and must be nothing other than the end of every act. Only then does the action correspond to the true dignity of the person" (cf. "Letter to Families," 12).

The Church is aware of the various difficulties married couples can encounter, especially in the present social context, not only in following but also

in the very understanding of the moral norm that concerns them. Like a mother,   **267**
the Church draws close to couples in difficulty to help them; but she does so
by reminding them that the way to finding a solution to their problems must
come through full respect for the truth of their love. "It is an outstanding
manifestation of charity toward souls to omit nothing from the saving doctrine
of Christ," Paul VI admonished (*Humanae Vitae*, 29).

The Church makes available to spouses the means of grace which Christ
offers in redemption and invites them to have recourse to them with ever
renewed confidence. She exhorts them in particular to pray for the gift of the
Holy Spirit, which is poured out in their hearts through the efficacy of their
distinctive sacrament. This grace is the source of the interior energy they need
to fulfill the many duties of their state, starting with that of being consistent
with the truth of conjugal love. At the same time, the Church urgently requests
the commitment of scientists, doctors, health care personnel, and pastoral workers to make available to married couples all those aids which prove an effective
support for helping them fully to live their vocation (cf. *Humanae Vitae*,
23–27). . . .

DOCUMENT 2 / Natural Family Planning

SOURCE: Pope John Paul II, "The Christian Family in the Modern World" (Nov. 22, 1981), *Vatican Council II*, Vol. 2, pp. 840–41.

In this perspective the Second Vatican Council clearly affirmed that "when there is a question of harmonizing conjugal love with the responsible transmission of life, the moral aspect of any procedure does not depend solely on sincere intentions or on an evaluation of motives. It must be determined by objective standards. These, based on the nature of the human person and his or her acts, preserve the full sense of mutual self-giving and human procreation in the context of true love. Such a goal cannot be achieved unless the virtue of conjugal chastity is sincerely practiced."

It is precisely by moving from "an integral vision of man and of his vocation, not only his natural and earthly, but also his supernatural and eternal vocation," that Paul VI affirmed that the teaching of the Church "is founded upon the inseparable connection, willed by God and unable to be broken by man on his own initiative, between the two meanings of the conjugal act: the unitive meaning and the procreative meaning." And he concluded by re-emphasizing that there must be excluded as intrinsically immoral "every action which, either in anticipation of the conjugal act, or in its accomplishment, or in the development of its natural consequences, proposes, whether as an end or as a means, to render procreation impossible."

When . . . by means of recourse to periods of infertility, the couple respect the inseparable connection between the unitive and procreative meanings of human sexuality, they are acting as "ministers" of God's plan and they "benefit from" their sexuality according to the original dynamism of "total" self-giving, without manipulation or altercation.

In the light of the experience of many couples and of the data provided by the different human sciences, theological reflection is able to perceive and is called to study further the difference, both anthropological and moral, between contraception and recourse to the rhythm of the cycle: it is a difference which is much wider and deeper than is usually thought, one which involves in the final analysis two irreconcilable concepts of the human person and of human sexuality. The choice of the natural rhythms involves accepting the cycle of the person, that is the woman, and thereby accepting dialogue, reciprocal respect, shared responsibility, and self-control. To accept the cycle and to enter into dialogue means to recognize both the spiritual and corporal character of conjugal communion, and to live personal love with its requirement of fidelity. In this context the couple comes to experience how conjugal communion is enriched with those values of tenderness and affection which constitute the inner soul of human sexuality in its physical dimension also. In this way sexuality is respected and promoted in its truly and fully human dimension, and is never "used" as an "object" that, by breaking the personal unity of soul and body, strikes at God's creation itself at the level of the deepest interaction of nature and person.

DOCUMENT 3 / Natural Family Planning

Source: Pope John Paul II, "Natural Family Planning" (Dec. 13, 1985), *The Pope Speaks* 31: no. 1, 1986, pp. 60–62.

. . . In the series of training meetings which you have attended, expertly qualified persons have instructed you on the knowledge of the body and its rhythms of fertility, on the moral and personal motivations of the regulation of birth, on the human conditions, physical and psychic, necessary for understanding and living marriage according to the design of divine providence. . . .

PASS ON TEACHINGS

. . . As we read in *Familiaris Consortio*, "the moral order cannot be something oppressive for man, something impersonal; on the contrary, responding as it does to the most profound exigencies of man created by God, it places itself at the service of his full humanity, with that delicate and binding love with which God himself inspires, sustains, and guides every creature toward its happiness."

. . . Undoubtedly your talk is a difficult one, because the information and knowledge of the natural methods for a responsible parenthood must be based on a correct anthropology, and therefore they require an education to self-control, and accordingly an esteem for chastity and an appreciation for the spiritual dimension of love which integrates in itself and sublimates the drives of instinct and the inclinations of sentiment. Even the commitment to self-denial is thus invested with the finality of expressing an authentic personal love, capable of a daily asceticism, and of mutual understanding and patience.

WITNESS TO CHASTITY

It is necessary to view marriage, and consequently the use of sexuality, in the light of the paschal mystery of Christ, which logically implies suffering and sacrifice, victory and joy, because it illuminates, purifies, elevates, and saves. Paul VI in the encyclical *Humanae Vitae* wrote as follows: "For if with the aid of reason and of free will they are to control their natural drives, there can be no doubt at all of the need for self-denial. Only then will the expression of love, particular to married life, conform to right order. And this is especially true as regards the practice of periodic continence. But self-discipline of this kind is a shining witness to the chastity of husband and wife and, so far from being a hindrance to their love of one another, transforms it by giving it a more truly human character. And if this self-discipline does demand that they persevere in their purpose and efforts, it has at the same time the salutary effect of enabling husband and wife to develop to the full their personalities and be enriched with spiritual blessings."

270

Instruction regarding natural methods is thus inseparable from a con- sciously developed interior life, nourished by prayer and confidence in God, and it also implies a constant education to recourse to the help of grace, to the frequent use of the sacraments of the Eucharist and of reconciliation, to a sense of responsibility in the field of charity. Indeed, what is involved is not merely a question of the biological and psychological order, but an entire conception and practice of life grounded in the "Word of God," which throws light on man's nature and destiny—a life therefore, set in the perspective of eternity.

In the "Final Report" of the recent Extraordinary Synod, celebrated twenty years after the conclusion of the Second Vatican Council, the Synod Fathers wrote among other things: "Everywhere on earth today the transmission to the young of the faith and the moral values deriving from the Gospel is in danger. Often, knowledge of the faith and the acceptance of the moral order are reduced to the minimum. Therefore, a new effort in evangelization and in integral and systematic catechesis is required."

COURAGE OF RESPONSIBILITY

You too must accept then with courage the responsibility of this new effort in the integral affirmation of the moral doctrine of the Church, for the Christian formation of the youth and of families. . . .

DOCUMENT 4 / Natural Family Planning

SOURCE: Pope John Paul II, "Responsible Procreation" (June 8, 1984), *The Pope Speaks* 29: no. 3, 1984, pp. 244–47.

. . . During these days of your congress you have set up a dialogue between science, ethics, and theology on a subject of decisive importance: responsible procreation. This dialogue answers an urgent need of our time, one that is recognized by scientists themselves: the need for scientific knowledge and its applications to be ruled from within by ethics.

This "rule by ethics" does not, of course, in any way detract from the epistemological independence of scientific knowledge. Rather, it assists science in fulfilling its most profound vocation of service to the human vocation of service to the human person. All knowledge of truth—including scientific truth—is a good of the human person and for the whole of humanity. . . .

VALUE OF RESPONSIBLE PROCREATION

You scientists here present have concentrated your research upon a precise point: knowledge of the fertile and infertile periods in the woman's cycle, in order to discover diagnostic methods of discerning them with certainty.

. . . Philosophical and theological ethics take up scientific knowledge in such a way that this latter becomes the path whereby the freedom of the human person achieves responsible procreation. Only in this way do married couples, possessing the necessary knowledge, accomplish a "harmonization" of all the dimensions of their humanity, and safeguard the whole truth of married love. You are aware that each individual scientist, philosopher, or theologian, according to his or her own competence, is directed toward the same objective: the moral value of responsible procreation, and each complements the others, in a precise hierarchy.

The experience which you are having during these present days must continue. The teaching of natural methods is extremely vital for the human and Christian well-being of so many couples. Hence, it must never be something purely technical. It must be rooted in true science and in a complete view of the human person.

A PASTORAL CONCERN

In your congress you have rightly given ample time to anthropological reflection, both philosophical and theological, because in the end all the matters which you have discussed and will discuss come back to one question: Who is man?—man in the unity of his relationship with God in the goodness of the married relationship. When the answer to this question is obscured, the ethics of marriage is deprived of its basis.

On the other hand, the full truth of the creation and redemption is a light 273 of incomprehensible brightness that places the ethics of marriage in proper perspective.

Your work is, therefore, in the service of the human person, in a civilization that has often replaced the criterion of what is good with the criterion of what is useful. Strive to pursue it in great unity among yourselves, with courage, for the truth and the good are stronger than error and evil.

I wish to call special attention to the pastoral implications of your studies of responsible procreation and your promotion of the natural methods of family planning. The theological study is basic because "the concrete pedagogy of the Church must always remain linked to its doctrine and never separated from it." Moreover, this study leads to a clearer understanding that natural family planning is not an end in itself but is one of the many dimensions of the Church's pastoral concern for married couples.

. . . In your own work with married couples, I urge you always to maintain a special sensitivity to their needs, their fidelity to the Church, and the sacrifices they so willingly make in proclaiming the Lord's message in and through their conjugal love and family life. The Church does not claim that responsible parenthood is easy, but the grace of the Sacrament of Marriage gives Christian couples a readiness and a capacity to live out their commitments with fidelity and joy.

PROVIDENTIAL THAT VARIOUS NATURAL METHODS EXIST

At the same time, the use of the natural methods gives a couple an openness to life, which is truly a splendid gift of God's goodness.

It also helps them deepen their conjugal communication and draw closer to one another in their union—a closeness that lasts throughout their lives.

We must also be convinced that it is providential that various natural family planning methods exist so as to meet the needs of different couples. The Church does not give exclusive approval to any one natural method, but urges that all be made available and be respected. The ultimate reason for any natural method is not simply its biological effectiveness or reliability, but its consistence with a Christian view of sexuality as expressive of conjugal love. For sexuality reflects the innermost being of the human person as such, and is realized in a truly human way only if it is an integral part of the love by which a man and woman commit themselves totally to one another until death.

In this pastoral effort, then, it is important that the various natural family planning groups should work together and share their research and studies so as to manifest a unity of purpose and commitment. In this way the Church is better able to present to the world the values of the natural methods, and reduce the strong emphasis on contraception, sterilization, and abortion that we often encounter in the world.

At the heart of this work in natural family planning must be a Christian view of the human person and the conviction that married couples can really attain, through God's grace and commitment to the natural methods, a deeper and stronger conjugal unity. Their unity, mutual respect, and self-control are achieved in their practice of natural family planning. . . .

DOCUMENT 5 / Natural Family Planning

SOURCE: National Conference of Catholic Bishops Committee on Pro-Life Activities, "Human Sexuality From God's Perspective," *Origins* 23 no. 10 (Aug. 12, 1993), pp. 164–66.

Natural Family Planning

As we reflect on the teaching of *Humanae Vitae*, we recognize the advances in natural family planning and the efforts of scientists, pastors and married couples committed to "instilling conviction and offering practical help to those who wish to live out their parenthood in a truly responsible way" (*Familiaris Consortio*, 35). With proper instruction, married couples can readily understand the cycle of fertility, and they are able to plan and space births in a way that is both consistent with God's law and supportive of their own intimacy and unity. Natural family planning, as Pope John Paul II reminds us, "involves accepting dialogue, reciprocal respect, shared responsibility and self-control" (ibid., 32). And as Paul VI noted in *Humanae Vitae*, its benefits to married couples are many:

"It demands continual effort, yet, thanks to its beneficent influence, husband and wife fully develop their personalities, being enriched with spiritual values. Such discipline bestows upon family life fruits of serenity and peace, and facilitates the solution of other problems; it favors attention for one's partner, helps both parties to drive out selfishness, the enemy of true love, and deepens their sense of responsibility. By its means, parents acquire the capacity of having a deeper and more efficacious influence in the education of their offspring" (no. 21).

Natural family planning gives couples a richer appreciation of human sexuality and of their own marital relationship, and it strengthens their openness to childbearing.

39: Nursing

DOCUMENT 1:

SOURCE: Pope Pius XII, "The Nursing Vocation" (May 21, 1952), *The Human Body: Papal Teachings*, pp. 189–93.

... Nevertheless, the care of the sick is not the exclusive prerogative of religious, but seeks out from the ranks of the laity a whole army of competent and generous assistants. Just as this care of the sick sprang from the spirit of Christianity, so now it must be fed on and nourished by this spirit.

It is the importance of an office which determines the responsibility of the person who exercises it. Now the nurse must answer not for any material business, but for a man who lives, one whose very life is more or less gravely affected, one who depends—completely—on the knowledge, ability, delicacy, and patience of doctor and nurse. In fact, under a certain aspect, he depends even more on the nurse than on the doctor, as an eminent surgeon once pointed out: "It is to the nurse that the patient is entrusted for the greater part of the day; it is the nurse who receives the patient after the operation, and who, by unobtrusive, modest, and effective aid, makes possible the success of the efforts of doctor and surgeon."

Your profession therefore supposes in you qualities over and above the ordinary: a solid professional formation, which means a technical knowledge soundly absorbed and constantly kept up-to-date, an acute intelligence, capable of constantly grasping developments, applying new methods, and utilizing new instruments and medicines.

Besides this, a calm, competent, attentive, conscientious temperament. You must specialize in self-mastery: a harsh gesture can bring new suffering for the patient, make a doctor feel ill at ease, inspire fear in the heart of the sick. The nurse must remain unruffled in receiving unreasonable complaints and requests from patients, and when faced with unforeseen emergencies. The nurse must foresee and prepare in time all that is needed for the care of the sick person, a duty which can be quite complicated. Nothing must be forgotten; at the same time, all the precautions imposed by hygiene and prudence must be taken. Time tables must be faithfully observed, doses scrupulously administered. The nurse must be as well a scrupulous observer, who can make known to the doctor the reactions of the patient and symptoms recognized from experience. Add to these qualities attention in the reception of orders, and promptness in their execution.

The nurse must possess as well a no less imposing array of moral qualities: an unassuming, sensitive and fine tact, which can understand the sufferings

276 of the sick and forestall their needs, which can distinguish what must be said from that which is better left unspoken; tactful, too, in the relations with the doctor, whose authority must always be respected and upheld, and with fellow nurses, particularly those who are younger, who must never be embarrassed or shamed, but rather aided when the need arises.

Your profession demands a complete dedication to the patient, be he rich or poor, be he a pleasant person or not. Thus a nurse is not like the clerk in the office, who can leave without a worry at the day's end. You may be called in for urgent cases, and your work promises days so full that there is no possibility of rest or relaxation.

Patience, too, is part of this total dedication. There are some who can rise to great heights now and then in extraordinary circumstances, but who tire and are irritated by the constant small bothers which occur day in and day out.

The crown, finally, of all the moral virtues of the nurse is discretion. The nurse must observe strictly the professional secret. Nothing the patient has said in confidence or in delirium may be revealed, nor anything which will harm his reputation or family.

There are other nobler virtues, too, on which Christian faith confers a special splendor. We are referring to respect for the sick, truthfulness, and moral firmness respect for him who at times loses many of the qualities which earn our respect: courage, calmness, lucidity; respect for his body, too, which is the temple of the Holy Spirit, redeemed with the precious blood of Christ, destined to rise again and enjoy eternal life; truthfulness in contacts with doctors, with patients, and their families: these must all be able to trust implicitly in the nurse's word. This matter is important not only for the health of the body, but for that of the soul: to delay by reticence a patient's preparation for his passing into eternity could easily be a grave sin.

. . . Nevertheless, you certainly cannot be equal to the task which your office and your obligations impose, if you do not possess the moral energies which derive from and are nourished by a deep and living faith. Were you to consider your work in practice simply as an occupation, honorable enough certainly, but a thing purely human, and if you do not draw especially from the Eucharistic fount, the water of Christian fortitude, you will not be able for long to remain faithful to your duties.

For in your life, there are so many sacrifices to be made, so many dangers to be overcome, that it would be impossible without supernatural help, to triumph constantly over human weakness. You must cultivate the spirit of self-denial, purity of heart, delicacy of conscience, so that your service may be truly that act of supernatural charity which the Christian faith asks of you. As we remarked at the very beginning, you must serve Jesus Christ himself in the sick: it is he who begs your care, just as one day he begged the Samaritan woman a glass of water. And to you we repeat those words spoken to her, to lead her to overcome her sense of surprise: "If thou knowest what it is God gives, and Who this is that is saying to you, Give Me to drink, it would have been for thee to ask Him instead, and He would have given thee living water. . . ."

DOCUMENT 2 / Nursing

SOURCE: Pontifical Council Cor Unum, *Questions of Ethics Regarding the Fatally Ill and the Dying*, Vatican Press, 1981, pp. 20–23.

7.4.1 THE IMPORTANCE OF THEIR RESPONSIBILITIES

Despite the fact that many doctors tend to look upon them as purely auxiliary, nurses have a fundamental role of mediation between doctors and patients. Although nurses are, it is true, by no means free of the danger of avoiding the patient during the final stages of his illness, they are nevertheless responsible for actions that can often be of crucial importance. They must decide, for example, whether or not to call the doctor when they find that the patient has suddenly become worse; or must decide whether or not to give the patient a calming substance the doctor has left it up to their judgment to use at an appropriate moment, etc. Fortunately, in many hospitals today, a true feeling of teamwork between doctors and nurses is beginning to prevail. Their close collaboration is essential to the relief and proper care of each patient.

7.4.2 COOPERATION AND CONSCIENCE

At times, especially when she or he works in non-Christian hospitals or for non-Christian doctors, the nurse is brought up against a moral dilemma posed by an order given by the doctor, the execution of which would gravely endanger, if not actually put an end to, the patient's life.

First and foremost, the nurse must adhere to the absolute prohibition against performing an act whose only purpose is to kill. Neither the doctor's order, nor the request of the family, nor even the plea of the patient can free the nurse from responsibility for such an act. Where actions are concerned which in themselves are not toward killing (even though the nurse knows that an impermissible result is being aimed at), the case is different if the nurse performs these actions by order of the doctor. Examples of this are: doing something which will shorten the life of the patient, suspending a treatment which is not "extraordinary," depriving of consciousness a patient who has not been able to fulfill his obligations. The nurse may not take the initiative for such actions. The only possible way to look at a nurse's performing them is as their being a "material cooperation" excusable only by necessity when examined in the light: 1) of the gravity of the action; 2) of the nurse's participation in the whole process and the obtaining of the immoral goal; 3) and of reasons which might have led the nurse to obey the order: fear of something personal being done to her or to him if the order is not carried out; an important personal good to be protected by not exposing oneself to the risk of being dismissed. Insofar as her or his status permits, the nurse who finds her or himself involved in practices of which one's conscience cannot approve, will make every effort possible to bear witness to her or his personal convictions. **277**

278 Catholic chaplains and physicians are in duty bound to help nurses face up to such difficult situations, in every way they can.

7.4.3 ETHICAL TRAINING IN NURSING SCHOOLS

All that we have reported in Section 7.1 concerning the necessity of ethical training for doctors, pharmacologists, et. al., holds true in the case of nursing schools as well. Catholic nursing schools have the right and the duty to defend, through their teaching, the ethical principles of the Church's Magisterium, particularly in courses which treat of the exercise of the nurse's profession: the value of each human individual, respect for life, morality and marriage, and so on. It is the duty of Catholic nursing schools to make this ethical orientation clear to all students applying for entrance. The schools further have the right to demand of all students their acceptance of these principles and their attendance at courses specializing in the teaching of professional ethics. The students must arrive at the conviction that here is an essential element, a condition sine qua non, of the proper training of a responsible nurse. Nor should this teaching be limited to a casuistical presentation of the subject. Rather, the professors will in every way seek to inculcate a profound familiarity with such fundamental notions as life, death, the personal vocation which a nurse has, and so on.

7.4.4 TRAINING FOR THE NURSING OF THE INCURABLY ILL

The familiarization of hospital personnel with the demands made by death and by the care of the dying does not take place only at the intellectual level. The actual face-to-face encounter with suffering, with a patient's anxiety, with death, can be a source of great anguish. Here is one of the main reasons why many professional people today are beginning to avoid having anything personal to do with the incurably ill, and are abandoning them to their loneliness. Thus must be added to the teaching of the theory and study of professional ethics an education in how to relate to people, and especially to the incurably ill. If this is not taught, then any teaching of ethics is in danger, in the long run, of not being applied to the real situations encountered professionally.

40: Ordinary and Extraordinary Means to Prolong Life

DOCUMENT 1:

SOURCE: Pope John Paul II, "The Gospel of Life" (Mar. 25, 1995), *Origins* 24: no. 42, Apr. 6, 1995, p. 712.

65. . . . Euthanasia must be distinguished from the decision to forgo so-called "aggressive medical treatment, " in other words, medical procedures which no longer correspond to the real situation of the patient either because they are by now disproportionate to any expected results or because they impose an excessive burden on the patient and his family. In such situations when death is clearly imminent and inevitable, one can in conscience "refuse forms of treatment that would only secure a precarious and burdensome prolongation of life, so long as the normal care due to the sick person in similar cases is not interrupted." Certainly there is a moral obligation to care for oneself and to allow oneself to be cared for, but this duty must take account of concrete circumstances. It needs to be determined whether the means of treatment available are objectively proportionate to the prospects for improvement. To forgo extraordinary or disproportionate means is not the equivalent of suicide or euthanasia; it rather expresses acceptance of the human condition in the face of death.

DOCUMENT 2 / Ordinary and Extraordinary Means to Prolong Life

SOURCE: Pope Pius XII, "The Prolongation of Life" (Nov. 24, 1957), *The Pope Speaks* 4: no. 4, 1958, pp. 395–96.

BASIC PRINCIPLES

... Natural reason and Christian morals say that man (and whoever is entrusted with the task of taking care of his fellowman) has the right and the duty in case of serious illness to take the necessary treatment for the preservation of life and health. This duty that one has toward himself, toward God, toward the human community, and in most cases toward certain determined persons derives from well-ordered charity, from submission to the Creator, from social justice, and even from strict justice, as well as from devotion toward one's family.

But normally one is held to use only ordinary means—according to circumstances of persons, places, times and culture—that is to say, means that do not involve any grave burden for oneself or another. A more strict obligation would be too burdensome for most people and would render the attainment of the higher, more important good too difficult. Life, health, all temporal activities are in fact subordinated to spiritual ends. On the other hand, one is not forbidden to take more than the strictly necessary steps to preserve life and health, as long as he does not fail in some more serious duty. ...

... The rights and duties of the doctor are correlative to those of the patient. The doctor, in fact, has no separate or independent right where the patient is concerned. In general he can take action only if the patient explicitly or implicitly, directly or indirectly, gives him permission. The technique of resuscitation which concerns us here does not contain anything immoral in itself. Therefore the patient, if he were capable of making a personal decision, could lawfully use it and, consequently, give the doctor permission to use it. On the other hand, since these norms of treatment go beyond the ordinary means to which one is bound, it cannot be held that there is an obligation to use them nor, consequently, that one is bound to give the doctor permission to use them.

The rights and duties of the family depend in general upon the presumed will of the unconscious patient if he is of age and *sui juris*. Where the proper and independent duty of the family is concerned, they are usually bound only to the use of ordinary means.

Consequently, if it appears that the attempt at resuscitation constitutes in reality such a burden for the family that one cannot in all conscience impose it upon them, they can lawfully insist that the doctor should discontinue these attempts, and the doctor can lawfully comply. There is not involved here a

case of direct disposal of the life of the patient, nor of euthanasia in any way: **281**
this would never be licit. Even when it causes the arrest of circulation, the
interruption of attempts at resuscitation is never more than an indirect cause
of the cessation of life, and one must apply in this case the principle of double
effect and of *voluntarium in causa*.

DOCUMENT 3 / Ordinary and Extraordinary Means to Prolong Life

SOURCE: National Conference of Catholic Bishops Committee for Pro-Life Activities, "Statement on Uniform Rights of the Terminally Ill Act" (Mar. 20, 1986), *Origins* 16: no. 12, Sept. 4, 1986, pp. 222–24.

In proposing a Uniform Rights of the Terminally Ill Act for enactment by state legislatures, the National Conference of Commissioners on Uniform State Laws has presented legislators with a new and complex challenge. Some of the provisions of the uniform act raise new and significant moral problems, highlighting the need for serious debate on the purpose and risks of legislation on this subject.

As Catholic bishops in the United States we feel a responsibility to contribute to this debate. We are concerned that legislation which is ethically unsound will further compromise the right to life and respect for life in American society. Moreover, we are confident that our Church's moral tradition can be of great assistance in determining the extent to which legislative proposals in this area are consistent with sound moral principles.

In keeping with this tradition we uphold the duty to preserve life while recognizing certain limits to that duty. We absolutely reject euthanasia, by which we mean "an act or an omission which of itself or by intention causes death, in order that all suffering may in this way be eliminated" (Vatican, "Declaration on Euthanasia," 1980). We maintain that one is obliged to use "ordinary" means of preserving life, that is, means which can effectively preserve life without imposing grave burdens on the patient—and we see the failure to supply such means as "equivalent to euthanasia" (USCC, "Ethical and Religious Directives for Catholic Health Facilities," 1975, para. 28). But we also recognize and defend a patient's right to refuse "extraordinary" means, that is, means which provide no benefit or which involve too grave a burden. In cases where patients cannot speak for themselves, we urge family members and physicians to be guided by these fundamental moral principles.

The task of judging how these principles can best be incorporated into social policy is complex and difficult. For example, various proposals giving legal force to an advance declaration or "living will" have been offered as ways of clarifying a terminally ill patient's legitimate right to refuse extraordinary medical treatment. From one perspective, clarification of this right seems increasingly necessary as physicians, concerned about legal liability, seek guidance concerning their legal rights and responsibilities. Indeed, public support for such legislation is due in large part to a concern that some physicians are resisting even morally appropriate requests for withdrawal of treatment when these requests have no explicit statutory recognition.

DOCUMENT 4 / Ordinary and Extraordinary Means to Prolong Life

Source: Congregation for the Doctrine of the Faith, "Declaration on Euthanasia" (May 5, 1980), *Vatican Council II*, Vol. 2, p. 515.

. . . Everyone has the duty to care for his or her own health or to seek such care from others. Those whose task it is to care for the sick must do so conscientiously and administer the remedies that seem necessary or useful.

However, is it necessary in all circumstances to have recourse to all possible remedies?

In the past, moralists replied that one is never obliged to use "extraordinary" means. This reply, which as a principle still holds good, is perhaps less clear today, by reason of the imprecision of the term and the rapid progress made in the treatment of sickness. Thus some people prefer to speak of "proportionate" and "disproportionate" means.

In any case, it will be possible to make a correct judgment as to the means by studying the type of treatment to be used, its degree of complexity or risk, its cost and the possibilities of using it, and comparing these elements with the result that can be expected, taking into account the state of the sick person and his or her physical and moral resources.

In order to facilitate the application of these general principles, the following clarifications can be added:

—If there are no other sufficient remedies, it is permitted with the patient's consent, to have recourse to the means provided by the most advanced medical techniques, even if these means are still at the experimental stage and are not without a certain risk. By accepting them, the patient can even show generosity in the service of humanity.

—It is also permitted, with the patient's consent, to interrupt these means, where the results fall short of expectations. But for such a decision to be made, account will have to be taken of the reasonable wishes of the patient's family, as also of the advice of the doctors who are specially competent in the matter. The latter may in particular judge that the investment in instruments and personnel is disproportionate to the results foreseen; they may also judge that the techniques applied impose on the patient strain or suffering out of proportion with the benefits which he or she may gain from such techniques.

—It is also permissible to make do with the normal means that medicine can offer. Therefore one cannot impose on anyone the obligation to have recourse to a technique which is already in use but which carries a risk or is burdensome. Such a refusal is not the equivalent of suicide; on the contrary, it should be considered as an acceptance of the human condition, or a wish to avoid the application of a medical procedure disproportionate to the results that can be expected, or a desire not to impose excessive expense on the family or the community.

41: Organ Donation and Transplantation

DOCUMENT 1:

SOURCE: Pope John Paul II, "The Gospel of Life" (Mar. 25, 1995), *Origins* 24: no. 42 (Apr. 6, 1995), pp. 718–19.

86. . . . It is in this context, so humanly rich and filled with love, that heroic actions too are born. These are the most solemn celebration of the Gospel of life, for they proclaim it by the total gift of self. They are the radiant manifestation of the highest degree of love, which is to give one's life for the person loved (cf. Jn 15:13). They are a sharing in the mystery of the cross, in which Jesus reveals the value of every person and how life attains its fullness in the sincere gift of self. . . . Over and above such outstanding moments, there is an everyday heroism made up of gestures of sharing, big or small, which build up an authentic culture of life. A particularly praiseworthy example of such gestures is the donation of organs, performed in an ethically acceptable manner, with a view to offering a chance of health and even of life itself to the sick who sometimes have no other hope.

DOCUMENT 2 / Organ Donation and Transplantation

SOURCE: Pope John Paul II, "Blood and Organ Donors" (Aug. 2, 1984), *The Pope Speaks* 30: no. 1, 1985, pp. 1–2.

... I am pleased with this initiative of yours, which is an indication of the vitality and sporting spirit that moved you to make this march. Above all I appreciate the purpose which has united and mobilized you, namely, to promote and encourage such a noble and meritorious act as donating your own blood or an organ to those of your brothers and sisters who have need of it. Such a gesture is the more laudable in that you are motivated, not by a desire for earthly gain or ends, but by a generous impulse of the heart, by human and Christian solidarity—the love of neighbor, which forms the inspiring motive of the Gospel message, and which has been defined, indeed, as the new commandment.

In giving blood or an organ of your body, may you always have this human and religious perspective: may your gesture be made as an offering to the Lord, who identified himself with those who suffer, either by sickness, accidents on the highway, or mishaps at work. May it be a gift made to the suffering Lord, who in his passion gave himself completely and poured out His blood for the salvation of mankind.

If you also include this supernatural intention, your humanitarian gesture, already so noble in itself, will be elevated and transformed into a splendid testimony of Christian faith, and your merit will certainly not be lost. . . .

DOCUMENT 3 / Organ Donation and Transplantation

SOURCE: Pope Pius XII, "Tissue Transplantation" (May 14, 1956), *The Human Body: Papal Teachings*, pp. 380–83.

RESPECT FOR THE DEAD BODY

In the first place, it is necessary to condemn a morally erroneous judgment which is formed in the soul of a person but usually influences his external conduct and consists in putting the corpse of a human being on the same plane as that of an animal or even a simple "thing." The dead body of an animal can be used in almost all its parts. The same can be said in regard to the dead body of a human being considered from a purely material aspect, that is to say, from the standpoint of the elements of which it is composed. For some people this attitude constitutes the final criterion of thought and the ultimate principle of action.

Such an attitude implies an error in judgment and a rejection of psychology and of the religious and moral sense. For the human corpse deserves to be regarded entirely differently. The body was the abode of a spiritual and immortal soul, an essential constituent of a human person whose dignity it shared. Something of this dignity still remains in the corpse. We can say also that, since it is a component of man, it has been formed "to the image and likeness" of God, which extends far beyond the general vestiges of resemblance to God that are found in animals without intelligence and even in purely material and inanimate creatures. In a way the words of the apostle Paul apply even to a corpse: "Do you not know that your members are the temple of the Holy Spirit who is in you?"

Finally, the dead body is destined for resurrection and eternal life. This is not true of the body of an animal, and it proves that it is not sufficient to visualize "therapeutic purposes" for a proper evaluation and treatment of the human corpse.

On the other hand, it is equally true that medical science and the training of future physicians demand a detailed knowledge of the human body, and that cadavers are needed for study. What we have just said does not forbid this. A person can pursue this legitimate objective while fully accepting what we have just said.

It also follows from this that a person may will to dispose of his body and to destine it to ends that are useful, morally irreproachable and even noble (among them the desire to aid the sick and the suffering). One may make a decision of this nature with respect to his own body with full realization of the reverence which is due to it, and with full attention to the words which the apostle Paul spoke to the Corinthians. This decision should not be condemned, but positively justified. . . .

Unless circumstances impose an obligation, we must respect the liberty and spontaneity of the parties involved. Ordinarily the deed cannot be presented as a duty or as an obligatory act of charity. In proposing it, an intelligent reserve must certainly be maintained in order to avoid serious internal and external conflicts.

Moreover, must one, as is often done, refuse on principle all compensation? This question remains unanswered. It cannot be doubted that grave abuses could occur if a payment is demanded. But it would be going too far to declare immoral every acceptance or every demand of payment. The case is similar to blood transfusions. It is commendable for the donor to refuse recompense; it is not necessarily a fault to accept it.

The removal of the cornea, through perfectly lawful in itself, can become illicit if the rights and the feelings of the third parties charged with the care of the body are violated. These are primarily the near relatives, but they could be other persons by virtue of public or private rights. It would not be humane to ignore sentiments so profound in the interest of medicine or of "therapeutic aims."

Generally speaking, doctors should not be permitted to undertake excisions or other operations on a corpse without the permission of those charged with its care, and perhaps even in the face of objections previously expressed by the person in question. Nor would it be fair for the bodies of poor patients in public clinics and hospitals to be regularly destined to the service of doctors and surgeons, while the bodies of wealthier patients are not. Money and social status should not intervene when it is a question of sparing such delicate human feelings.

On the other hand, the public must be educated. It must be explained with intelligence and respect that to consent explicitly or tacitly to serious damage to the integrity of the corpse in the interest of those who are suffering is not a violation of the reverence due to the dead since it is justified by valid reasons. In spite of everything, this consent can involve sadness and sacrifice for the near relatives, but this sacrifice is glorified by the aureole of merciful charity toward some suffering brothers.

Public authorities and the laws which concern the use of corpses should, in general, be guided by these same moral and humane considerations, since they are based on human nature itself, which takes precedence over society in the order of causality and in dignity. In particular, public authorities have the duty to supervise their enforcement and above all to take care that a "corpse" shall not be considered and treated as such until death has been sufficiently proved.

On the other hand, public authorities are empowered to protect the lawful interests of medicine and of medical education. If it is suspected that death was due to a criminal cause, or if there is danger to the public health, the corpse must be delivered to the authorities. All this can and should be done without neglect of the respect due to the deceased and to the rights of the next of kin. Finally, public authorities can contribute effectively toward convincing people of the necessity and of the moral lawfulness of certain regulations regarding dead bodies and thus prevent or dispel the occasion of conflicts, both internal and external, in the individual, the family, and society.

DOCUMENT 4 / Organ Donation and Transplantation

SOURCE: Pope John Paul II, "Many Ethical, Legal, and Social Questions Must Be Examined in Greater Depth" (June 20, 1991), *Dolentium Hominum*, n.3, Vatican Press, 1992, pp. 12–13.

... Among the many remarkable achievements of modern medicine, advances in the fields of immunology and of surgical technology have made possible the therapeutic use of organ and tissue transplants. It is surely a reason for satisfaction that many sick people, who recently could only expect death or at best a painful and restricted existence, can now recover more or less fully through the replacement of a diseased organ with a healthy donated one. We should rejoice that medicine, in its service to life, has found in organ transplantation a new way of serving the human family, precisely by safeguarding that fundamental good of the person.

1. This splendid development is not, of course, without its dark side. There is still much to be learned through research and clinical experience, and there are many questions of an ethical, legal, and social nature which need to be more deeply and widely investigated. There are even shameful abuses which call for determined action on the part of medical associations and donor societies, and especially of competent legislative bodies. Yet in spite of these difficulties we can recall the words of the fourth century Doctor of the Church, Saint Basil the Great: "As regards medicine, it would not be right to reject a gift of God (that is, medical science), just because of the bad use that some people make of it ...; we should instead throw light on what they have corrupted" ("Great Rules," 55:3, cf. MIGNE, PG 31:1048).

With the advent of organ transplantation, which began with blood transfusions, man has found a way to give of himself, of his blood and of his body, so that others may continue to live. Thanks to science and to the professional training and commitment of doctors and health care workers, whose collaboration is less obvious but no less indispensable for the outcome of complicated surgical operations, new and wonderful challenges are presented. We are challenged to love our neighbor in new ways; in evangelical terms, to love "to the end" (Jn 13:1), yet within certain limits which cannot be exceeded, limits laid down by human nature itself.

2. Above all, this form of treatment is inseparable from a human act of donation. In effect, transplantation presupposes a prior, explicit, free, and conscious decision on the part of the donor or of someone who legitimately represents the donor, generally the closest relatives. It is a decision to offer, without reward, a part of one's own body for the health and well-being of another person. In this sense, the medical action of transplantation makes possible the donor's act of self-giving, that sincere gift of self which expresses our constitutive calling to love and communion.

Love, communion, solidarity, and absolute respect for the dignity of the **289** human person constitute the only legitimate context of organ transplantation. It is essential not to ignore the moral and spiritual values which come into play when individuals, while observing the ethical norms which guarantee the dignity of the human person and bring it to perfection, freely and consciously decide to give a part of themselves, a part of their own body, in order to save the life of another human being.

3. In effect, the human body is always a personal body, the body of a person. The body cannot be treated as a merely physical or biological entity, nor can its organs and tissues ever be used as items for sale or exchange. Such a reductive materialist conception would lead to a merely instrumental use of the body, and therefore of the person. In such a perspective, organ transplantation and the grafting of tissue would no longer correspond to an act of donation but would amount to the dispossession or plundering of a body.

Furthermore, a person can only donate that of which he can deprive himself without serious danger or harm to his own life or personal identity, and for a just and proportionate reason. It is obvious that vital organs can only be donated after death. But to offer in life a part of one's body, an offering which will become effective only after death, is already in many cases an act of great love, the love which gives life to others. Thus, the progress of the biomedical sciences has made it possible for people to project beyond death their vocation to love. By analogy with Christ's Paschal Mystery, in dying death is somehow overcome and life restored.

For Christians, Jesus' offering of himself is the essential point of reference and inspiration of the love underlying the willingness to donate an organ, which is a manifestation of generous solidarity, all the more eloquent in a society which has become excessively utilitarian and less sensitive to unselfish giving.

4. Much more could be added, including a meditation on doctors and their assistants, who make possible this striking form of human solidarity. A transplant, and even a simple blood transfusion, is not like other operations. It must not be separated from the donor's act of self-giving, from the love that gives life. The physician should always be conscious of the particular nobility of this work. He becomes the mediator of something especially significant, the gift of self which one person has made—even after death—so that another might live. The difficulty of the operation, the need to act swiftly, the need for complete concentration on the task, should not make the physician lose sight of the mystery of love involved in what he is doing.

Nor should the recipients of organ transplants forget that they are receiving a unique gift from someone else: the gift of self made by the donor, a gift which is certainly to be considered an authentic form of human and Christian solidarity. At the approach of the Third Millennium, in a period of great historic promise, yet one in which threats against life are becoming ever more powerful and deadly, as in abortion and euthanasia, society needs these concrete gestures of solidarity and self-giving love.

5. In conclusion, let us remember those words of Jesus narrated by the Evangelist and physician Luke: "give, and it will be given to you; good measure,

290   pressed down, shaken together, running over, will be put into your lap" (Lk 6:38). We shall receive our supreme reward from God according to the genuine and effective love we have shown to our neighbor.

May the Lord of heaven and earth sustain you in your endeavors to defend and serve life through the wonderful means which medical science places at your disposal. May he bless you and your loved ones with peace and joy.

42: Pain Relief

DOCUMENT 1:

Source: Pope John Paul II, "The Gospel of Life" (Mar. 25, 1995), *Origins* 24: no. 42 (Apr. 6, 1995), p. 712.

65. . . . In modern medicine, increased attention is being given to what are called "methods of palliative care," which seek to make suffering more bearable in the final stages of illness and to ensure that the patient is supported and accompanied in his or her ordeal. Among the questions which arise in this context is that of the licitness of using various types of painkillers and sedatives for relieving the patient's pain when this involves the risk of shortening life. While praise may be due to the person who voluntarily accepts suffering by forgoing treatment with painkillers in order to remain fully lucid and, if a believer, to share consciously in the Lord's passion, such "heroic" behavior cannot be considered the duty of everyone. Pius XII affirmed that it is licit to relieve pain by narcotics even when the result is decreased consciousness and a shortening of life, "if no other means exist, and if, in the given circumstances, this does not prevent the carrying out of other religious and moral duties." In such a case, death is not willed or sought, even though for reasonable motives one runs the risk of it. There is simply a desire to ease pain effectively by using the analgesics which medicine provides. All the same, "it is not right to deprive the dying person of consciousness without a serious reason": As they approach death people ought to be able to satisfy their moral and family duties, and above all they ought to be able to prepare in a fully conscious way for their definitive meeting with God.

DOCUMENT 2 / Pain Relief

Source: Congregation for the Doctrine of the Faith, "Declaration on Euthanasia" (May 5, 1980), *Vatican Council II*, Vol. 2, p. 514.

. . . But the intensive use of painkillers is not without difficulties, because the phenomenon of habituation generally makes it necessary to increase their dosage in order to maintain their efficacy. At this point it is fitting to recall a declaration by Pius XII, which retains its full force; in answer to a group of doctors who had put the questions: "Is the suppression of pain and consciousness by the use of narcotics . . . permitted by religion and morality to the doctor and the patient (even at the approach of death and if one foresees that the use of narcotics will shorten life)?", the Pope said: "If no other means exist, and if, in the given circumstances, this does not prevent the carrying out of other religious and moral duties: Yes." In this case, of course, death is in no way intended or sought, even if the risk of it is reasonably taken; the intention is simply to relieve pain effectively, using for this purpose painkillers available to medicine.

However, painkillers that cause unconsciousness need special consideration. For a person not only has to be able to satisfy his or her moral duties and family obligations; he or she also has to prepare himself or herself with full consciousness for meeting Christ. Thus Pius XII warns: "It is not right to deprive the dying person of consciousness without a serious reason."

DOCUMENT 3 / Pain Relief

SOURCE: Pontifical Council Cor Unum, *Questions of Ethics Regarding the Fatally Ill and the Dying*, Vatican Press, 1981, pp. 1–13.

4. THE USE OF PAINKILLERS IN TERMINAL CASES
4.1 There Are Various Ways to Ease Suffering.

The use of painkillers affecting the central nervous system involves the risk of secondary effects: they can affect respiratory functions, alter the state of consciousness, cause dependency, and, losing their effect, necessitate larger and larger doses. This is why it is always better not to use them so long as the patient's suffering can be relieved by other means.

These latter are not few in number: remedies such as aspirin, the immobilization of certain parts of the body, various radiation therapies, even surgical operations . . . and, above all, combating the solitude and anguish of the patient simply with the presence of another human being. There are also quite new methods coming into use which enable the patient to acquire a certain mastery of his own body.

4.2 The Use of Painkillers Acting on the Central Nervous System

In many cases, however, the relief of sometimes truly unbearable suffering does require the use of painkillers acting on the central nervous system (for example, morphine along with other narcotics) at least at the present state of medical knowledge and techniques.

There exists no reason to refuse to make use of such drugs, especially as their side effects can be greatly reduced if they are used judiciously, that is, in appropriate dosages and at accurately determined intervals. For the using of drugs against pain, while still keeping the patient as conscious as possible, requires a perfect knowledge of these products: the ways to give them, their secondary effects, and their contraindications. When decisions are being made concerning them, it becomes important for the pharmacologist to be consulted and, even, actually to be with the patient.

4.3 The Necessity of a Human Presence

When speaking of narcotics, we must warn against the temptation of believing that they are a sufficient remedy for suffering. Human suffering very frequently contains an element of anguish, of fear in the face of the unknown brought out by severe illness and the nearness of death. Drugs can diminish anguish but, more often than not, are powerless to relieve it completely. It is only a human presence, discreet and attentive, that can procure the relief so much needed, by allowing the sick person to express his thoughts and by giving him human and spiritual comfort.

294 4.4 Is It Permissible to Put the Sick Person into a State of Unconsciousness?

We can now approach the question of whether it is right, when death is very near, to use narcotics to put the patient into a state of unconsciousness. In certain cases, the use of them for this purpose is necessary, and Pope Pius XII has recognized the moral rightness of doing so under certain conditions. (Allocution of Feb. 24, 1957).

The problem is, however, that there exists a great temptation to have recourse to narcosis as a general practice, doubtless, at times, out of pity, but often more or less deliberately, in order to save the doctors, nurses, family, and others around the patient the emotional wear and tear of being with a person on the verge of death. This clearly indicates that it is not the good of the patient which is being sought; rather, it is the protection of people who are perfectly well but who are members of a society that is afraid of death, that flees death by any means at its disposal.

Yet systematic narcosis deprives the dying patient of the possibility of "living out his death." It deprives him of arriving at a serene acceptance of it, of achieving a state of peace; of sharing, perhaps, a last intense relationship between a person reduced to that last of human poverties and another person who will have been privileged by thus knowing him. And if the dying person is a Christian, he is being deprived of experiencing his death in communion with Christ.

What is therefore important is to protest vigorously against any systematic plunging into unconsciousness of the fatally ill and to demand, on the contrary, that medical and nursing personnel learn how to listen to the dying. They must learn how to create relationships among themselves which will sustain them through their days and nights with the dying, and which can help them to help families be with their near and dear one during the last phase of life.

DOCUMENT 4 / Pain Relief

SOURCE: Pope Pius XII, "Christian Principles and the Medical Profession" (Nov. 12, 1944), *The Human Body: Papal Teachings*, pp. 56–58.

... Physical pain has no doubt a natural and salutary function as well: it is a danger signal which gives warning that some hidden sickness has been born and is developing, perhaps secretly; and thus it induces one to seek the remedy. But in the course of his scientific research the doctor inevitably comes upon suffering and death like a locked door to which his mind does not hold the key. In the exercise of his profession, they loom inexorably and mysteriously, a law in the face of which his art often stands helpless and his compassion sterile. He can make his diagnosis according to the principles of the laboratory and clinic, plan the treatment in accordance with all the demands of science ... ; in the depths of his being, as man and scientist, he feels that the explanation of that mystery continues to elude him. He suffers; a consuming anguish grips him until he asks of faith the answer which though now incomplete—it is complete in the mysterious designs of God and will be revealed as such in eternity—has yet the power of bringing him peace of soul.

And this is the answer faith gives. God, when he created man, had by a gift of grace made him exempt from that natural law which governs every living material being. God had not wished to include in man's destiny suffering and death. They were introduced by sin. But he, the Father of mercy, took them into his own hands, made them pass through the body, the veins, the heart of his beloved Son, God like himself, become man for the salvation of the world. And thus suffering and death became for every man who accepts Christ a means of redemption and sanctification. And thus man's pilgrimage here below, continually shadowed by the sign of the cross and the law of suffering and death, develops and purifies the soul, and leads it to happiness without end in eternal life.

To suffer ... to die .... It is truly, to use the bold phrase of the Apostle of the Gentiles, the "folly of God"—a folly which is wiser than all the wisdom of men. In the pale radiance of this weak faith, the poor poet sang:

L'homme est un apprenti, la douleur est son maître,
Et nul ne se connait tant qu'il n'a pas souffert.

In the light of revelation, the holy author of the *Imitation of Christ* could pen the sublime twelfth chapter of his second book, *De regia via sanctae crucis*, all aglow with the most wonderful understanding of the noblest Christian conception of life.

In the face of the insistent problem of pain, what reply can the doctor give, for his own satisfaction first, and to the unhappy person whom sickness has reduced to a blind torpor and in whom rises a vain sense of rebellion against suffering and death? Only a heart impregnated with a deep and living

296 faith will find the words which carry the sincerity and deep conviction capable of rendering acceptance in the words of the divine Master: "It is necessary to suffer and to die, and so enter into glory." The doctor will fight against sickness and death with all the means and methods of his science and art, but not with the desperate resignation of pessimism, nor yet with the "exasperated resolution" which a certain modern philosophy has seen fit to exalt, but with the calm peace of one who sees and knows what suffering and death mean in the salvific designs of the omniscient and infinitely good and merciful Lord.

43: Pharmacology

DOCUMENT 1:

SOURCE: Pope Pius XII, Vatican Secretariat of State, "The Responsibility of the Pharmacist" (Sept. 1954), *The Human Body: Papal Teachings*, pp. 301–02.

The dignity of a profession is deduced from the nobility, extension, and value of the interests with which it is entrusted. Among the natural goods in man's possession, certainly health takes first place. The possibility of utilizing all the other energies given by nature depends on health. And so the pharmacist, cooperating as he does with the doctor in taking care of life, helps to preserve one of man's most precious gifts. His Catholic faith teaches him something more: that the body which he cures with his medicines will rise again and share in an eternal destiny. This, then, is the solid basis of the dignity of the profession of the pharmacist, a dignity, too, which is not without its formidable responsibilities in the search for new formulae, in the handling and application of remedies, some of which are particularly delicate. This dignity is the common privilege—though in a different measure—both of the great laboratories which turn out pharmaceutical products, and of the modest country chemist. As well as health, there are at times other sacrosanct gifts at stake: the honor of the sick man and of his family, and the most precious good of the physician himself—his good reputation, which is often dependent on the knowledge, ability, and discretion of the pharmacist.

On this point, the Holy Father spoke in 1950, in his address to an earlier congress: "Your responsibility extends still further. The good or bad effect of a remedy has a moral as well as a technical aspect, a morality which must be emphasized more today because of the prevailing waywardness of consciences."

The pharmacist, in order to act without hesitation and to defend himself from solicitations which come generally from his clients, should be well acquainted with Catholic morality, and the matters with which it is in accord or discord. This morality in its turn merely confirms and elevates the natural law. Furthermore, the pharmacist will need a sound formation in medical ethics, which will enable him to apply the laws and principles. But above all, he needs an upright Christian conscience, the immediate judge and guide in all his actions.

On the other hand, the pharmacist more than most others is in direct contact with the day-to-day life of the people, especially in their most distressing moments, when affection is more deeply felt and relationships are more cordial. In this he can be a great force in forming public opinion on certain pressing

298   problems. His upright behavior, his charity towards his fellow men, his cultural, religious, social formation will make him, under the guidance of Providence, a professional man of outstanding dignity.

Let the nobility and majesty of their mission inspire the delegates at the Saragossa Congress. Let love for their neighbor, in imitation of the love of Jesus Christ, stimulate them in their professional studies and activity.

His Holiness implores of God an abundant stream of grace upon all the members of this illustrious assembly, that there may flow therefrom fruits as abundant as they are precious. At the same time, he imparts to all his paternal apostolic benediction.

44: Population

DOCUMENT 1:

Source: Vatican Council II, "Pastoral Constitution on the Church in the Modern World" (Dec. 7, 1965), *Vatican Council II*, Vol. 1, pp. 996–97.

SOME USEFUL NORMS

87. International cooperation is vitally necessary in the case of those peoples who very often in the midst of many difficulties are faced with the special problems arising out of rapid increases in population. There is a pressing need to harness the full and eager cooperation of all, particularly of the richer countries, in order to explore how the human necessities of food and suitable education can be furnished and shared with the entire human community. Some peoples could improve their standard of living considerably if they were properly trained to substitute new techniques of agricultural production for antiquated methods and adapt them prudently to their own situation. The social order would also be improved and a fairer distribution of land ownership would be assured.

The government has, assuredly, in the matter of the population of its country, its own rights and duties, within the limits of its proper competence, for instance as regards social and family legislation, the migration of country-dwellers to the city, and information concerning the state and needs of the nation. Some men nowadays are gravely disturbed by this problem; it is to be hoped that there will be Catholic experts in these matters, particularly in universities, who will diligently study the problems and pursue their researches further.

Since there is widespread opinion that the population expansion of the world, or at least some particular countries, should be kept in check by all possible means and by every kind of intervention by public authority, the Council exhorts all men to beware of all solutions, whether uttered in public or in private or imposed at any time, which transgress the natural law. Because in virtue of man's inalienable right to marriage and the procreation of children, the decision regarding the number of children depends on the judgment of the parents and is in no way to be left to the decrees of public authority. Now, since the parents' judgment presupposes a properly formed conscience, it is of great importance that all should have an opportunity to cultivate a genuinely human sense of responsibility which will take account of the circumstances of time and situation and will respect the divine law; to attain this goal a change for the better must take place in educational and social conditions, and, above all, religious formation, or at least full moral training, must be available. People should be discreetly informed of scientific advances in research into methods of birth regulation, whenever the value of these methods has been thoroughly proved and their conformity with the moral order established.

DOCUMENT 2 / Population

Source: Pope John Paul II, "Population Development" (June 7, 1984), *The Pope Speaks* 29: no. 3, 1984, pp. 248–52.

. . . It is readily apparent that the worldwide population situation is very complex and varies from region to region.

Behind the demographic facts there are many interrelated issues that have to do with improving the circumstances of living so that people can live in dignity, justice, and peace, so that they can exercise the God-given right to form families, to bear and bring up children, and so that they can pursue their eternal destiny, which is union with the loving God who has created them. Thus, the Catholic Church takes positive note of the concern for improving systems of education and health care, recognizing the roles of aging persons, obtaining greater opportunities for people to be active participants in the development process, and in constructing a new global economic system based on justice and equity.

The Church recognizes the role of governments and of the international community to study and to face with responsibility the population problem in the context of and with a view to the common good of individual nations and of all humanity.

But demographic policies must not consider people as mere numbers, or only in economic terms, or with any kind of prejudice. They must respect and promote the dignity and the fundamental rights of the human person and of the family.

The dignity of the human person—of each and every person—and his or her uniqueness and capacity to contribute to the well-being of society are of primary importance to the Church, when entering into discussions about population, for the Church believes that human dignity is based on the fact that God has created each person, that we have been redeemed by Christ, and that, according to the divine plan, we shall rejoice with God forever.

The Church must always stand as a sign and safeguard of the transcendent character of the human person, restoring hope to those who might otherwise despair of anything better than their present lot. This conviction of the Church is shared by others and is in harmony with the most secret desires of the human heart and responds to the deepest longings of the human person. The dignity of the person, then, is a value of universal importance, one that is upheld by people of differing religious, cultural, and national backgrounds.

This emphasis on the value of the person demands respect for human life, which is always a splendid gift of God's goodness. Against the pessimism and selfishness which cast a shadow over the world, the Church stands for life and calls for ever greater efforts to correct those situations which endanger or diminish the value and appropriate enjoyment of human life.

RECALLS APOSTOLIC EXHORTATION

Thus, I recall the words of my apostolic exhortation *Familiaris Consortio* which reflect the consensus of the 1980 World Synod of Bishops on the family in the modern world:

"The Church is called upon to manifest anew to everyone, with clear and stronger conviction, her will to promote human life by every means and to defend it against all attacks, in whatever condition or state of development it is found.

"Thus the Church condemns as a grave offense against human dignity and justice all those activities of governments or other public authorities which attempt to limit in any way the freedom of couples in deciding about children. Consequently, any violence applied by such authorities in favor of contraception or, still worse, of sterilization and procured abortion must be altogether condemned or forcefully rejected.

"Likewise to be denounced as gravely unjust are cases where, in international relations, economic help given for the advancement of peoples is made conditional on programs of contraception, sterilization, and procured abortion. . . ."

ROLE OF WOMEN IMPORTANT

Special attention should be given to the role of women in modern society. Improving the status of women is important. In this regard we should not overlook the contributions that women make in the home and in their unique capacity to nurture the infant and guide the child in the earliest phase of education. This particular contribution of women is often ignored or diminished in favor of economic considerations or employment opportunities, and sometimes even in order to decrease the number of children. Continued efforts should be made to ensure the full integration of women in society, while giving due recognition to their important social role as mothers. This should include maternal and child health care, proper maternal leave, and family income supplements.

The Church is also aware of the initiatives in favor of the aging sponsored by the UNFPA (United Nations Fund for Population Activities). The number of aging persons is increasing in most countries. Their needs are often overlooked and also the contribution they make to society. They bring experience, wisdom, and a special patience to the solution of human problems, and they can and should be active members of contemporary society.

Much attention is given to the relationship of population to development. It is widely recognized that a population policy is only one part of an overall development strategy. Once again, the Church emphasizes that the needs of families should be a primary consideration in development strategies, that families should be encouraged to assume responsibility for transforming society and be active participants in the development process.

Yet, development itself should be more than a pursuit of material benefits; it should involve a more comprehensive approach that respects and satisfies the spiritual as well as the material needs of each person and of the whole of

302   society. In a word, development strategies should be based on a just worldwide socioeconomic order directed toward an equitable sharing of created goods, respectful stewardship of the environment and natural resources, and a sense of moral responsibility and cooperation among nations in order to achieve peace, security, and economic stability for all.

Above all, development should not be interpreted simply in terms of population control, nor should governments or international agencies make development assistance dependent on the achievement of family planning goals. . . .

DOCUMENT 3 / Population

SOURCE: Pope John Paul II, "The Gospel of Life" (Mar. 25, 1995), *Origins* 24: no. 42, Apr. 6, 1995, pp. 695, 720.

16. . . . Today not a few of the powerful of the earth act in the same way. They too are haunted by the current demographic growth and fear that the most prolific and poorest peoples represent a threat for the well-being and peace of their own countries. Consequently, rather than wishing to face and solve these serious problems with respect for the dignity of individuals and families and for every person's inviolable right to life, they prefer to promote and impose by whatever means a massive program of birth control. Even the economic help which they would be ready to give is unjustly made conditional on the acceptance of an anti-birth policy.

91. Today an important part of policies which favor life is the issue of population growth. Certainly public authorities have a responsibility to "intervene to orient the demography of the population." But such interventions must always take into account and respect the primary and inalienable responsibility of married couples and families, and cannot employ methods which fail to respect the person and fundamental human rights, beginning with the right to life of every innocent human being. It is therefore morally unacceptable to encourage, let alone impose, the use of methods such as contraception, sterilization and abortion in order to regulate births. The ways of solving the population problem are quite different. Governments and the various international agencies must above all strive to create economic, social, public health, and cultural conditions which will enable married couples to make their choices about procreation in full freedom and with genuine responsibility. They must then make efforts to ensure "greater opportunities and a fairer distribution of wealth so that everyone can share equitably in the goods of creation. Solutions must be sought on the global level by establishing a true economy of communion and sharing of goods, in both the national and international order." This is the only way to respect the dignity of persons and families as well as the authentic cultural patrimony of peoples.

303

DOCUMENT 4 / Population

Source: Pontifical Council for the Family, "Population Trends: Ethical and Pastoral Dimensions," *Origins* 24: no. 10 (Aug. 4, 1994), pp. 174–86.

In publishing this text the Pontifical Council for the Family wishes to present points for consideration concerning population realities. The first part of this document examines population trends. The second part describes attitudes regarding demographic realities. The third part sets out ethical principles in the light of which the Church analyzes these realities. This examination forms the basis for proposing pastoral guidelines.

... Far from being indifferent to various population trends, the Church closely evaluates their significance and complexity. Nevertheless she proclaims that among the attitudes which are envisaged, all are not morally acceptable.

... The anxiety of those who always speak about a "world population crisis" does not seem justified by the diversified trends actually found among populations in the different countries of the world. This anxiety really expresses a kind of ideology of fear of the future and mistrust of man ...

... First of all, the Church forcefully calls attention to the covert appearance of a new form of poverty. It is expressed precisely in negative attitudes regarding life and family. These attitudes lead to forgetting solidarity; they drive man back into solitude, they are not sufficiently open to future generations nor are they sensitive enough to what the lack of people involves. These attitudes reveal the worst kind of poverty: moral poverty.

... The Church is also aware of the reality of population changes in developing nations. She affirms the vocation of every person and nation to development .... Underdevelopment is not inevitable. Forces can be put into motion which allow each person and country to develop their potentialities and thus overcome underdevelopment. Among others, universal access to knowledge is an absolute priority, so that all people and all nations themselves find satisfactory solutions to the basic problems of subsistence and development within the framework of international solidarity.

With regard to demographic realities, the search for a truly human response is clarified by the Church's teaching on the common good on what is surplus and on the universal destination of goods. Seeing the universal common good as requiring effective solidarity among people could guide the efforts of each to the benefit of all. No one—whether individual or nation—is justified in putting his particular good over the demands of the common good of the human family.

... In its teaching on the universal destination of goods, the Church recalls that, according to the Creator's plan, the whole of humanity's goods—spiritual and intellectual included—are at the disposal of the human community, both present and future, and each generation should act as its responsible stewards.

The principle of subsidiarity also applies to the demographic domain. As recent popes have indicated, the Church recognizes a right of public authorities, within the limit of their competence, to intervene regarding population matters, but she also affirms that in this area the state is not to arrogate to itself the responsibilities of which couples ought not to be deprived.

. . . Two other ethical principles must be recalled, because the Church begins with these when she speaks out on population trends. The first is concerned with the sacred nature of human life and the responsibility of couples for the transmission of life. Created in the image and likeness of God, the origin of all life, men and women are called to be partners with the Creator in transmitting the sacred gift of human life. Within the communion of life and love which is marriage, they form the family, which is the basic cell of society. . . .

. . . The second principle regards the inherent right of parenthood. In the Charter of the Rights of the Family, the Church affirms:

"The spouses have the inalienable right to found a family and to decide on the spacing of births and the number of children to be born, taking into full consideration their duties toward themselves, their children already born, the family and society, in a just hierarchy of values and in accordance with the objective moral order, which excludes contraception, sterilization, and abortion."

. . . Free to choose the number of children they desire, the couple must be equally free to use natural methods for the responsible regulation of their fertility, for serious reasons and in conformity with the teaching of the Church. These various methods deserve to be known and spread widely. Couples must be offered the means to freely exercise their responsible motherhood and father-hood. The artificial methods of birth control as well as sterilization do not respect the human person of a woman and man because they eliminate or impede fertility, which is an integral part of the person.

The Church vigorously encourages the relevant experts, especially demog-raphers, economists, and political experts, to carry out deeper scientific research on demographic realities. All associations and organizations committed to re-spect for the human person and the family must make provision for a correct knowledge of facts and demographic diversity in their reflection and activities. They should provide a reasoned rejection of the ideology which is expressed as a fear of life and the future. This task also involves organizations working for justice and peace in solidarity.

On their part, all educational institutions are asked to include systematic and critical reflection on demographic realities in their program. All these efforts should be crowned with the resolve to provide objective information for opinion makers and the mass medica as well as public opinion.

Only when the rights of the family are recognized and promoted can there exist an authentic development which respects women and children and gives attention to the rich diversity of cultures. In the context of this authentic human development, there is a fundamental moral truth which cannot be

306 changed either by laws or population policies, whether these be evident or hidden. This fundamental truth is that human life must be respected from conception until natural death. The quality of a society is not only shown by the respect it has for the woman. Its quality is also shown by the respect or contempt a society has for life and human dignity.

DOCUMENT 5 / Population

SOURCE: John Paul II, "Population Conference Draft Document Criticized," *Origins* 23: no. 41 (Mar. 31, 1994), pp. 716–719.

. . . The global population situation is very complex. There are variations not simply from continent to continent, but even from one region to another. U.N. studies tell us that a rapid decrease in the global rate of population growth is expected to begin during the 1990s and carry on into the new century. At the same time, growth rates remain high in some of the least-developed nations of the world, while population growth has declined appreciably in the industrialized developed nations. . . .

. . . In accordance with its specific competence and mission, the Holy See is concerned that proper attention should be given to the ethical principles determining actions taken in response to the demographic, sociological, and public policy analyses of the data on population trends. Therefore, the Holy See seeks to focus attention on certain basic truths: that each and every person— regardless of age, sex, religion or national background—has a dignity and worth that is unconditional and inalienable; that human life itself from conception to natural death is sacred; that human rights are innate and transcend any constitutional order; and that the fundamental unity of the human race demands that everyone be committed to building a community which is free from injustice and which strives to promote and protect the common good. These truths about the human person are the measure of any response to the findings which emerge from the consideration of demographic data. It is in the light of authentic human values—recognized by peoples of diverse cultures, religious and national backgrounds across the globe—that all policy choices must be evaluated. No goal or policy will bring positive results for people if it does not respect the unique dignity and objective needs of those same people.

3. There is widespread agreement that a population policy is only one part of an overall development strategy. Accordingly, it is important that any discussion of population policies should keep in mind the actual and projected development of nations and regions. At the same time, it is impossible to leave out of account the very nature of what is meant by the term development. All development worthy of the name must be integral, that is, it must be directed to the true good of every person and of the whole person. True development cannot consist in the simple accumulation of wealth and in the greater availability of goods and services, but must be pursued with due consideration for the social, cultural, and spiritual dimensions of the human being. Development programs must be built on justice and equality, enabling people to live in dignity, harmony, and peace. They must respect the cultural heritage of peoples and nations and those social qualities and virtues that reflect the God-given dignity of each and every person and the divine plan which calls all persons

308 to unity. Importantly, men and women must be active agents of their own development, for to treat them as mere objects in some scheme or plan would be to stifle that capacity for freedom and responsibility which is fundamental to the good of the human person.

4. Development has been and remains the proper context for the international community's consideration of population issues. Within such discussions there naturally arise questions relating to the transmission and nurturing of human life. But to formulate population issues in terms of individual "sexual and reproductive rights" or even in terms of "women's rights" is to change the focus which should be the proper concern of governments and international agencies. I say this without in any way wishing to reduce the importance of securing justice and equity for women.

Moreover, questions involving the transmission of life and its subsequent nurturing cannot be adequately dealt with except in relation to the good of the family: that communion of persons established by the marriage of husband and wife which is, as the Universal Declaration of Human Rights affirms, "the natural and fundamental group unit of society" (art. 16.3). The family is an institution founded upon the very nature of the human person, and it is the proper setting for the conception, birth, and upbringing of children. At this moment in history, when so many powerful forces are arrayed against the family, it is more important than ever that the Conference on Population and Development should respond to the challenge implicit in the United Nations' designation of 1994 as the International Year of the Family by doing everything within its power to ensure that that family receives from "society and the state" that protection to which the same universal declaration says it is "entitled" (ibid.). Anything less would be a betrayal of the noblest ideals of the United Nations.

5. Today the duty to safeguard the family demands that particular attention be given to securing for husband and wife the liberty to decide responsibly, free from all social or legal coercion, the number of children they will have and the spacing of their births. It should not be the intent of governments or other agencies to decide for couples, but rather to create the social conditions which will enable them to make appropriate decisions in the light of their responsibilities to God, to themselves, to the society of which they are a part, and to the objective moral order. What the Church calls responsible parenthood is not a question of unlimited procreation or lack of awareness of what is involved in rearing children, but rather the empowerment of couples to use their inviolable liberty wisely and responsibly, taking into account social and demographic realities as well as their moral criteria. All propaganda and misinformation directed at persuading couples that they must limit their family to one or two children should be steadfastly avoided, and couples that generously choose to have large families are to be supported.

In defense of the human person, the Church stands opposed to the imposition of limits on family size and to the promotion of methods of limiting births which separate the unitive and procreative dimensions of marital intercourse, which are contrary to the moral law inscribed on the human heart or which constitute an assault on the sacredness of life. Thus sterilization, which is more **309** and more promoted as a method of family planning, because of its finality and its potential for the violation of human rights, especially of women, is clearly unacceptable; it poses a most grave threat to human dignity and liberty when promoted as part of a population policy. Abortion, which destroys existing human life, is a heinous evil, and it is never an acceptable method of family planning, as was recognized by consensus at the Mexico City U.N. International Conference on Population (1984).

. . . As well as reaffirming the fundamental role of the family in society, I wish to draw special attention to the status of children and women, who all too often find themselves the most vulnerable members of our communities. Children must not be treated as a burden or inconvenience, but should be cherished as bearers of hope and signs of promise for the future. The care which is essential for their growth and nurture comes primarily from their parents, but society must help by sustaining the family in its needs and in its efforts to maintain the caring environment in which children can develop. Society ought to promote "social policies which have the family as their principal object, policies which assist the family by providing adequate resources and efficient means of support, both for bringing up children and for looking after the elderly, so as to avoid distancing the latter from the family unit and in order to strengthen relations between generations" (*Centesimus Annus*, 49). A society cannot say that it is treating children justly or protecting their interests if its laws do not safeguard their rights and respect the responsibility of parents for their well-being.

It is sad reflection on the human condition that still today, at the end of the 20th century, it is necessary to affirm that every woman is equal in dignity to man and a full member of the human family, within which she has a distinctive place and vocation that is complementary to but in no way less valuable than man's. In much of the world much still has be done to meet the educational and health needs of girls and young women so that they may achieve their full potential in society. . . .

45: Proxy Consent

DOCUMENT 1:

Source: Congregation for the Doctrine of the Faith, "Declaration on Euthanasia" (May 5, 1980), *Vatican Council II*, Vol. 2, pp. 513–15.

. . . It may happen that, by reason of prolonged and barely tolerable pain, for deeply personal or other reasons, people may be led to believe that they can legitimately ask for death or obtain it for others. Although in these cases the guilt of the individual may be reduced or completely absent, nevertheless the error of judgment into which the conscience falls, perhaps in good faith, does not change the nature of this act of killing, which will always be in itself something to be rejected. The pleas of gravely ill people who sometimes ask for death are not to be understood as implying a true desire for euthanasia; in fact it is almost always a case of an anguished plea for help and love. What a sick person needs, besides medical care, is love, the human and supernatural warmth with which the sick person can and ought to be surrounded by all those close to him or her, parents and children, doctors and nurses.

DUE PROPORTION IN THE USE OF REMEDIES

Today it is very important to protect, at the moment of death, both the dignity of the human person and the Christian concept of life, against a technological attitude that threatens to become an abuse. Thus, some people speak of a "right to die," which is an expression that does not mean the right to procure death either by one's own hand or by means of someone else, as one pleases, but rather the right to die peacefully with human and Christian dignity. From this point of view, the use of therapeutic means can sometimes pose problems.

In numerous cases, the complexity of the situation can be such as to cause doubts about the way ethical principles should be applied. In the final analysis, it pertains to the conscience either of the sick person, or of those qualified to speak in the sick person's name, or of the doctors to decide in the light of moral obligations and of the various aspects of the case.

Everyone has the duty to care for his or her own health or to seek such care from others. Those whose task it is to care for the sick must do so conscientiously and administer the remedies that seem necessary or useful. . . .

DOCUMENT 2 / Proxy Consent

SOURCE: Pope Pius XII, "The Intangibility of the Human Person" (Sept. 13, 1952), *The Human Body: Papal Teachings*, p. 201.

THE INTERESTS OF THE PATIENT

. . . The frontier is the same as for the patient: it is the one fixed by the judgment of right reason, and it is traced by the demands of the moral law, which is derived from the natural finality or purpose stamped on beings, and from the scale of values expressed by the very nature of things. The boundaries are the same for the doctor as for the patient, because, as we have already said, the doctor, as does the private individual, disposes of rights, and those rights alone, which are granted by the patient, and because the patient cannot give more than he possesses himself.

What we have already said is true also of the legal representative of anyone incapable of disposing of himself and of his affairs, for example, children who have not arrived at the age of reason, the feeble of mind, the insane. Such legal representatives, appointed by a private decision or by public authority, do not possess over the body and the life of their subordinates any other rights than they themselves would have, if they were capable of it, and to the same extent. They cannot then give the doctor permission to dispose of them outside of these limits.

DOCUMENT 3 / Proxy Consent

SOURCE: Pope Pius XII, "The Prolongation of Life" (Nov. 24, 1957), *The Pope Speaks* 4: no. 4, 1958, p. 397.

A DOCTOR'S RIGHTS AND DUTIES

... The rights and duties of the doctor are correlative to those of the patient. The doctor, in fact, has no separate or independent right where the patient is concerned. In general he can take action only if the patient explicitly or implicitly, directly or indirectly, gives him permission. The technique of resuscitation which concerns us here does not contain anything immoral in itself. Therefore the patient, if he were capable of making a personal decision, could lawfully use it and, consequently, give the doctor permission to use it. On the other hand, since these forms of treatment go beyond the ordinary means to which one is bound, it cannot be held that there is an obligation to use them nor, consequently, that one is bound to give the doctor permission to use them.

... The rights and duties of the family depend in general upon the presumed will of the unconscious patient if he is of age and *sui juris*. Where the proper and independent duty of the family is concerned, they are usually bound only to the use of ordinary means.

Consequently, if it appears that the attempt at resuscitation constitutes in reality such a burden for the family that one cannot in all conscience impose it upon them, they can lawfully insist that the doctor should discontinue these attempts, and the doctor can lawfully comply. There is not involved here a case of direct disposal of the life of the patient, nor of euthanasia in any way: this would never be licit. Even when it causes the arrest of circulation, the interruption of attempts at resuscitation is never more than an indirect cause of the cessation of life, and one must apply in this case the principle of double effect and of *voluntarium in causa*.

46: Principle of Cooperation

DOCUMENT 1:

Source: Pope John Paul II, "The Gospel of Life" (Mar. 25, 1995), *Origins* 24: no. 42, Apr. 6, 1995, pp. 715–16.

74. . . . In order to shed light on this difficult question, it is necessary to recall the general principles concerning cooperation in evil actions. Christians, like all people of good will, are called upon under grave obligation of conscience not to cooperate formally in practices which, even if permitted by civil legislation, are contrary to God's law. Indeed, from the moral standpoint, it is never licit to cooperate formally in evil. Such cooperation occurs when an action, either by its very nature or by the form it takes in a concrete situation, can be defined as a direct participation in an act against innocent human life or a sharing in the immoral intention of the person committing it. This cooperation can never be justified either by invoking respect for the freedom of others or by appealing to the fact that civil law permits it or requires it. Each individual in fact has moral responsibility for the acts which he personally performs; no one can be exempted from this responsibility, and on the basis of it everyone will be judged by God himself (cf. Rom 2:6; 14:12).

To refuse to take part in committing an injustice is not only a moral duty; it is also a basic human right. Were this not so, the human person would be forced to perform an action intrinsically incompatible with human dignity, and in this way human freedom itself, the authentic meaning and purpose of which are found in its orientation to the true and the good, would be radically compromised. What is at stake therefore is an essential right which, precisely as such, should be acknowledged and protected by civil law. In this sense, the opportunity to refuse to take part in the phases of consultation, preparation, and execution of these acts against life should be guaranteed to physicians, health care personnel, and directors of hospitals, clinics, and convalescent facilities. Those who have recourse to conscientious objection must be protected not only from legal penalties, but also from any negative effects on the legal, disciplinary, financial, and professional plane.

47: Principle of Double Effect

DOCUMENT 1:

SOURCE: Congregation for the Doctrine of the Faith, "Instruction on Respect for Human Life in Its Origin and on the Dignity of Procreation" (Feb. 22, 1987), *Origins* 16: no. 40, Mar. 19, 1987, p. 711.

The obligation to avoid disproportionate risks involves an authentic respect for human beings and the uprightness of therapeutic intentions. It implies that the doctor "above all ... must carefully evaluate the possible negative consequences which the necessary use of a particular exploratory technique may have upon the unborn child and avoid recourse to diagnostic procedures which do not offer sufficient guarantees of their honest purpose and substantial harmlessness. And if, as often happens in human choices, a degree of risk must be undertaken, he will take care to assure that it is justified by a truly urgent need for the diagnosis and by the importance of the results that can be achieved by it for the benefit of the unborn child himself."

DOCUMENT 2 / Principle of Double Effect

SOURCE: Pope Pius XII, "The Attempt on Innocent Human Life" (Nov. 26, 1951), *The Human Body: Papal Teachings*, p. 182.

. . . Deliberately we have always used the expression "direct attempt on the life of an innocent person," "direct killing." Because if, for example, the saving of the life of the future mother, independently of her pregnant condition, should urgently require a surgical act or other therapeutic treatment which would have an accessory consequence, in no way desired nor intended, but inevitable, the death of the fetus, such an act could no longer be called a direct attempt on an innocent life. Under these conditions the operation can be lawful, like other similar medical interventions—granted always that a good of high worth is concerned, such as life, and that it is not possible to postpone the operation until after birth of the child, nor to have recourse to other efficacious remedies. . . .

DOCUMENT 3 / Principle of Double Effect

SOURCE: Pope Pius XII, "The Prolongation of Life" (Nov. 24, 1957), *The Pope Speaks* 4: no. 4, 1985, p. 397.

. . . Consequently, if it appears that the attempt at resuscitation constitutes in reality such a burden for the family that one cannot in all conscience impose it upon them, they can lawfully insist that the doctor should discontinue these attempts, and the doctor can lawfully comply. There is not involved here a case of direct disposal of the life of the patient, nor of euthanasia in any way: this would never be licit. Even when it causes the arrest of circulation, the interruption of attempts at resuscitation is never more than an indirect cause of the cessation of life, and one must apply in this case the principle of double effect and of *voluntarium in causa.*

48: Principle of Totality

DOCUMENT 1:

SOURCE: Pope Pius XII, "Christian Principles and the Medical Profession" (Nov. 12, 1944), *The Human Body: Papal Teachings*, pp. 54–56.

. . . In forming man, God regulated each of his functions, assigning them to the various organs. In this way, he distinguished those which are essential to life from those which contribute only to the integrity of the body, however precious be the activity, well-being, and beauty of this last. At the same time, God fixed, prescribed, and limited the use of each organ. He cannot therefore allow man now to arrange his life and the functions of his organs according to his own taste, in a manner contrary to the intrinsic and immanent function assigned them. Man, in truth, is not the owner of his body nor its absolute lord, but only its user. A whole series of principles and norms derives from this fact, governing the use of the body with its members and organs, and the right to dispose of them: principles and norms to which are equally subject the individual concerned and the doctor called in for consultation.

SOCIETY AND THE INDIVIDUAL
. . . Regarding the body, the life, and the corporal integrity of the individual, the juridical position of society differs essentially from that of the individual himself. Man's power over his members and organs is a direct—though not unlimited—power; because these are parts which go to make up his physical being. Their association in the one being has for a goal only the well-being of the whole physical organism, and hence it is clear that each of these organs and members can be sacrificed if it puts the whole organism in danger, a danger which cannot in any other way be averted. Quite different is the case with society, which is not a physical being, but a simple community of purpose and action. In virtue of this it can demand of those who make it up and who are called its members all those services essential for the true common good.

Such are the foundations on which must rest every judgment on the moral value of acts and operations concerning the human body, human life, and corporal integrity of the person, which public authority allows or imposes.

DOCUMENT 2 / Principle of Totality

SOURCE: Pope Pius XII, "The Intangibility of the Human Person" (Sept. 14, 1952), *The Human Body: Papal Teachings*, pp. 199–207.

... The patient has not the right to involve his physical and psychic integrity in medical experiments or researches when these interventions entail, either immediately or subsequently, acts of destruction, or of mutilization and wounds, or grave dangers.

Furthermore, in exercising his right to dispose of himself, of his faculties and organs, the individual must observe the hierarchy of the scale of values—and within an identical order of values, the hierarchy of individual goods, to the extent demanded by the laws of morality. So, for example, man cannot perform upon himself or allow medical operations, either physical or somatic, which beyond doubt do remove serious defects or physical or psychic weaknesses, but which entail at the same time permanent destruction of, or a considerable and lasting lessening of, freedom, that is to say, of the human personality in its particular and characteristic function. Thus is man degraded to the level of a being purely sensitive to acquired reflexes, or of an automaton. Such a reversal of values the moral law does not support; therefore here it establishes the limits and frontiers of the "medical interests of the patient."

Take the following example: in order to rid himself of repressions, inhibitions, and psychic complexes, man is not free to awaken in himself for therapeutic ends each and every sexual appetite, which moves, or is moved, in his being and sends its impure waves through his unconscious or subconscious self. He cannot make them the object of his conduct or of his fully conscious desires, with all the upheavals and repercussions involved in such a proceeding. For man, and for the Christian, there exists a law of integrity and personal purity, of personal esteem for himself, which forbids him to plunge himself thus wholly into the world of sexual representations and tendencies. The "medical and psychotherapeutical interests of the patient" find here a moral limit. It is not proved, nay it is even untrue, that the pansexual method of a certain school of psychoanalysis is an integrant indispensable part of all serious psychotherapy worthy of the name; that the fact of having neglected this method in the past has caused serious psychic harm, errors in doctrine and in its application in the field of education, of psychotherapy, and not least in the pastoral field; that there is a pressing need of making good this deficiency, and of initiating all those occupied in psychic questions in its guiding principles, and even, if necessary, in the practical management of this technique of sexuality.

The community is the great medium ordained by nature and by God to regulate the exchanges by which mutual needs are met, to help each one to develop his personality according to his individual social capacity. The community, considered as a whole, is not a physical unity which subsists in **319** itself. Its individual members are not integrating parts of it. The physical organism of living beings, of plants, animals, or men, possesses as a whole a unity which subsists in itself. Each of the members, for example, the hand, the foot, the heart, the eye, is an integrant part, destined by its whole being to be a part of one complete organism. Outside the organism it has not of its own nature any meaning, any purpose: its being is wholly absorbed in the complete organism with which it is linked.

A quite different state of affairs obtains in the moral community and in each organism of a purely moral character. The whole has not here a unity which subsists in itself, but a simple unity of purpose and of action. In the community the individuals are only collaborators and instruments for the realization of the ends of the community.

What follows with regard to the physical organism? The master, the person who uses this organism, which possesses a subsisting unity, can dispose directly and immediately of the integrant parts, the members and the organs, within the framework of their natural finality. Likewise he can intervene, when and as far as the well-being of the whole demands, to paralyze, destroy, mutilate, separate its members. In contrast, however, when the whole does not possess a unity except of finality and of action, its head, that is to say, in the present case the public authority, retains without doubt a direct authority, and the right to impose its demands on the activity of the parts, but in no case can it dispose directly of its physical being. Moreover, every direct injury attempted against its essential being by public authority is a departure from that sphere of activity which rightly belongs to it.

... We feel that we must throw light yet again on the subject treated in this part, in the light of the principle to which appeal is usually made in cases such as these. We refer to the principle of totality. It declares that the part exists for the whole, and that, consequently, the good of the part remains subordinated to the good of the whole: that the whole is that which determines the part and can dispose of it in its own interest. The principle springs from the essence of notions and of things, and must thereby have absolute value.

Certainly, one must respect the principle of totality in itself. However, to be able to apply it correctly, we must first of all explain certain presuppositions. The fundamental presupposition is to make clear the *quaestio facti*—the question of fact: do the objects to which the principle is applied stand in relationship of whole to part? A second presupposition: to clarify the nature, the extent, and the closeness of this relationship. Does it fall within the sphere of essence, or only the part under a definite aspect, or in every respect? And in the field where it applies, does it absorb the part completely, or does it leave to the part a certain degree of limited finality, a limited independence? The reply to these questions can never be inferred from the principle of totality itself: that would look very like a vicious circle. The reply must depend on other facts, and on other sources of knowledge. The principle of totality itself affirms nothing except this: where the relationship of whole to part is verified, and in the exact degree to which it is verified, the part is subordinated to the whole, which

320   later can in its own interest dispose of the part. Too frequently, alas, in resorting to the principle of totality, these considerations are left aside: not only in the domain of theoretical study and the field of application of the law, of sociology, of physics, of biology, of medicine, but also in logic, psychology, and metaphysics.

49: Psychotherapy

DOCUMENT 1:

Source: John Paul II, "The Moral Component of the Therapeutic Task," *Origins* 22: no. 31, (Jan. 14, 1993), p. 540.

. . . By its very nature your work often brings you to the threshold of the human mystery. It involves a sensitivity to the often tangled workings of the human mind and heart, and an openness to the ultimate concerns which give meaning to people's lives. These are areas of utmost importance to the Church, and they call to mind the urgent need for a constructive dialogue between science and religion for the sake of shedding greater light on the mystery of man in its fullness. The Church's own history of commitment to caring for the sick, especially the poor and the marginated, is rooted in the conviction that the human person is a unity of body and spirit, possessing an inviolable dignity as one made in the image of God and called to a transcendent destiny. For this reason, the Church is convinced that no adequate assessment of the nature of the human person or the requirements for human fulfillment and psychosocial well-being can be made without respect for man's spiritual dimension and capacity for self-transcendence. Only by transcending themselves and living a life of self-giving and openness to truth and love can individuals reach fulfillment and contribute to building an authentic human community.

Your association is rightly concerned to promote human dignity and the inviolability of individuals and of their freedom. The foundations of human dignity are to be found in the truth about man and in his human freedom to form his instincts and passions according to the objective requirements of the moral order. As the Scriptures suggest, there is an unbreakable link between authentic freedom and truth (cf. Jn 10:47); indeed, "freedom attains its full development only by accepting the truth" (*Centesimus Annus*, 46). It follows that no genuine therapy or treatment for psychic disturbances can ever conflict with the moral obligation of the patient to pursue the truth and to grow in virtue. This moral component of the therapeutic task makes great demands upon psychiatrists, who must be committed to attaining a more adequate grasp of the truth of their own lives and to showing profound respect for the dignity of their patients.

Psychiatrists must also feel themselves responsible for the social ramifications of their practice. This is especially true today, when there is ever more clearly a relationship between the appearance and aggravation of certain illnesses and mental disturbances and the crisis of value which society is experiencing. You and your associates will make an important contribution to the

322   future of society by seeking to point out, in the light of a dispassionate commitment to truth, the limits of certain models of social life which can lead to the manipulation of persons and to an unhealthy conditioning of human freedom. In your work to overcome the stigma which has often been associated with mental illness, to end the abuse of psychiatry for ideological reasons, and to strengthen the family as the basic unit of society, as well as in your efforts to draw society's attention to the special needs of the poor, the homeless and the abused, you can be certain of the Church's appreciation and ready cooperation.

The task of healing others and ensuring their psychosocial equilibrium is indeed important and delicate. Together with scientific knowledge there is need of great wisdom in those who devote themselves to this work. Assuring you once more of the Church's esteem, I cordially invoke upon you and the members of your associations the abundant blessings of almighty God.

DOCUMENT 2 / Psychotherapy

SOURCE: John Paul II, "The Image of God in People with Mental Illness," *Origins* 26: no. 30 (Jan. 16, 1997), pp. 495–97.

I am pleased with this meeting which allows me to offer you my greetings, distinguished participants in the international conference sponsored by the Pontifical Council for Pastoral Assistance to Health Care Workers on the problem of mental illness, with the significant title, "In the Image and Likeness of God: Always? Illness of the Human Mind."

Distinguished ladies and gentlemen, present among you are researchers, scientists, specialists in the field of the biomedical sciences, theologians, moralists, jurists, psychologists, sociologists, and health care workers. Together you represent a heritage of humanity and wisdom, of science and experience which can produce very useful advice for the understanding, treatment, and care of the mentally ill.

The Church looks on these persons with special concern as she looks on any other human being affected by illness. Instructed by the divine teacher's words, she believes that "man, made in the image of the Creator, redeemed by the blood of Christ, and made holy by the presence of the Holy Spirit has as the ultimate purpose of his life to live 'for the praise of God's glory' (Eph 1:12), striving to make each of his actions reflect the splendor of that glory" (*Veritatis Splendor*, 10).

Man Is Created in God's Image and Likeness

The Church is deeply convinced of this truth, even when man's mental faculties—the noblest, because they testify to his spiritual nature—seem severely limited and even impeded by a pathological process. She therefore reminds the political community of its duty to recognize and celebrate the divine image in man with actions that support and serve all those who find themselves in a condition of serious mental illness. This is a task which science and faith, medicine and pastoral care, professional skill and a sense of common brotherhood must help to carry out through an investment of adequate human, scientific, and socioeconomic resources.

The title of the congress invites us to examine further this line of reflection which has just been outlined. Indeed, while on the one hand it again offers an authoritative affirmation of the Bible, on the other it raises a disturbing question.

The conviction that man has been created in the image and likeness of God is one of the pillars of Christian anthropology. This is what is written in the first chapter of Genesis (1:26). Philosophical and theological reflection have identified in man's mental faculties, that is, in his reason and in his will, a privileged sign of this affinity with God. These faculties, in fact, enable man to know the Lord and to establish a relationship of dialogue with him. In discussing this, St. Thomas 323

324   points out, "person signifies what is most perfect in all nature, that is, a subsistent individual of a rational nature" (*Summa Theol.* I, q. 29, a. 3).

It should be made clear however that the whole man, not just his spiritual soul, including his intelligence and free will, but also his body, shares in the dignity of "the image of God." In fact, the human body "is a human body precisely because it is animated by a spiritual soul, and it is the whole human person that is intended to become, in the body of Christ, a temple of the Spirit" (*Catechism of the Catholic Church*, no. 364). "Do you not know," the apostle writes, "that your bodies are members of Christ?. . . You are not your own. . . . So glorify God in your body" (1 Cor 6:15, 19–20). Hence the need to respect one's own body, and also the body of every other person, especially the suffering (cf. *Catechism of the Catholic Church*, no. 1004).

By Grace Man Becomes a Child of God

Precisely because man is a person, his dignity is unique among all creatures. Every individual man is an end in himself and can never be used as a mere means for reaching other goals, not even in the name of the well-being and progress of the community as a whole. By creating man in his own image, God wished to make him share in his lordship and his glory. When he entrusted him with the task of caring for all creation, he took into account his creative intelligence and his responsible freedom.

The Second Vatican Council, delving into the mystery of man under the guidance of Christ's words (cf. Jn 17:21–22), opened up to us horizons inaccessible to human reason. In the constitution *Gaudium et Spes*, "a certain parallel between the union existing among the divine persons and the union of the sons of God in truth and love" (no. 24) is explicitly mentioned. When God turns his gaze on man, the first thing he sees and loves in him is not the deeds he succeeds in doing, but his own image, an image that confers on man the ability to know and love his own creator, to rule over all earthly creatures, and to use them for God's glory (cf. ibid., no. 12). And this is why the Church recognizes the same dignity in all human beings and the same fundamental value, regardless of any other circumstantial consideration. Therefore, regardless too—and this is most important—of the fact that this ability cannot be utilized because impeded by mental illness.

This conception of man as the image and likeness of God is not only confirmed by the New Testament revelation, but supremely enriched by it. St. Paul says: "But when the time had fully come, God sent forth his Son, born of woman, born under the law, to redeem those who were under the law, so that we might receive adoption as sons" (Gal 4:4–5). By grace, therefore, man truly shares in this divine sonship, becoming a child of God in the Son.

The Second Vatican Council teaches that Christ is "the image of the invisible God" (Col 1:15). He is the perfect man, who has restored in the children of Adam that likeness to God which had been disfigured ever since the first sin. Human nature, by the very fact that it was assumed, not absorbed, in him, has been raised in us also to a dignity beyond compare. For by his incarnation, the Son of God has in a certain way united himself with each man" (*Gaudium et Spes*, 22).

At this point we feel the whole weight of the disturbing question which appears in the theme: Always? This is a provocative question which is not only asked at the ontological level—here faith and reason converge in recognizing the full human dignity of the mentally ill—as much as at the deontological level. One can in fact ask whether the way a mentally ill person is treated by his peers in daily life corresponds fully and adequately to what he is in God's plan.

That question, "Always?," must spur both the personal and the collective conscience to a sincere reflection on our behavior toward those persons who are suffering from mental illness. Is it not true that all too often these persons encounter indifference and neglect, when not also exploited and abused?

Through God's grace there is also another side to the coin. I stressed this in the encyclical *Evangelium Vitae,* recalling "all those daily gestures of openness, sacrifice, and unselfish care which countless people lovingly make in families, hospitals, orphanages, homes for the elderly, and other centers or communities which defend life" (27). But we cannot close our eyes to certain forms of behavior which seem to ignore human dignity and to trample on his inalienable rights.

Mentally Ill Always Bear God's Image and Likeness

We Christians especially cannot do so. In this regard the Gospel speaks clearly. Christ not only took pity on the sick and healed many of them, restoring health to both their bodies and their minds; his compassion also led him to identify with them. He declares: "I was sick and you visited me" (Mt 25:36). The disciples of the Lord, precisely because they were able to see the image of the "suffering" Christ in all people marked by sickness, opened their hearts to them, spending themselves in various forms of assistance.

Well, Christ took all human suffering on himself, even mental illness. Yes even this affliction, which perhaps seems the most absurd and incomprehensible, configures the sick person to Christ and gives him a share in his redeeming passion.

Thus the response to the theme's question is clear: whoever suffers from mental illness "always" bears God's image and likeness in himself, as does every human being. In addition, he "always" has the inalienable right not only to be considered as an image of God and therefore as a person, but also to be treated as such.

It is everyone's duty to make an active response. Our actions must show that mental illness does not create insurmountable distances, nor prevent relations of true Christian charity with those who are its victims. Indeed, it should inspire a particularly attentive attitude toward these people who are fully entitled to belong to the category of the poor to whom the kingdom of heaven belongs (cf. Mt 5:3).

Distinguished ladies and gentlemen, I have recalled these fundamental and comforting truths, well aware that I am speaking to people who fully understand them. I gladly take this opportunity to express to you my full appreciation of your valuable work and to encourage you to continue a service with such lofty humanitarian importance.

DOCUMENT 3 / Psychotherapy

SOURCE: Pope Pius XII, *On Psychotherapy and Religion* (Apr. 13, 1953), National Catholic Welfare Conference, Washington, DC, pp. 3–10.

2. . . . Science affirms that recent observations have brought to light the hidden layers of the psychic structure of man and tries to understand the meaning of these discoveries, to interpret them and render them capable of use. People speak of dynamisms, determinisms, and mechanisms hidden in the depths of the soul, endowed with immanent laws whence are derived certain modes of acting. Undoubtedly these begin to operate within the subconscious or the unconscious, but they also penetrate into the realms of the conscious and determine it. People claim to have devised methods that have been tried and recognized as adequate to scrutinize the mystery of the depths of the soul, to elucidate them and put them back on the right road when they are exercising a harmful influence.

3. . . . Theoretical and practical psychology, the one as much as the other, should bear in mind that they cannot lose sight of the truths established by reason and by faith, nor of the obligatory precepts of ethics.

4. . . . Briefly, we intend to outline the fundamental attitude which is imposed upon the Christian psychologist and psychotherapeutist.

5. This fundamental attitude can be summed up in the following formula: psychotherapy and clinical psychology must always consider man (1) as a psychic unit and totality, (2) as a structured unit in itself, (3) as a social unit, and (4) as a transcendent unit, that is to say, in man's tending towards God.

I. MAN AS A PSYCHIC UNIT AND TOTALITY

6. Medicine has learned to consider the human body as a mechanism of great precision, whose parts fit into each other and are connected to each other. The place and the characteristics of these parts are dependent on the whole. They serve its existence and its functions. But this conception is more applicable still to the soul, whose delicate wheels have been assembled with much more care. The various psychic faculties and functions form part of the whole spiritual being and subordinate themselves to its final end.

7. It is useless to develop this point further. But you, psychologists and psychic healers, must bear this fact in mind: the existence of each psychic faculty and function is explained by the end of the whole man. What constitutes man is principally the soul, the substantial form of his nature. From it, ultimately, flows all the vital activity of man. In it are rooted all the psychic dynamisms with their own proper structure and their organic law. It is the soul which nature charges with the government of all man's energies, insofar as these have not yet acquired their final determination.

326

8. Given this ontological and psychological fact, it follows that it would be a departure from reality to attempt in theory or in practice, to entrust the determining role of the whole to one particular factor, for example, to one of the elementary psychic dynamisms and thus install a secondary power at the helm. Those psychic dynamisms may be in the soul, in man. They are not, however, the soul nor the man. They are energies of considerable intensity perhaps, but nature has entrusted their direction to the center-post, to the spiritual soul endowed with intellect and will, which is normally capable of governing these energies. That these energies may exercise pressure upon one activity does not necessarily signify that they compel it. To deprive the soul of its central place would be to deny an ontological and psychic reality.

9. It is not possible, therefore, when studying the relationship of the ego to the dynamisms that compose it, to concede unreservedly in theory the autonomy of man—that is, of his soul—but to go on immediately to state that in the reality of life this theoretical principle appears to be very frequently set aside or minimized to the extreme.

10. In the reality of life, it is argued, man always retains his freedom to give his internal consent to what he does, but in no way the freedom to do it. The autonomy of free will is replaced by the heteronomy of instinctive dynamism. That is not the way in which God fashioned man.

11. Original sin did not take away from man the possibility or the obligation of directing his own actions himself through his soul. It cannot be alleged that the psychic troubles and disorders which disturb the normal functioning of the psychic being represent what usually happens. The moral struggle to remain on the right path does not prove that it is impossible to follow that path, nor does it authorize any drawing back.

II. MAN AS A STRUCTURED UNIT

12. Man is an ordered unit and whole, a microcosm, a sort of state whose charter, determined by the end of the whole, subordinates to this end the activity of the parts according to the true order of their value and function. This charter is, in the final analysis, of an ontological and metaphysical origin, not a psychological and personal one. There are those who have thought it necessary to accentuate the opposition between the metaphysical and the psychological. A completely wrong approach! The psychic itself belongs to the domain of the ontological and metaphysical. . . .

15. . . . The study of the constitution of real man, ought, in fact, to take as object "existential" man, such as he is, such as his natural dispositions, the influences of his milieu, education, his personal development, his intimate experiences and external events have made him. It is only man in the concrete that exists. And yet, the structure of this personal ego obeys in the smallest detail the ontological and metaphysical laws of human nature of which we have spoken above. They have formed it and thus should govern and judge it. The reason behind this is that "existential" man identifies himself in his intimate structure with "essential" man.

328   16. The essential structure of man does not disappear when individual notes are added to it. It is not further transformed in another human nature. But the charter, of which we spoke just now, rests precisely in its principal terms on the essential structure of real man, man in the concrete.

17. Consequently, it would be erroneous to establish for real life norms which would deviate from natural and Christian morality, and which, for want of a better word, could be called "personalist" ethics. The latter would without doubt receive a certain "orientation" from the former, but this would not admit any strict obligation. The law of the structure of man in the concrete is not to be invented but applied. . . .

III. MAN AS A SOCIAL UNIT

24. . . . What has just been said of inconsiderate initiation for therapeutic purposes is valid also for certain forms of psychoanalysis. One should not come to regard them as the only means of relieving or of curing psychical sexual troubles. The trite principle that sexual trouble of the unconscious, as all other inhibitions of identical origin, can be suppressed only by their being brought to the level of consciousness, is not valid if it is generalized without distinction. The indirect treatment also has its efficacy and often it suffices to a large extent. As to the use of the psychoanalytic method in the sexual domain, our allocution of Sept. 13, already cited, has already pointed out the moral limits. In truth, one cannot consider as licit, without further consideration, the evocation to the level of consciousness of all the representations, emotions, and sexual experiences which lie dormant in the memory and the unconscious, and which are thus actualized in the psychic. If the protests arising from a sense of human and Christian dignity are heeded, who would risk making the claim that this manner of treatment does not imply both immediate and future moral danger, when, even if the therapeutic necessity of unlimited exploration be affirmed, this necessity is not, after all, established?

25. Error by excess: It consists in emphasizing the exigency of a total surrender of the ego and of its personal affirmation. With regard to this, we wish to consider two points: a general principle and a point of therapeutic practice.

26. From certain psychological explanations, the thesis is formulated that the unconditioned extroversion of the ego constitutes the fundamental law of congenital altruism and of its dynamic tendencies. This is a logical, psychological, and ethical error. There exists in fact a defense, an esteem, a love, and a service of one's personal self, which is not only justified but demanded by psychology and morality. It is a natural evidence and a lesson of the Christian faith (cf. St. Thomas, *Summa Theol.*, 2a2ae q.26, article 4, in c). Our Lord taught: "Thou shalt love thy neighbor as thyself" (Mk 12:31). Christ, then, proposes as the rule of love of neighbor charity towards oneself, not the contrary. Applied psychology would undervalue this reality if it were to describe all consideration of the ego as psychic inhibition, error, return to a state of former development, under the pretext that it is contrary to the natural altruism of the psychic being.

27. The point about psychotherapeutic practice that we mentioned concerns an essential interest of society: the safeguarding of secrets which the use

of psychoanalysis endangers. It is not at all excluded that a fact or knowledge   **329**
which is secret and repressed in the subconscious provokes serious psychic
conflicts. If psychoanalysis disclosed the cause of this trouble, it will want,
according to its principle, to draw out entirely this unconscious element and
make it conscious in order to remove the obstacle. But there are secrets which
must on no account be divulged, even to a doctor, even in spite of grave
personal inconveniences. The secret of Confession may never be revealed. It
is equally forbidden for the professional secret to be communicated to another,
including a doctor. The same is true of other secrets. One may invoke the
principle: "for a proportionately grave reason it is permitted to reveal a secret
to a prudent man and one capable of keeping a secret." This principle is correct
within narrow limits for certain kinds of secrets. It is not right to make use of
it indiscriminately in psychoanalytic practice.

28. As regards morality, for the common good in the first place, the
principle of discretion in the use of psychoanalysis cannot be sufficiently emphasized. Obviously it is not primarily a question of the discretion of the psychoana-
lyst, but of that of the patient, who frequently has no right whatever to give
away his secrets. . . .

DOCUMENT 4 / Psychotherapy

SOURCE: Pope Pius XII, "The Intangibility of the Human Person" (Sept. 13, 1952), *The Human Body: Papal Teachings*, pp. 200–01.

THE INTERESTS OF THE PATIENT

... Take the following example: in order to rid himself of repressions, inhibitions, and psychic complexes, man is not free to awaken in himself for therapeutic ends each and every sexual appetite, which moves, or is moved, in his being and sends its impure waves through his unconscious or subconscious self. He cannot make them the object of his conduct or of his fully conscious desires, with all the upheavals and repercussions involved in such a proceeding. For man, and for the Christian, there exists a law of integrity and personal purity, of personal esteem for himself, which forbids him to plunge himself thus wholly into the world of sexual representations and tendencies. The "medical and psychotherapeutical interests of the patient" find here a moral limit. It is not proved, nay it is even untrue, that the pansexual method of a certain school of psychoanalysis is an integrant indispensable part of all serious psychotherapy worthy of the name; that the fact of having neglected this method in the past has caused serious psychic harm, errors in doctrine and in its application in the field of education, of psychotherapy, and not least in the pastoral field; that there is a pressing need of making good this deficiency, and of initiating all those occupied in psychic questions in its guiding principles, and even, if necessary, in the practical management of this technique of sexuality.

We speak of this, because, today, these assertions are uttered all too often, with an apodictic assurance. It would be better, in the domain of the instinctive life, to give more attention to the indirect treatment and to the action of the conscious psychism on the whole imaginative and affective activity. This technique avoids signal deviations. It tends to enlighten, to heal, to direct. It influences also the dynamic in sexuality, on which so much stress in laid, which ought to reside—and does, in fact, reside—in the unconscious or the subconscious.

50: Public Policy

DOCUMENT 1:

Source: John Paul II, "The Gospel of Life" (Mar. 25, 1995), *Origins* 24: no. 42, Apr. 16, 1995, pp. 720, 722–23.

90. . . . If charity is to be realistic and effective, it demands that the Gospel of life be implemented also by means of certain forms of social activity and commitment in the political field as a way of defending and promoting the value of life in our ever more complex and pluralistic societies. Individuals, families, groups, and associations, albeit for different reasons and in different ways, all have a responsibility for shaping society and developing cultural, economic, political, and legislative projects which, with respect for all and in keeping with democratic principles, will contribute to the building of a society in which the dignity of each person is recognized and protected and the lives of all are defended and enhanced.

This task is the particular responsibility of civil leaders. Called to serve the people and the common good, they have a duty to make courageous choices in support of life, especially through legislative measures. In a democratic system where laws and decisions are made on the basis of the consensus of many, the sense of personal responsibility in the consciences of individuals invested with authority may be weakened. But no one can ever renounce this responsibility, especially when he or she has a legislative or decision-making mandate, which calls that person to answer to God, to his or her own conscience, and to the whole of society for choices which may be contrary to the common good. Although laws are not the only means of protecting human life, nevertheless they do play a very important and sometimes decisive role in influencing patterns of thought and behavior. I repeat once more that a law which violates an innocent person's natural right to life is unjust and, as such, is not valid as a law. For this reason I urgently appeal once more to all political leaders not to pass laws which, by disregarding the dignity of the person, undermine the very fabric of society.

98. In a word, we can say that the cultural change which we are calling for demands from everyone the courage to adopt a new lifestyle consisting in making practical choices—at the personal, family, social, and international level—on the basis of a correct scale of values: the primacy of being over having, of the person over things. This renewed lifestyle involves a passing from indifference to concern for others, from rejection to acceptance of them. Other people are not rivals from whom we must defend ourselves, but brothers

332   and sisters to be supported. They are to be loved for their own sakes, and they enrich us by their very presence.

      In this mobilization for a new culture of life no one must feel excluded. Everyone has an important role to play. Together with the family, teachers and educators have a particularly valuable contribution to make. Much will depend on them if young people, trained in true freedom, are to be able to preserve for themselves and make known to others new, authentic ideals of life and if they are to grow in respect for and service to every other person in the family and in society. . . .

DOCUMENT 2 / Public Policy

SOURCE: Congregation for the Doctrine of the Faith, "Instruction on Respect for Human Life in Its Origin and on the Dignity of Procreation" (Feb. 22, 1987), *Origins* 16: no. 40, Mar. 19, 1987, pp. 708–10.

III. MORAL AND CIVIL LAW
The Values and Moral Obligations that Civil Legislation Must Respect and Sanction in this Matter

The inviolable right to life of every innocent human individual and the rights of the family and of the institution of marriage constitute fundamental moral values because they concern the natural condition and integral vocation of the human person; at the same time they are constitutive elements of civil society and its order.

For this reason the new technological possibilities which have opened up in the field of biomedicine require the intervention of the political authorities and of the legislator, since an uncontrolled application of such techniques could lead to unforeseeable and damaging consequences for civil society. Recourse to the conscience of each individual and to the self-regulation of researchers cannot be sufficient for ensuring respect for personal rights and public order. If the legislator responsible for the common good were not watchful, he could be deprived of his prerogatives by researchers claiming to govern humanity in the name of the biological discoveries and the alleged "improvement" processes which they would draw from those discoveries. "Eugenism" and forms of discrimination between human beings could come to be legitimized. This would constitute an act of violence and a serious offense to the equality, dignity, and fundamental rights of the human person.

The intervention of the public authority must be inspired by the rational principles which regulate the relationships between civil law and moral law. The task of the civil law is to ensure the common good of people through the recognition of and the defense of fundamental rights and through the promotion of peace and of public morality. In no sphere of life can the civil law take the place of conscience or dictate norms concerning things which are outside its competence. It must sometimes tolerate, for the sake of public order, things which it cannot forbid without a greater evil resulting. However, the inalienable rights of the person must be recognized and respected by civil society and the political authority. These human rights depend neither on single individuals nor on parents; nor do they represent a concession made by society and the state. They pertain to human nature and are inherent in the person by virtue of the creative act from which the person took his or her origin.

Among such fundamental rights one should mention in this regard: a) every human being's right to life and physical integrity from the moment of conception until death; b) the rights of the family and of marriage as an

334 institution and, in this area, the child's right to be conceived, brought into the world, and brought up by his parents. To each of these two themes it is necessary here to give some further consideration.

In various states certain laws have authorized the direct suppression of innocents. The moment a positive law deprives a category of human beings of the protection which civil legislation must accord them, the state is denying the equality of all before the law. When the state does not place its power at the service of the rights of each citizen, and in particular of the more vulnerable, the very foundations of a state based on law are undermined. The political authority consequently cannot give approval to the calling of human beings into existence through procedures which would expose them to those very grave risks noted previously. The possible recognition by positive law and the political authorities of techniques of artificial transmission of life and the experimentation connected with them would widen the breach already opened by the legalization of abortion.

As a consequence of the respect and protection which must be ensured for the unborn child from the moment of his conception, the law must provide appropriate penal sanctions for every deliberate violation of the child's rights. The law cannot tolerate—indeed it must expressly forbid—that human beings, even at the embryonic stage, should be treated as objects of experimentation, be mutilated or destroyed with the excuse that they are superfluous or incapable of developing normally.

The political authority is bound to guarantee to the institution of the family, upon which society is based, the juridical protection to which it has a right. From the very fact that it is at the service of people, the political authority must also be at the service of the family. Civil law cannot grant approval to techniques of artificial procreation which, for the benefit of their parties (doctors, biologists, economic or governmental powers), take away what is a right inherent in the relationship between spouses; and therefore civil law cannot legalize the donation of gametes between persons who are not legitimately united in marriage.

Legislation must also prohibit, by virtue of the support which is due to the family, embryo banks, postmortem insemination and "surrogate motherhood."

It is part of the duty of the public authority to ensure that the civil law is regulated according to the fundamental norms of the moral law in matters concerning human rights, human life, and the institution of the family. Politicians must commit themselves, through their interventions upon public opinion, to securing in society the widest possible consensus on such essential points and to consolidating this consensus wherever it risks being weakened or is in danger of collapse.

In many countries the legalization of abortion and juridical tolerance of unmarried couples make it more difficult to secure respect for the fundamental rights recalled by this instruction. It is to be hoped that states will not become responsible for aggravating these socially damaging situations of injustice. It is rather to be hoped that nations and states will realize all the cultural, ideological, and political implications connected with the techniques of artificial pro-

creation and will find the wisdom and courage necessary for issuing laws   335
which are more just and more respectful of human life and the institution of
the family.

The civil legislation of many states confers an undue legitimation upon
certain practices in the eyes of many today; it is seen to be incapable of guaranteeing that morality which is in conformity with the natural exigencies of the
human person and with the "unwritten laws" etched by the Creator upon the
human heart. All men of good will must commit themselves, particularly within
their professional field and in the exercise of their civil rights, to ensuring the
reform of morally unacceptable civil laws and the correction of illicit practices.
In addition, "conscientious objection" vis-à-vis such laws must be supported
and recognized. A movement of passive resistance to the legitimation of practices contrary to human life and dignity is beginning to make an ever sharper
impression upon the moral conscience of many, especially among specialists
in the biomedical sciences.

DOCUMENT 3 / Public Policy

SOURCE: Archbishop John Quinn, "The Several Meanings of 'Religion and Politics'" (Sept. 20, 1984), *Origins* 14: no. 14, Sept. 20, 1984, pp. 221–22.

ROLE OF THE CHURCH IN THE PUBLIC-POLICY DEBATE

The Church enters the public-policy debate both as a social institution and as a community of believers. When it does so, the relationship of church and state arises as a religious issue for the Church and as a constitutional issue for the state.

Until the rise of the democratic and pluralist societies, the relationship of church and state was largely a matter of the relationship of pope and emperor. But with the advent of the pluralist democracies a new factor enters the picture: new emphasis is given to the fact that the Church also relates to and has a role in society. And so the problematic can no longer be contained simply in the formula "church-state." We must also speak of the Church and society. Society is a larger reality than the state. The state is only one component of society, which includes such realities as the family, labor unions, universities, corporations, and all sorts of various other associations.

The Church's role in society, as distinguished from its relationship to the state, derives not only from its doctrinal position—the universal mandate to preach the Gospel to all nations. It derives also from the guarantees of our Constitution.

The so-called "separation clause," which I believe should more accurately be called the "antiestablishment clause," stands between two extremes. It holds that religious institutions should expect neither favoritism nor discrimination in the exercise of their civic or religious responsibilities. Religious organizations must earn their way into the public debate by the quality of their positions. But the First Amendment is not designed to silence or exclude the religious voice. The fundamental and important distinction between society and state reinforces the right and responsibility of religious groups to participate in the public arena.

Furthermore, within the wider society the constitutional tradition reserves a crucial role for voluntary associations. These groups, organized for public purposes but independent of the state, play an essential role in a democracy. In the American political system religious organizations are classified as voluntary associations.

There is much evidence to indicate that the framers of the Constitution and its amendments envisioned limiting the power of government and maximizing freedom, and that one of the chief concerns in the First Amendment is to ensure freedom for religion in the nation.

To considerations of the antiestablishment clause we must add the "free   **337** exercise" clause. In light of this, religious freedom implies and includes the right of free association, the right of freedom of expression, and the right to establish educational and social service institutions and programs.

In a freed, pluralist society, then, the Church has the right to make and to express moral judgments about public policy for two reasons: first, to guide and help in the formation of the conscience of believers; and second, to contribute to the public-policy debate by creating space for the moral dimension of these issues and by helping to set the correct terms for that public debate.

In short, whatever may be said about the separation of church and state, it can never be a pretext for the separation of the Church from society.

PERSONAL CONSCIENCE AND THE OFFICEHOLDER

In "A Man for All Seasons," Thomas More says, "I believe when statesmen forsake their own private conscience for the sake of their public duties . . . they lead their country by a short route to chaos."

We are not living in 16th-century England and the problems are more complex. Nevertheless the words of Thomas More are a reminder that holders of public office have sometimes to confront severe dilemmas of conscience.

While the nuclear issue has placed the focus on the church-state issue, the abortion issue has served to place the focus on the question of personal conscience and public office.

If there is anything which can be affirmed with confidence, it is that this tension between private conscience and public office has never received more attention and yet is becoming more and more confused and confusing in the public forum.

I do not claim to have all the answers to this vexing issue. But it does seem to me that if we are to adopt any sensible attitude about it we ought to begin by recognizing that the formulation "religion and politics" has several meanings. It may mean the relationship of church and state. It may refer to the relationship of the Church and society. Or, finally, it may mean the role of private conscience in the conduct of public office.

While I acknowledge with respect other religious traditions, I cannot speak for them and thus I hope you will understand if I speak from my own tradition. As far as Catholic moral analysis goes, from medieval times to the present century the great emphasis in Church documents had to do with the respective rights and duties of the Church and state. But with Pope Leo XIII, around the turn of the century there arose a developing moral doctrine of the rights and duties of the citizen, including the role of the conscience of the citizen. Pius XII in the '40s carried this further, asserting that the individual as citizen is the foundation, the end, and the agent of political society.

John Paul II was clearly in this tradition when, speaking to the United Nations in 1978, he said: "Each one of you . . . represents a particular state, system, and political structure, but what you represent above all are individual human beings. . . . All political activity . . . in the final analysis . . . comes from

338   man, is exercised by man, and is for man." In other words, the dignity of the individual human person and citizen holds a priority for political systems, which exist to serve the dignity of the person endowed with inalienable rights, among which the rights of conscience must be considered preeminent.

How, then, can we come to grips at all with the very complex issue of the rights of conscience of an officeholder in a pluralist society? It would seem to me that we ought to begin by recognizing a clear difference between the moral law and civil law. It is a fundamental postulate of Catholic moral doctrine that the moral law covers every aspect of human behavior, public, private, internal, professional, national, and international. On the other hand, civil law does not cover all aspects of human behavior, least of all the interior, and it should not. Then what aspects of human behavior should be covered by civil law?

In general, I think we would agree that civil law ought to cover those things which affect the public order and the public interest of society. These things must be open to legislation and public-policy determination.

But what are such issues? Almost everyone would agree that the defense of the nation would be such an issue. But on the other side of the coin we seem to have developed a national consensus that the prohibition of drinking is not an appropriate object of civil law. Even so, some aspects of drinking are regarded as appropriate concerns of law, for example, driving while drunk. But it is how, not whether, one drinks that is the agreed object of public concern.

But when it comes to abortion, we have not reached a national consensus on the basic question of whether it is a public issue and therefore to be regulated by law or whether it is a private issue and therefore subject only to the dictates of personal conscience. For those who describe themselves as pro-choice, abortion is a matter of private morality and the state should not control or regulate a woman's choice to have a child.

In Catholic moral doctrine, abortion is an issue of public morality. The reason is that for us the issue is not the simple issue of the woman's right to have a child or not. For us there are three actors, not one. For us it is an issue of the conflict of rights, the rights of the woman and the rights of the unborn child, and we reason that where there is a conflict of rights there is a legitimate place for the state to be involved. Our formulation of the issues, then, involves the woman, the child, and the state, and for us it is an issue of public, not merely private, morality.

The problem we presently encounter in the public discussion of this issue derives at least to some degree from the failure to define the terms accurately. If an officeholder believes that abortion is wrong, but doesn't oppose it through the legitimately available democratic processes, then in effect that officeholder is saying that he or she believes it is a matter of private morality, a unitary issue of the right of a woman to have or not to have a child.

But if an officeholder believes that abortion is wrong, that it involves a conflict of the rights of the woman and the rights of the child and that the destruction of the unborn child has a significant impact on the public good, then that officeholder in effect believes that it is a matter of public morality.

In this case, logic as well as conscience would indicate that such an officeholder   **339**
should make use of the democratic processes to control and regulate abortion
and should use the right of free speech to persuade public opinion in favor of
his or her position. This cannot reasonably or justly be alleged as "imposing
one's personal views" on others. For as John Courtney Murray quite rightly
stated, "Any minority group has the right to work toward the elevation of
public morality in the pluralist society, through the use of the methods of
persuasion and pacific argument."

Abortion is not the only important issue of concern to the Church. But it
is unique for various reasons. One is that the position adopted publicly by
some—private objection to abortion but public support of abortion—is almost
never applied to other issues such as the killing of the whales or the deployment
of the MX missile. Principled private objection to these is usually accompanied
by public opposition as well. If an officeholder truly believes that human life
is being destroyed through abortion, that that life has rights just as the mother
has rights, then logic and conscience would demand that the officeholder make
efforts to bring about the repeal of laws favoring abortion and the enactment
of laws protecting unborn human life.

Surely it is not advantageous to the nation to encourage the idea that we
want officeholders who keep their deepest personal convictions separate from
the way they fulfill their public responsibilities. Edmund Burke said something
to the effect that "I owe my constituents not only the obligation of representing
them and their wishes, but also of bringing my best judgment to bear on
the issues."

The last word has not yet been said on the great issues of religion and
politics or conscience and public office. I have tried to probe them a bit today.
It is the essence of a pluralist society that we should have different views of
religion and morality. Though imperfect and incomplete, I hope that my words
today have made at least some small contribution to the dialogue.

51: Rape

DOCUMENT 1:

Source: Pennsylvania Catholic Conference, "Guidelines for Catholic Hospitals Treating Victims of Sexual Assault," *Origins* 22: no. 47 (May 6, 1993), p. 810.

One of the most violent and traumatic crimes is that of sexual assault. As a presence of Christ's healing, Catholic hospitals are called to treat persons who have been sexually assaulted with compassion, sensitivity, and respect. In caring for victims of sexual assault, Catholic hospitals are committed to quality holistic care by meeting their physical, psychological, emotional, social, and spiritual needs.

1. The first consideration in sexual assault cases should be for the total well-being of the person:
   a. Services of a chaplain or other suitable counselor should be made available.
   b. The victim should be treated with respect and compassion.
   c. No judgment on the victim's responsibility should be stated or implied by word or by action.
   d. The privacy and dignity of the person must, at all times, be respected.
2. Since the sperm in the case of rape is the result of unjust aggression, steps may be taken to prevent conception.
3. Any medical procedure, the purpose and/or effect of which is abortive, is never permissible.
   Hygienic procedures, including vaginal douching, are morally permitted since they are not abortifacient in effect.
4. A pregnancy test is essential to determine existence of pregnancy:
   a. If the pregnancy test is positive, no antiovulant drugs may be used.
   b. If the pregnancy test is negative, it is essential that hospital personnel question the patient to ascertain the time of ovulation within the menstrual cycle.
   c. If the patient has just ovulated, an antiovulant drug may not be administered. The use of a contraceptive steroid is permissible only to prevent ovulation.
5. Prophylaxis for venereal disease may be implemented.
6. Legal procedures should be followed when they do not conflict with the moral standards:
   a. Specific circumstances of the sexual assault may be ascertained and recorded.

b. Physical evidence of sexual assault may be gathered by means of   **341**
swabs, smears, aspirations, and other standard procedures.

c. Visual and tactile evidence of trauma may be noted, recorded,
and treated.

d. Material evidence of sexual assault from clothing, hair, and other
sources may be retained as evidence.

7. The above guidelines are given primarily from a moral perspective.
No judgment is made or implied concerning the acceptable medical
regimen or legal protocol.

8. Catholic hospitals, to the extent they have the capability of providing
treatment, accept victims of sexual assault. It is strongly recommended
that the sexually assaulted person be advised of these standing policies,
particularly the ethical restrictions which prevent Catholic hospitals
from using abortifacient procedures.

DOCUMENT 2 / Rape

Source: Joint Committee on Bioethical Issues of the Bishops' Conferences of Scotland, Ireland, England and Wales, "Use of the 'Morning-After Pill' in Cases of Rape" (Jan. 31, 1986), *Origins* 15: no. 39, Mar. 13, 1986, pp. 633, 635–38.

The British bishops have approved use of the "morning-after pill" in cases of rape if physicians determine that the victim has not ovulated. A report on this question was approved by the bishops of England and Wales during their November meeting and published Jan. 31 in *Briefing 86,* a publication of the England and Wales bishops' conference. But if administered after ovulation, the effect of the pill would be abortifacient, the report said. It also discussed use of an intrauterine device [IUD] in cases of rape. "There seems to be little or no basis on which an IUD could rightly be inserted at any time later than about half an hour after a sexual assault to counter the effects of the assault. The evidence suggests that, in practice, the only relevant operation of an ordinary IUD inserted after sexual assault would be as an abortifacient." The report examined the relationship between Church teaching on contraception and the administration of hormones after a rape. It said: "Consistent with Catholic teaching, there appears to be only one type of circumstance in which 'postcoital pills' might rightly be prescribed, administered, or taken. There do not appear to be any circumstances in which an IUD might rightly be used postcoitally." The report was drafted and released by a joint bioethics committee for the bishops of England and Wales, Scotland, and Ireland. The text of the report follows.

I. HOW DOES IT WORK?

There are two methods of preventing or terminating pregnancies in the immediate aftermath of intercourse, in current medical practice:

1. the insertion of an intrauterine device (IUD) or, more usually,
2. the administration of hormones.

The postcoital insertion of the IUD brings about changes in the womb which prevent the embryo from implanting; so the effects of such insertion will in practice be abortifacient in character.

The effect of administering hormones—large doses of estrogen or estrogen-progestogen combinations—will differ according to the stage of the menstrual cycle when they are given. If administered early in the cycle, they should prevent ovulation and therefore conception. If given about the time of ovulation, they could immobilize the sperm in the genital tract and thereby inhibit fertilization. If given after ovulation, their effects upon the female reproductive tract

are such that the survival of any embryo will be put at risk, whether directly   **343**
or by prevention of implantation or by inducing early menstruation as a result
of a sudden fall in the steroid level.

II. WHAT IS ADMINISTERED AND WHEN?

In a sense there is no such thing as the postcoital contraceptive pill, since
the ordinary contraceptive pills are used for this purpose. Indeed, pharmaceutical companies generally do not provide data sheets or promotional information
on postcoital contraceptive pill use nor may their representatives discuss or
encourage the use of their hormonal products for this purpose. Similarly the
British National Formulary does not include advice to doctors on the use of
pills for postcoital contraception.

The use of "the pill" for normal contraceptive purposes involves a dosage
of 30 micrograms of estrogen daily. In postcoital usage the dosage is 100 micrograms of estrogen given within 72 hours of intercourse and repeated 12
hours later.

The DHSS Handbook of Contraceptive Practice (1978) states that "owing
to the high estrogen medication this method should only be used as an emergency and not as regular contraceptive practice."

To increase the availability of this "emergency" service the Family Planning Association, in its publication Family Planning Today, has circularized
30,000 general practitioners with details of postcoital contraceptive pill prescription. The information is being disseminated in this manner because the majority
of pharmaceutical companies that manufacture the hormonal preparations used
as postcoital contraceptive pills have not applied for product licenses to use
these products for this purpose.

The British *Journal of Family Planning,* in commending this method to
general practitioners in 1983, indicated an almost boundless range of situations
when this treatment would be appropriate—indeed any act of intercourse
when pregnancy is unwanted. It should be and is widely inferred that talk of
"emergency use" means only that this is not recommended as a regular method
of contraception.

The British Pregnancy Advisory Service makes it a condition of giving
treatment that the woman seeking it should undertake that:

"a. Should treatment fail she will consider seeking an abortion.

"b. Should the treatment fail and she continues with a pregnancy, she
will not hold BPAS responsible for any defect or malformation in any child
born to her.

"c. She promises to return for the follow-up visit."

Further, they advise:

"Patients with moral or religious objections to induced abortion should
be carefully counseled before postcoital treatment, since they may wish to give
serious consideration to the possibility of requesting an abortion under the
1967 Abortion Act should the treatment fail."

As already noted, the pharmaceutical companies will not underwrite the
use of hormonal preparations as postcoital contraceptive pills; they are keenly

344   aware of their exposure to the risk of expensive litigation. General practitioners, aware of the dangers inherent in the use of hormonal preparations as postcoital contraceptive pills, have understandably been reluctant to prescribe them for this purpose without the manufacturer's support. This, then, is the situation in which attempts are being made to persuade general practitioners that no medico-legal implications need follow prescriptions of postcoital contraceptive pills if recognized and approved medical practice is followed. The practitioner is counseled to obtain an accurate menstrual and coital history, blood pressure measurement, pelvic examination, immediate and adequate counseling concerning the side effects and dangers of the treatment, and the booking of an appropriate follow-up appointment. Full case notes, recording the "emergency" consultation, will be needed to protect the practitioner from legal liability in the event of complications which may follow the prescription of postcoital contraceptive pills.

III. IS IT LEGAL?

On the assumption that the whole law relating to abortion is contained in Sections 58 and 59 of the Offenses Against the Person Act 1891, the question is whether one who takes, administers, or supplies either pills or an IUD for use after intercourse, in the belief that conception (fertilization) may well have occurred and with the intention to cause the loss of any embryo, intends to "procure a miscarriage."

(The assumption that there is no common-law rule protecting the embryo during the first weeks or months of its life is very commonly made but may be open to challenge.)

Until very recently it has been universally accepted that the law is as stated by Professor Glanville Williams (longtime president of the Abortion Law Reform Association) in his book The Sanctity of Life and the Criminal Law (London, 1958), at page 141:

"At present both English law and the law of the great majority of the United States may regard any interference with pregnancy, however early it may take place, as criminal, unless for therapeutic reasons. The fetus is a human life to be protected by the criminal law from the moment when the ovum is fertilized."

But the advent of in vitro fertilization and of techniques for inducing very early abortion have made it seem convenient to propose that conception is not complete until implantation and that until that time the woman is not pregnant and, at any rate, cannot miscarry. This contention has been adopted by the Department of Health and Social Security, and, in May 1983, the attorney general informed Parliament that he proposed to institute no proceedings relating to the supply of "postcoital medications which are intended to be taken by women following unprotected intercourse to inhibit implantation in the womb of any fertilized ovum."

There are strong grounds for doubting the historical and legal accuracy of the arguments used by the attorney general in explaining his announcement. But if he is and remains unwilling to authorize either a prosecution or a civil (relator) action, it will be very difficult to test his view in the courts.

IV. WHAT ARE THE ETHICAL IMPLICATIONS?

Consistent with Catholic teaching, there appears to be only one type of circumstance in which "postcoital pills" might rightly be prescribed, administered, or taken. There do not appear to be any circumstances in which an IUD might rightly be used postcoitally. In this section we explain and amplify these conclusions.

A. Preventing Conception After Sexual Assault

A woman who is the victim of rape is "entitled to defend herself against the continuing effects of such an attack and to seek immediate medical assistance with a view to preventing conception": "Abortion and the Right to Live: A Joint Statement of Catholic Archbishops of Great Britain," no. 21 (Jan. 24, 1980, Catholic Truth Society).

Such efforts to prevent conception following rape need not be, morally speaking, acts of contraception such as have been excluded from Christian life by the constant and very firm teaching of the Church. Rather, they can be undertaken as efforts to remove or neutralize the assailant's sperm or seminal fluid, whose continuing presence in the victim's body is a continuation of the assault which violated her bodily integrity. To seek or make such efforts does not constitute a choice of the sort described and condemned by the Second Vatican Council, Paul VI, and John Paul II in their expositions of the Christian teaching on contraception.

"In the exposition of Vatican II, the morally essential character of contraception is its failure or refusal 'to preserve the full sense (sensus, meaning) of self-giving and human procreation' (*Gaudium et Spes*, 51). In the teaching of Paul VI, too, the point is the preservation of the 'inseparable connection . . . between the two meanings of the conjugal act: the unitive meaning and the procreative meaning.' And he identified the acts to be excluded as those which propose (whether as an end or as a means) to impede procreation 'either in anticipation, or in the accomplishment, or in the development of the natural consequences, of the conjugal act' (*Humanae Vitae*, 12, 14)."

John Paul II further explains why resort to contraception by married couples degrades human sexuality by separating "the two meanings that God the Creator has inscribed in the being of man and woman and in the dynamism of their sexual communion."

For "thus the innate language that expresses the total reciprocal self-giving of husband and wife is overlaid, through contraception, by an objectively contradictory language, namely, that of not giving oneself totally to the other. This leads not only to a positive refusal to be open to life but also to a falsification of the inner truth of conjugal love, which is called upon to give itself in personal totality" (*Familiaris Consortio*, 32).

In short, the wrongfulness of contraception (in the morally relevant sense of the word contraception) has to do with the character of the double choice it involves: both to bring oneself into an intimate bodily relationship of sexual communion with another human being and positively to exclude the transmission of new life that might otherwise complete their relationship. There is no

346 such double choice in the use of conception-preventing agents or procedures after a sexual assault. The woman has made no choice of sexual communion, and so her choice can now be directed to putting an end to the continuing invasion of her body and need not be a choice to repudiate the good of procreation by sexual communion.

B. Abortifacient Use

"In a very small number of cases, conception may in fact occur (after a rape). Then there exists a new being (with an) individuality, distinct from each of its parents and from any of their cells . . . . From that time, the requirements of the moral law, transcending even the most understandable emotional reactions, are clear: the newly conceived child cannot rightly be made to suffer the penalty of death for a man's violation of the woman" ("Abortion and the Right to Live," 21).

As the archbishops had earlier said, unborn children (including embryos at any stage after conception) have the right not to be made an object of attack:

"So the course of their development before birth must not be interfered with by any procedure or technical process carried out with the intention of preventing the continuation of that development. When we speak of abortion and condemn any attempt to procure it, we are referring to any procedure or technique which is adopted with that intention . . . . If a technique or device achieves such effects after conception, it is in fact an abortifacient, an abortion device, even if it is called by other names such as 'contraceptive' or 'menstrual extraction' and so on" ("Abortion and the Right to Live," 16).

What is excluded, therefore, is any intervention "with the intention of preventing the continuation of (embryonic) development" and any "interference with the (embryo) just in order to get rid of it . . . even if one did not positively want to kill it but acted regardless of the certainty or risk that it would thereby die" ("Abortion and the Right to Live," 16).

C. Distinguishing Conception-Preventing from Abortifacient Uses

As stated in Section I above, responsible scientific opinion at present accepts that the effect of large doses of estrogen or of estrogen-progestogen combinations varies according to the stage in the menstrual cycle at which they are administered. Three such stages can, for these purposes, be distinguished:

1. If administered prior to ovulation, the effect is normally to prevent ovulation and therefore fertilization; the cycle would be rendered anovular.

2. If administered just before ovulation, such doses may prevent conception not by preventing ovulation but either (a) by immobilizing sperm in the genital tract, or (b) by preventing those physiological changes in the sperm which are necessary for fertilization, or (c) by affecting the cells surrounding the ovum during the ovum's own process of preparation.

3. If administered after ovulation, the effect, if any, will be abortifacient; **347**
scientific opinion at present ascribes these effects to (a) alteration in
the environment of the fallopian tube, (b) inhibition of implantation
by creation of a hostile environment in the endometrium, and/or (c)
hormonal effects producing shedding of the endometrium and loss of
the implanted or unimplanted embryo.

A medical practitioner who accepts scientific opinions such as those just
mentioned and who is consulted by a woman after sexual assault upon her
may rightly prescribe such doses of estrogen or estrogen-progestogen if his
intention in so doing is to prevent or inhibit fertilization.

It is not morally permissible to prescribe such doses for the sake of their
abortifacient effects; nor will the upright and informed conscience be willing
to prescribe or take such doses where there is a substantial risk that their
effect will be abortifacient. It is sometimes possible to establish by inquiry or
examination that the woman is in the postovulatory stage of her cycle; in this
case, the only point of administering large doses of oral contraceptives would
be abortifacient.

Sometimes it may be impossible to discover even approximately the stage
of the woman's cycle. Such cases will no doubt be rare; but even when they
occur the matter has to be assessed on the basis of statistical probabilities.
Assuming that the woman could be anywhere along the, say, 24 days outside
the detectable period of menstruation and assuming that the effective life of
an ovum is about 12 hours, the assessable probability that the insemination
will have coincided with those 12 hours and that fertilization will have occurred
is about 2 percent. It follows that in such a case of blind administration, if
the estrogen or estrogen-progestogen dose is administered very soon after
intercourse, the likelihood that its effect will be abortifacient is about 2 percent.
(The likelihood at that stage of a contraceptive effect is about 4 percent; and
the dose is 94 percent likely to have neither effect.) But delay increases linearly
the likelihood that the dose will be (if anything) abortifacient. Thus at 12 hours
after intercourse, the effect is 4 percent likely to be abortifacient and 4 percent
likely to be contraceptive; at 24 hours the respective probabilities are 6 percent
abortifacient, 4 percent contraceptive; at 48 hours, 10 percent abortifacient and
3 percent contraceptive. Since sperm life is only about 72 hours, it is certain
that administration of the dose 72 hours or more after the sexual assault cannot
have any contraceptive effect and must be either futile or abortifacient.

D. IUD
There seems to be little or no basis on which an IUD could rightly be
inserted at any time later than about half an hour after a sexual assault, to
counter the effects of the assault. The evidence suggests that in practice the
only relevant operation of an ordinary IUD inserted after sexual assault would
be as an abortifacient; and the spermicidal effects of even a medicated IUD
could only be significant if the IUD were inserted within a half an hour of
the assault.

348 V. SUMMARY

1. "Postcoital contraception" is a term which covers (a) large and repeated doses of hormonal preparations usually used as ordinary oral contraceptives and (b) insertion of an intrauterine device; in each case, after intercourse or sexual assault.

2. Use of the IUD in this manner will always in practice be either abortifacient or futile.

3. Administration of hormones after intercourse or sexual assault will be abortifacient (or futile) if ovulation has taken place. If ovulation has not taken place, conceptions may be prevented in one or more ways, and there is little or no likelihood of any abortifacient effects.

4. Catholics may seek and administer hormonal postcoital contraception after insemination by sexual assault, provided (i) that there are no grounds for judging that ovulation preceded or will coincide with the administration of postcoital contraception, and (ii) that the postcoital contraceptive is administered urgently, within about a day, after the assault.

5. The medical and family-planning literature about postcoital contraception speaks of its appropriateness for "emergency" use. But this talk of emergency turns out to mean no more than postcoital contraception. It is (a) medically unsuitable for regular use by any one woman because of its vigorous hormonal effects upon her and (b) always carries a risk of damaging any unborn child which might survive the drugs or IUD. For both these reasons, the manufacturers of the preparations used for postcoital contraception do not recommend such use.

DOCUMENT 3 / Rape

SOURCE: Joint Committee on Bioethical Issues of the Bishops' Conferences of England and Wales, Scotland, and Ireland, "A Reply: Use of the 'Morning-After Pill' in Cases of Rape" (1986), *Origins* 16: no. 13, Sept. 11, 1986, pp. 237–38.

There have been misgivings about the report of a working party of the Catholic Bishops' Joint Committee on Bioethical Issues on the "morning-after pill."

Does the report commend the use of "the pill" after rape? Does it consider abortions acceptable provided they are reserved for rare cases? Or assume that doctors can rightly ignore the risk that a patient complaining of rape may be untruthful or already pregnant? Or overlook the variability of the ovulatory cycle? Or accept a 30 percent risk of causing abortion or some other form of "Russian roulette" with the unborn? Or consider the use of contraceptives acceptable provided they are reserved for "an emergency?"

The working party wishes to point out that the answer to all these questions is no.

The report accepts without any qualification whatsoever three truths constantly and very firmly taught by the Church:

i) The human embryo, at every stage from fertilization, must never be interfered with by any procedure or technical process (including administration of drugs) carried out with the intention of preventing the embryo's development or even of making its development less likely.

ii) Conjugal intercourse is the only morally acceptable sexual intercourse, and

iii) It is never right to take steps to impede the possible procreative consequences of an act of conjugal intercourse.

But it has long been common teaching of bishops and sound theologians that when a woman has been sexually violated (i.e., has been subjected to sexual intercourse without any choice of hers to engage in it, whether as an ends or as a means), she may rightly choose to put an end to the continuing invasion of her body by her assailant's bodily substances. And, in the opinion of the joint committee, she may also rightly choose to prevent ovulation; in the circumstance she is under no obligation to leave herself open to the possibility of conceiving. One means of effecting these self-defensive choices could in some circumstances be the medically supervised administration of the hormones commonly called the postcoital pill.

The possible presence of an unborn child changes the moral situation notably. Whatever the circumstances, it cannot be right for anyone to take any **349**

350 steps with the intention, even the part intention, of getting rid of an embryo whose presence is known, suspected, or even merely expected or feared.

Moreover, as the report clearly states, the upright and informed conscience will not be willing to accept any substantial risk of killing the embryo, even as a side effect of pursuing some other choice such as preventing ovulation or sperm transport. A side effect is an effect not chosen either as end or as means, but merely foreseen and in that sense accepted. But it can be wrong to accept side effects, e.g., when to do so would be unjust to a third party such as, in the present context, the embryo.

However, there are many legitimate activities which foreseeably cause some risk of serious or even fatal harm, a risk which in many cases is rightly accepted by upright and informed people as a possible side effect of their choices to engage in those activities. What sorts and degrees of risk are substantial and unjustified, e.g., because unfair to an innocent third party, must be judged in the circumstances by those who genuinely and fairly respect human good and impartially favor the lives of the innocent.

The report gives certain estimates of the statistical probabilities that administration of "the pill" to a woman after rape—in a case where nothing is known about the stage of her cycle—will be a) conception preventing, b) abortifacient, or c) neither. The report leaves to the conscience of upright Catholic medical practitioners the judgment whether, given these probabilities, it could be right to administer the pill in such a case. Responsible medical practitioners will not make such a decision on the basis of bare statistical probabilities, without regard to their assessment of the actual case before them. The report makes no criticisms of medical practitioners who decide that in all such cases the probability of an abortifacient effect is so high relative to the probability of a conception-preventing effect that it would not be fair and right to administer the pill.

Some commentators on the report have stated that there is "only" a 70 percent chance that the postcoital pill will prevent conception, and that therefore there is a 30 percent chance that it will be abortifacient. This comment is doubly mistaken. At many stages in the cycle the chance that the pill will prevent conception is nil or far below 70 percent. At some stages it may be above 70 percent. But even if there is a stage at which the probability of preventing conception is 70 percent, it is simply fallacious to assume that in the "remaining" 30 percent there is an abortifacient effect. For physiological reasons, it is very much more likely that in those cases the pill has neither effect, i.e., is futile.

Concern for the unborn and loyalty to Catholic teaching should not lead anyone to conceal the truth that for women in the predicament of rape there are possibly some effective self-defensive choices which, in some circumstances, they and/or their medical advisers might take in full conformity with all the truths which the Catholic Church upholds about strict respect, not only in attitude but also in each and every choice, for human life and for procreative significance of sexual communion.

52: Research* on Human Subjects

DOCUMENT 1:

SOURCE: Congregation for the Doctrine of the Faith, "Instruction on Respect for Human Life in Its Origin and on the Dignity of Procreation" (Feb. 22, 1987), *Origins* 16: no. 40, Mar. 19, 1987, pp. 697–711.

INTRODUCTION
1. Biomedical Research and the Teaching of the Church

The gift of life which God the Creator and Father has entrusted to man calls him to appreciate the inestimable value of what he has been given and to take responsibility for it. This fundamental principle must be placed at the center of one's reflection in order to clarify and solve the moral problems raised by artificial interventions on life as it originates and on the processes of procreation.

Thanks to the progress of the biological and medical sciences, man has at his disposal ever more effective therapeutic resources; but he can also acquire new powers, with unforeseeable consequences, over human life at its very beginning and in its first stages. Various procedures now make it possible to intervene not only in order to assist, but also to dominate the processes of procreation. These techniques can enable man to "take in hand his own destiny," but they also expose him "to the temptation to go beyond the limits of a reasonable dominion over nature." They might constitute progress in the service of man, but they also involve serious risks. Many people are therefore expressing an urgent appeal that in interventions on procreation the values and rights of the human person be safeguarded. Requests for clarification and guidance are coming not only from the faithful, but also from those who recognize the

---

*Since the terms *research* and *experimentation* are often used equivalently and ambiguously, it is deemed necessary to specify the exact meaning given them in this document.

1) By *research* is meant any inductive-deductive process which aims at promoting the systematic observation of a given phenomenon in the human field or at verifying a hypothesis arising from previous observations.

2) By *experimentation* is meant any research in which the human being (in the various stages of his existence: embryo, fetus, child, or adult) represents the object through which one intends to verify the effect, at present unknown or not sufficiently known, of a given treatment (e.g., pharmacological, teratogenic, surgical, etc.).

352 Church as "an expert in humanity" with a mission to serve the "civilization of love" and of life.

The Church's Magisterium does not intervene on the basis of a particular competence in the area of the experimental sciences; but having taken account of the data of research and technology, it intends to put forward, by virtue of its evangelical mission and apostolic duty, the moral teaching corresponding to the dignity of the person and to his or her integral vocation. It intends to do so by expounding the criteria of moral judgment as regards the applications of scientific research and technology, especially in relation to human life and its beginnings. These criteria are the respect, defense, and promotion of man, his "primary and fundamental right" to life, his dignity as a person who is endowed with a spiritual soul and with moral responsibility and who is called to beatific communion with God.

The Church's intervention in this field is inspired also by the love which she owes to man, helping him to recognize and respect his rights and duties. This love draws from the font of Christ's love: as she contemplates the mystery of the incarnate Word, the Church also comes to understand the "mystery of man"; by proclaiming the Gospel of salvation, she reveals to man his dignity and invites him to discover fully the truth of his own being. Thus the Church once more puts forward the divine law in order to accomplish the work of truth and liberation.

For it is out of goodness—in order to indicate the path of life—that God gives human beings his commandments and the grace to observe them; and it is likewise out of goodness—in order to help them persevere along the same path—that God always offers to everyone his forgiveness. Christ has compassion on our weaknesses. He is our Creator and Redeemer. May his Spirit open men's hearts to the gift of God's peace and to an understanding of his precepts.

2. Science and Technology at the Service of the Human Person

God created man in his own image and likeness: "Male and female he created them" (Gn 1:27), entrusting to them the task of "having dominion over the earth" (Gn 1:28). Basic scientific research and applied research constitute a significant expression of this dominion of man over creation. Science and technology are valuable resources for man when placed at his service and when they promote his integral development for the benefit of all; but they cannot of themselves show the meaning of existence and of human progress. Being ordered to man, who initiates and develops them, they draw from the person and his moral values the indication of their purpose and the awareness of their limits.

It would on the one hand be illusory to claim that scientific research and its applications are morally neutral; on the other hand one cannot derive criteria for guidance from mere technical efficiency, from research's possible usefulness to some at the expense of the others or, worse still, from prevailing ideologies. Thus science and technology require for their own intrinsic meaning an unconditional respect for the fundamental criteria of the moral law. That is to say, they must be at the service of the human person, of his inalienable rights and his true and integral good according to the design and will of God.

The rapid development of technological discoveries gives greater urgency to this need to respect the criteria just mentioned. Science without conscience can only lead to man's ruin. "Our era needs such wisdom more than bygone ages if the discoveries made by man are to be further humanized. For the future of the world stands in peril unless wiser people are forthcoming."

3. Anthropology and Procedures in the Biomedical Field

Which moral criteria must be applied in order to clarify the problems posed today in the field of biomedicine? The answer to this question presupposes a proper idea of the nature of the human person in his bodily dimension.

For it is only in keeping with his true nature that the human person can achieve self-realization as a "united totality," and this nature is at the same time corporal and spiritual. By virtue of its substantial union with a spiritual soul, the human body cannot be considered as a mere complex of tissues, organs, and functions, nor can it be evaluated in the same way as the body of animals; rather it is a constitutive part of the person who manifests and expresses himself through it.

The natural moral law expresses and lays down the purposes, rights, and duties which are based upon the bodily and spiritual nature of the human person. Therefore this law cannot be thought of as simply a set of norms on the biological level; rather it must be defined as the rational order whereby man is called by the Creator to direct and regulate his life and actions and in particular to make use of his own body.

A first consequence can be deduced from these principles: an intervention on the human body affects not only the tissues, the organs, and their function, but also involves the person himself on different levels. It involves, therefore, perhaps in an implicit but nonetheless real way, a moral significance and responsibility. Pope John Paul II forcefully reaffirmed this to the World Medical Association when he said:

"Each human person, in his absolutely unique singularity, is constituted not only by his spirit, but by his body as well. Thus, in the body and through the body one touches the person himself in his concrete reality. To respect the dignity of man consequently amounts to safeguarding this identity of the man *corpore et anima unus*, as the Second Vatican Council says (*Gaudium et Spes*, 14.1). It is on the basis of this anthropological vision that one is to find the fundamental criteria for decision making in the case of procedures which are not strictly therapeutic, as, for example, those aimed at the improvement of the human biological condition."

Applied biology and medicine work together for the integral good of human life when they come to the aid of a person stricken by illness and infirmity and when they respect his or her dignity as a creature of God. No biologist or doctor can reasonably claim, by virtue of his scientific competence,

354   to be able to decide on people's origin and destiny. This norm must be applied in a particular way in the field of sexuality and procreation, in which man and woman actualize the fundamental values of love and life.

God, who is love and life, has inscribed in man and woman the vocation to share in a special way in his mystery of personal communion and in his work as Creator and Father. For this reason marriage possesses specific goods and values in its union and in procreation which cannot be likened to those existing in lower forms of life. Such values and meanings are of the personal order and determine from the moral point of view the meaning and limits of artificial interventions on procreation and on the origin of human life. These interventions are not to be rejected on the grounds that they are artificial. As such, they bear witness to the possibilities of the art of medicine. But they must be given a moral evaluation in reference to the dignity of the human person, who is called to realize his vocation from God to the gift of love and the gift of life.

I. RESPECT FOR HUMAN EMBRYOS
4. How is One to Evaluate Morally Research and Experimentation on Human Embryos and Fetuses?

Medical research must refrain from operations on live embryos, unless there is a moral certainty of not causing harm to the life or integrity of the unborn child and the mother, and on condition that the parents have given their free and informed consent to the procedure. It follows that all research, even when limited to the simple observation of the embryo, would become illicit were it to involve risk to the embryo's physical integrity or life by reason of the methods used or the effects induced.

As regards experimentation, and presupposing the general distinction between experimentation for purposes which are not directly therapeutic and experimentation which is clearly therapeutic for the subject himself, in the case in point one must also distinguish between experimentation carried out on embryos which are still alive and experimentation carried out on embryos which are dead. If the embryos are living, whether viable or not, they must be respected just like any other human person; experimentation on embryos which is not directly therapeutic is illicit.

No objective, even though noble in itself such as a foreseeable advantage to science, to other human beings, or to society, can in any way justify experimentation on living human embryos or fetuses, whether viable or not, either inside or outside the mother's womb. The informed consent ordinarily required for clinical experimentation on adults cannot be granted by the parents, who may not freely dispose of the physical integrity or life of the unborn child. Moreover, experimentation on embryos and fetuses always involves risk, and indeed in most cases it involves the certain expectation of harm to their physical integrity or even their death.

To use human embryos or fetuses as the object or instrument of experimentation constitutes a crime against their dignity as human beings having a right to the same respect that is due to the child already born and to every human person.

The Charter of the Rights of the Family published by the Holy See affirms: "Respect for the dignity of the human being excludes all experimental manipulation or exploitation of the human embryo." The practice of keeping alive human embryos in vivo or in vitro for experimental or commercial purposes is totally opposed to human dignity.

In the case of experimentation that is clearly therapeutic, namely, when it is a matter of experimental forms of therapy used for the benefit of the embryo itself in a final attempt to save its life and in the absence of other reliable forms of therapy, recourse to drugs or procedures not yet fully tested can be licit.

The corpses of human embryos and fetuses, whether they have been deliberately aborted or not, must be respected just as the remains of other human beings. In particular, they cannot be subjected to mutilation or to autopsies if their death has not yet been verified and without the consent of the parents or of the mother. Furthermore, the moral requirements must be safeguarded that there be no complicity in deliberate abortion and that the risk of scandal be avoided. Also, in the case of dead fetuses, as for the corpses of adult persons, all commercial trafficking must be considered illicit and should be prohibited.

5. How is One to Evaluate Morally the Use for Research Purposes of Embryos Obtained by Fertilization "In Vitro?"

Human embryos obtained in vitro are human beings and subjects with rights. Their dignity and right to life must be respected from the first moment of their existence. It is immoral to produce human embryos destined to be exploited as disposable "biological material."

In the usual practice of in vitro fertilization, not all of the embryos are transferred to the woman's body; some are destroyed. Just as the Church condemns induced abortion, so she also forbids acts against the life of these human beings. It is a duty to condemn the particular gravity of the voluntary destruction of human embryos obtained "in vitro" for the sole purpose of research, either by means of artificial insemination or by means of "twin fission." By acting in this way the researcher usurps the place of God; and, even though he may be unaware of this, he sets himself up as the master of the destiny of others inasmuch as he arbitrarily chooses whom he will allow to live and whom he will send to death and kills defenseless human beings.

Methods of observation or experimentation which damage or impose grave and disproportionate risks upon embryos obtained in vitro are morally illicit for the same reasons. Every human being is to be respected for himself and cannot be reduced in worth to a pure and simple instrument for the advantage of others. It is therefore not in conformity with the moral law deliberately to expose to death human embryos obtained "in vitro." In consequence of the fact that they have been produced in vitro, those embryos which are not transferred into the body of the mother and are called "spare" are exposed to an absurd fate, with no possibility of their being offered safe means of survival which can be licitly pursued.

DOCUMENT 2 / Research on Human Subjects

Source: Pope John Paul II, "Medicines at the Service of Human Life" (Oct. 24, 1986), *Health Progress*, Apr. 1987, pp. 84, 93.

. . . In the present state of scientific knowledge, it is not possible to predict with sufficient accuracy the properties and the characteristics of new medical preparations. Before being used in treatment, they must be tested on laboratory animals. . . . In a second stage, before being made available for general use, medicines should be tested on the human being, on the sick, and sometimes even on a person in good health. Clinical experimentation is subject to strict laws and norms which regulate it and aim at offering all possible guarantees. We may at least hope that the day will come when the risks and the unknowns in the area of experimentation with medicines will be notably reduced. However, at any rate, great prudence is necessary to prevent the human person from ever becoming a mere object of experimentation, and at all costs avoiding danger to one's life, sanity, equilibrium, and health. . . .

Among the problems that remain unsolved are those which concern the situation of certain underdeveloped countries. Although access to health care is recognized as a fundamental right, large sections of humanity are still deprived of even the most elementary medical care. The problem is one of such dimensions that individual efforts, valuable and irreplaceable as they may be, are insufficient. At the present time, it is absolutely necessary for us to try to work together and to coordinate, at the international level, policies of aid and thus of concrete initiatives. . . .

Developed countries have the duty to place their experience, their technology, and a part of their economic wealth at the disposal of those that are less so. . . .

In this context, we cannot forget that there are still medicines which, for almost exclusively commercial reasons, have not been given serious attention and are not benefiting from research and scientific progress. These are often necessary not only for the treatment of certain rare diseases but also for those which strike millions of people in the poorer tropical zones. In this respect, it is necessary in the first place to discern the objectives and their order of priority, then to see how the economic and political barriers which impede the research, development, and production of such medicines might be overcome. . . .

DOCUMENT 3 / Research on Human Subjects

Source: Pope John Paul II, "Biological Experimentation" (Oct. 23, 1982), *The Pope Speaks* 28: no. 1, 1983, pp. 75–76.

RESPECT FOR THE PERSON

Consequently, I have no reason to be apprehensive for those experiments in biology that are performed by scientists who, like you, have a profound respect for the human person, since I am certain that they will contribute to the integral well-being of man.

On the other hand, I condemn, in the most explicit and formal way, experimental manipulations of the human embryo, since the human being, from conception to death, cannot be exploited for any purpose whatsoever. Indeed, as the Second Vatican Council teaches, man is "the only creature on earth which God willed for itself. . . ."

The experimentation which you have been discussing is directed to a greater knowledge of the most intimate mechanisms of life, by means of artificial models, such as the cultivation of tissues, and experimentation on some species of animals genetically selected. Moreover, you have indicated some experiments to be accomplished on animal embryos, which will permit you to know better how cellular differences are determined.

It must be emphasized that new techniques, such as the cultivation of cells and tissues, have had a notable development which permits very important progress in biological sciences, and they are also complementary to experimentation done on animals.

It is certain that animals are at the service of man and can, hence, be the object of experimentation. Nevertheless, they must be treated as creatures of God which are destined to serve man's good, but not to be abused by him. Hence the diminution of experimentation on animals, which has progressively been made ever less necessary, corresponds to the plan and well-being of all creation. . . .

"IN VITRO" EXPERIMENTS

. . . It is also to be hoped, with reference to your activities, that the new techniques of modification of the genetic code, in particular cases of genetic chromosomic diseases, will be a motive of hope for the great number of people affected by those maladies.

It can also be thought that, through the transfer of genes, certain specific diseases can be cured, such as sickle-cell anemia, which in many countries affects individuals of the same ethnic origin. It should likewise be recalled that some hereditary diseases can be avoided through progress in biological experimentation.

358   The research of modern biology gives hope that the transfer and mutations of genes can ameliorate the condition of those who are affected by chromosomic diseases; in this way the smallest and weakest of human beings can be cured during their intrauterine life or in the period immediately after birth. . . .

DOCUMENT 4 / Research on Human Subjects

SOURCE: Pope John Paul II, "A Patient Is a Person" (Oct. 27, 1980), *The Pope Speaks* 26: no. 1, 1981, pp. 3–4.

EXPERIMENTATION

. . . I come now to experimentation, a subject much discussed nowadays. Here again, the acknowledgment of the person's dignity and of the ethical norms based on that dignity, when taken as the supreme value that inspires scientific research, has quite specific consequences at the level of moral obligations.

Pharmacologico-clinical research may not be initiated unless all precautions have been taken to assure that the intervention will not be positively harmful. To this end, the preclinical phase of research must provide the broadest possible documentation of the possible toxicological effects of the drug.

It is evident as well that the patient must be informed of the fact that the experiment is being tried, and of its purpose and possible dangers, so that he or she may give or refuse consent with full awareness and freedom. A doctor has only such authority and rights over a patient as the latter chooses to yield.

INHERENT LIMIT OF EXPERIMENTATION

Moreover, the consent given by the patient is not unlimited in its scope. Except in special cases, the essential purpose of the patient in cooperating with the experiment is the improvement of his or her health. Any such experiment derives its primary justification from the way it serves the interests of the individual, not of the collective.

This does not mean, however, that, provided his or her own substantial integrity is preserved, the patient may not legitimately accept a share of risk as a way of making a personal contribution to the progress of medicine and thus to the common good. Medical science exists in the community as a force that is meant to liberate human beings from the infirmities which encumber them and from the psychic and somatic weaknesses that lay them low. Such a gift of oneself, within the limits set by the moral law, can, therefore, be a highly meritorious proof of love and an occasion for spiritual growth of such magnitude as to offset the dangers of a possible physical diminution that is not substantial in kind.

A RE-PERSONALIZATION OF MEDICINE

These reflections on drug research and medical therapy can be applied to other areas of medicine. More often than people realize, it is possible, in the very act of helping the sick, to violate their personal right to psychophysical

360   integrity by inflicting a de facto violence. This may be done by diagnostic inquiries that use complicated and, not infrequently, traumatizing procedures; by surgical treatment which today engages in very bold forms of dismantling and reconstruction; by organic transplants; by applied medical research; and by the very organization of hospitals. . . .

DOCUMENT 5 / Research on Human Subjects

SOURCE: Pope Pius XII, "The Intangibility of the Human Person" (Sept. 3, 1952), *The Human Body: Papal Teachings*, pp. 196–97, 199, 201–04, 207–08.

MEDICAL SCIENCE

Scientific knowledge has its own value in the domain of medical science—not less than in the domains of the other sciences, such as, for example, physics, chemistry, cosmology, psychology—a value which should by no means be minimized, and is imposed quite independently of the usefulness and of the use made of the acquired knowledge. Moreover, knowledge as such and the fullness of knowledge of all truth are the occasion of no moral objection. In virtue of the same principle, research and the acquisition of truth with a view to arriving at new knowledge and a new, more vast, more profound comprehension of this same truth are in themselves in harmony with the moral order.

This does not mean, however, that every method, even a method well established by scientific research and technique, offers a moral guarantee, or further, that every method becomes lawful by the fact that it increases and deepens our knowledge. Sometimes it happens that one method cannot be put into operation without infringing on the rights of another, or violating some absolute moral value. In this case, advancement of knowledge is the goal seen and aimed at—all well and good; but this method is not morally admissible. Why is this? Because science is not the highest value to which all the other orders of values—or in a single scale of values, all the particular values—should be subjected. Science itself then, along with its researches and attainments, must be inserted in the order of values. Here, well-defined frontiers present themselves which even medical science cannot transgress without violating higher moral rules. The relationship of confidence between doctor and patient, the right of the patient to life, physical and spiritual, in its psychic or moral integrity—here, amongst others, are values which rule scientific interests. The statement will be made clearer still by what follows. . . .

THE INTERESTS OF THE PATIENT

. . . The patient has not the right to involve his physical and psychic integrity in medical experiments or researches, when these interventions entail, either immediately or subsequently, acts of destruction, or of mutilation and wounds, or grave dangers. . . .

. . . A third set of interests are adduced for the moral justification of the rights of medicine in its use of new experiments and interventions, of new methods and processes: the interests of the community, of human society, the *bonum commune*, the common good, as philosophers and sociologists put it.

362   It is beyond doubt that such a common good exists: nor can it be contested that it calls for and justifies further researches. The two sets of interests already named, those of science and those of the patient, are closely bound up with the general interest.

THE COMMON GOOD

However, for a third time the question arises: Are the medical interests of the community, in their content and extension, limited by any moral boundaries? Are there "full powers" for every serious experiment on living human beings? Are barriers raised in the interest of science or of the individual? Or, to state it another way: Can the public authority, whose function it is to care for the common good, give the doctor the power to make experiments on the individual in the interests of science and the community, in order to invent and try out new methods and processes when these experiments infringe on the right of the individual to dispose of himself? Can the public authority, in the interests of the community, really limit or suppress the rights of the individual over his body and his life, his corporal and psychological integrity?

To anticipate an objection: it is always understood that it is a matter of serious research, of honest effort to promote scientific theory and practice; not some maneuver, which serves as a scientific pretext to cover other ends and to realize them with impunity.

As for the questions already mentioned, many have reckoned, and still do today, that the answer must be in the affirmative. In support of this attitude they argue that the individual is subordinate to the community, that the good of the individual must yield to that of the community, and be sacrificed to it. They add that the sacrifice of the individual to the ends of scientific research and exploration ultimately benefits the individual.

The great postwar trials have brought to light a frightful quantity of documents testifying to the sacrifice of the individual to "medical interests of the community." In these acts are found testimonies and reports which show how, with the assent, and sometimes even by formal command of the public authority, certain centers demanded a regular supply of men from concentration camps for their medical experiments. We learn how men were delivered up to the centers; so many men, so many women, so many for this experiment, so many for that. There exist reports on the progress and result of these experiments, on the objective and subjective symptoms observed on those undergoing the experiment through its different phases. One cannot read these notes without being seized with a deep compassion for the victims, many of whom met their death in the process. One recoils before such an aberration of the human mind and heart. Yet, we can also add: those responsible for such atrocities have done nothing if not to supply an affirmative answer to the questions which we have put, and to show the practical consequence of such action.

Are the interests of the individual at this point subordinated to common interests of medicine, or do we find here a transgression, albeit in good faith, of the most basic demands of the natural law, a transgression which cannot be permitted for any reason of medical research?

One's eyes must be firmly shut to reality, if one believes that at the present hour there is to be found no one in the medical world holding and defending the ideas which are at the origin of the deeds which we have quoted. It is enough to follow for a time the reports on the medical trials and experiments to be convinced of the contrary. One wonders involuntarily what authorized this doctor or the other to do such a thing, and whence could he have any such authority. With calm objective statement, the experiment is described in its progress and effects; notes are made on what is established as true and what is not so. On the question of its moral lawfulness, not a word. This question remains, however, and passing it over in silence does not suppress it.

Insofar as, in the cases mentioned, the moral justification of the intervention is based on the mandate of the public authority, and therefore from the subordination of the individual to the community, of the individual good to the social good, it rests on a mistaken application of the principle. It must be pointed out that man, as a person, in the final reckoning, does not exist for the use of society; on the contrary, the community exists for man. . . .

. . . Our purpose was to draw your attention to certain principles of deontology which define the boundaries and limits of research and experimentation in new medical methods applied immediately to living human beings.

In the field of science, it is an obvious law that the application of new methods to the living person must be preceded by research on the dead body or the laboratory model, and by experimenting on animals. Sometimes, however, this procedure is shown to be impossible, inadequate, or, in practice, unable to be followed. Then medical research will make its attempt on its immediate object, the living human being, in the interests of science, of the patient, of the community. This is not to be dismissed without ado, but it is necessary to stop at the moral limits which we have explained.

Doubtless, before authorizing new methods according to moral law, the total exclusion of all danger and of every risk cannot be demanded. This is beyond the possibilities of human nature, would paralyze all scientific research, and would very often turn to the detriment of the patient. The appreciation of the element of danger must be left, in these cases, to the judgment of an experienced and competent doctor. There is, however, as our explanations have shown, a degree of danger which the moral law cannot permit. It may happen in doubtful cases, when the known methods have failed, that a new and insufficiently tried method offers, along with elements of great danger, appreciable chances of success. If the patient gives his consent, the application of the process in question is lawful. But this method of action cannot be established as a line of treatment for normal cases.

It will perhaps be objected that the ideas developed here will constitute a grave obstacle to research and scientific work. Nonetheless, the line we have drawn is not definitely an obstacle to progress. The same holds good in the field of medicine as in the other fields of research, experiment, and human activity. The mighty laws of morality force the swiftly rolling wave of human thought and will to flow like a mountain stream in a course well defined. They contain it for its own greater and effective usefulness. They dam its flood and

364 save it from overflowing and from working havoc, which could never find compensation in the specious good which it might pursue. In appearance, moral demands are a curb. In reality, they make their own contribution to the better and nobler achievements produced by man for the benefit of science, of the individual, and of the community. . . .

53: Right to Health Care

DOCUMENT 1:

SOURCE: National Conference of Catholic Bishops, "Pastoral Letter on Health and Health Care" (Nov. 16–19, 1981), *Origins* 11: no. 25, Dec. 3, 1981, pp. 400–02.

3. PROPHETIC ROLE

... We believe and hope that American society will move toward the establishment of a national policy which guarantees adequate health care for all while maintaining a pluralistic approach. As this develops, the role of Catholic institutions in the health field will change. They will take an even greater responsibility in fulfilling the prophetic role of promoting basic Christian values, championing the cause of the poor and neglected in society, and finding new ways to blend personal care and technological skills in health care service.

Service to the poor is one particularly important way of fulfilling this prophetic role. Here again we commend to all the emphatic words of Pope John Paul II:

"Social thinking and social practice inspired by the Gospel must always be marked by a special sensitivity toward those who are most in distress, those who are extremely poor, those suffering from all the physical, mental, and moral ills that afflict humanity including hunger, neglect, unemployment, and despair....

"But neither will you recoil before the reforms—even profound ones— of attitudes and structures that may prove necessary in order to re-create over and over again the conditions needed by the disadvantaged if they are to have a fresh chance in the hard struggle of life. The poor of the United States and of the world are your brothers and sisters in Christ. You must never be content to leave them just the crumbs from the feast. You must take of your substance and not just of your abundance in order to help them. And you must treat them like guests at your family table."

All those in the health apostolate who heed this call and follow the example of Jesus will continue to serve the poor, the frail elderly, the powerless, and the alienated. Sometimes this will be at great sacrifice, and it will demand both courage and imagination. For example, when locating or relocating facilities, leaders in the health apostolate can offer special insights for health care improvement in drastically underserved inner-city and rural areas, especially among Hispanics, blacks, and native Americans and other minorities.

Many of those whom the Catholic institution seeks to serve are reluctant or unable to seek help. They may be intimidated by the formality of a hospital, or live in an isolated area, or speak no English. Some may cling to an exaggerated

366 ideal of self-reliance. Catholic health care institutions should take the initiative in reaching out to these needy people. They should not hesitate, moreover, to initiate social action programs on behalf of their patients or potential patients and their families. Such programs will sometimes involve advocacy in the cause of justice for the underprivileged. This will include working for changes in reimbursement methodologies which penalize and threaten the existence of hospitals which seek to serve the poor.

A second important way of fulfilling the Church's prophetic role in the health care field is the development of alternative models of health care. For example, community clinics, "satellite" clinics, and other new models of health care delivery which meet the needs of the indigent, the underserved, and the poor should be supported and developed. Hospices, which offer humane, personal care for the terminally ill, are also a welcome development in recent years. These services exemplify the all-important integration of the spiritual, physical, psychological, and social dimensions of health care.

We likewise encourage further innovation in personal health education programs and in preventive health care services. For example, programs of health screening for the elderly which are conducted in local parishes or in congregate housing have proven to be both effective and desirable. Home health care for the frail elderly and disabled and new developments in long term care facilities are also welcome signs of innovation. We trust that Catholic health care facilities will continue to be leaders in the promotion of these and other alternatives in the years ahead. . . .

PUBLIC POLICY

It is appropriate in this context to call attention to the significant impact that public policy has on health care in our society. The government, working for the common good, has an essential role to play in ensuring that the right of all people to adequate health care is protected. The function of government reaches beyond the limited resources of individuals and private groups. Private agencies and institutions alone are unable to develop a comprehensive national health policy, or to ensure that all Americans have adequate health insurance, or to command the vast resources necessary to implement an effective national health policy. These functions are in large part the responsibility of government. However, in accord with the traditional Catholic principle of subsidiarity, we believe voluntary institutions must continue to play an essential role in our society.

Christian people have a responsibility to participate actively in the shaping and executing of public policy that relates to health care. On this issue, as on all issues of basic human rights, the Church has an important role to play in bringing Gospel values to the social and political order. In our statement on political responsibility issued earlier, we outline this role in more detail:

"The Church's responsibility in the area of human rights includes two complementary pastoral actions: the affirmation and promotion of human rights and the denunciation and condemnation of violations of these rights. In addition, it is the Church's role to call attention to the moral and religious dimensions of secular issues, to keep alive the values of the Gospel as a norm for social

and political life, and to point out the demands of the Christian faith for a just
transformation of society. Such a ministry on the part of every Christian and
the Church inevitably involves political consequences and touches upon public affairs."

We urge Catholics to fulfill their political responsibility in the area of
health care policy by educating themselves on the issues and by making their
views known. Acting both individually and collectively through parishes, Catholic organizations, and other appropriate networks, they can make a valuable
contribution toward the development of a just and humane national health
policy.

PRINCIPLES FOR PUBLIC POLICY

In the interest of providing a sound framework for discussion and policy
development, we affirm the following principles which we believe should be
reflected in a national health policy. These principles are consistent with and
flow from a recent constructive dialogue between the Catholic Health Association, the National Conference of Catholic Charities, and the USCC.

1. Every person has a basic right to adequate health care. This right flows
from the sanctity of human life and the dignity that belongs to all human
persons, who are made in the image of God. It implies that access to that
health care which is necessary and suitable for the proper development and
maintenance of life must be provided for all people, regardless of economic,
social, or legal status. Special attention should be given to meeting the basic
health needs of the poor. With increasingly limited resources in the economy,
it is the basic rights of the poor that are frequently threatened first. The Church
should work with government to avoid this danger.

2. Pluralism is an essential characteristic of the health care delivery system
of the United States. Any comprehensive health system that is developed,
therefore, should use the cooperative resources of both the public and private
sectors, the voluntary, religious, and nonprofit sectors. In any national health
system, provision should be made for the protection of conscience in the delivery of care. This applies not only to individual and institutional providers, but
also to consumers.

3. The benefits provided in a national health care policy should be sufficient to maintain and promote good health as well as to treat disease and
disability. Emphasis should be placed on the promotion of health, the prevention
of disease, and the protection against environmental and other hazards to
physical and mental health. If health is viewed in an integrated and comprehensive manner, the social and economic context of illness and health care must
become an important focus of concern and action. Toward this end, public
policy should provide incentives for preventive care, early intervention, and
alternative delivery systems. All of these actions should be carried out in
the context of our fundamental commitment to the sanctity and dignity of
human life.

4. Consumers should be allowed a reasonable choice of providers, whether
they be individual providers, groups, clinics, or institutions. Likewise, to

368 enhance personal and family responsibility in health care, public policy should ensure broad consumer participation in the planning and decision making that affects health maintenance and health care delivery both in the community and in institutions.

5. Health care planning is an essential element in the development of an efficient and coordinated health care system. Public policy should ensure that uniform standards are part of the health care delivery system. This is the joint responsibility of the private and public sectors. They should work cooperatively to ensure the provision of standards that will help to achieve equity in the range and quality of services and in the training of providers.

6. Methods of containing and controlling costs are an essential element of national health policy. Incentives should be developed at every level for administering health care efficiently, effectively, and economically.

Following on these principles and on our belief in health care as a basic human right, we call for the development of a national health insurance program. It is the responsibility of the federal government to establish a comprehensive health care system that will ensure a basic level of health care for all Americans. The federal government should also ensure adequate funding for this basic level of care through a national health insurance program. . . .

DOCUMENT 2 / Right to Health Care

SOURCE: National Conference of Catholic Bishops, "Economic Justice for All: Catholic Social Teaching and the U.S. Economy" (June 3, 1986), *Origins* 16: no. 3, June 5, 1986, pp. 50, 53.

1. CHARACTERISTICS OF POVERTY

a. Children in Poverty

173. Poverty strikes some groups more severely than others. Perhaps most distressing is the growing number of children who are poor. Today one in every four American children under the age of 6 and one in every two black children under 6 are poor. The number of children in poverty rose by 4 million over the decade between 1973–1983, with the result that there are now more poor children in the United States than at any time since 1965. The problem is particularly severe among female-headed families, where more than half of all children are poor. Two-thirds of black children and nearly three-quarters of Hispanic children in such families are poor.

174. Most poor families with children receive no government assistance, have no health insurance, and cannot pay medical bills. Less than half are immunized against preventable diseases such as diphtheria and polio. Poor children are disadvantaged even before birth; their mothers' lack of access to high-quality prenatal care leaves them at much greater risk of premature birth, low-birth weight, physical and mental impairment, and death before their first birthday. . . .

3. GUIDELINES FOR ACTION

208. Public-assistance programs should be designed to assist recipients, wherever possible, to become self-sufficient through gainful employment. Individuals should not be worse off economically when they get jobs than if they relied only on public assistance. Under current rules, people who give up welfare benefits to work in low-paying jobs soon lose their Medicaid benefits. To help recipients become self-sufficient and reduce dependency on welfare, public-assistance programs should work in tandem with job-creation programs that include provisions for training, counseling, placement, and child care. Jobs for recipients of public assistance should be fairly compensated so that workers receive the full benefits and status associated with gainful employment.

209. Welfare programs should provide recipients with adequate levels of support. This support should cover basic needs in food, clothing, shelter, health care, and other essentials. At present only 4 percent of poor families with children receive enough cash welfare benefits to lift them out of poverty. The combined benefits of AFDC and food stamps typically come to less than three-fourths of the official poverty level. Those receiving public assistance should not face the prospect of hunger at the end of the month, homelessness, sending children to school in ragged clothing, or inadequate medical care. . . .

DOCUMENT 3 / Right to Health Care

Source: United States Catholic Conference, "The Right to Health Care" (Sept. 3, 1985), *Origins* 15: no. 12, Sept. 5, 1985, pp. 86ff.

... The fact that at least 35 million Americans cannot afford adequate health care should be a deep concern to the Church and to our whole society. Affordable health care has been a major objective of labor unions and working people throughout the century in both bargaining agreements and public policy. Decades of steady progress are now being eroded as discussion of health care issues focus almost exclusively on cost containment.

Earlier gains in rates of health insurance coverage are being eroded as unemployment and labor force realignments leave a larger proportion of working people and their families with minimal or no protection. Fewer of the poor are now eligible for Medicaid; only half of those with incomes below the federal poverty standard can receive benefits. Millions of others with incomes just above the poverty line have no group insurance and cannot afford private plans.

By the latest official estimates, 35 million Americans have neither the financial resources nor public or private health insurance to pay for adequate health care. Half of those with incomes below the federal poverty standard have no insurance and are ineligible for Medicaid. Others with slightly higher incomes still cannot afford the cost of private health insurance and are ineligible for coverage under employer-sponsored plans.

The poor and uninsured in our country have often depended on care from publicly funded health services: public hospitals, community health centers, maternal and child health projects. Unfortunately, at a time when the number of poor and uninsured has been rising, care from those sources has diminished as many public facilities have closed or cut back on hours of services. While some individual hospitals have increased aid to the poor, on the whole the private sector has not filled the gap. In fact, the combined effect of cost-containment efforts and increased competition has actually reduced care for the poor among private hospitals. In some states there appears to be a clear relationship between the growth of investor-owned health facilities and reduced access to care for the poor and uninsured.

Even government insurance programs do not fully protect access to care for those of the poor and the elderly who are covered. The number of physicians who refuse to accept new Medicaid patients is rising, leaving poor sick people with Medicaid cards that are worthless until they become sick enough that they cannot be turned away from hospital emergency rooms. Elderly Medicare patients increasingly find that hospitals are eager to discharge them, regardless of their ability to manage alone at home or the availability of nursing home or home-care services.

Health care delivery systems are changing too. The tremendous growth in investor-owned facilities for nonhospital emergency and surgical care is troubling. As such systems become the norm and begin to dominate the market for certain kinds of services, those who cannot pay and have no insurance will find fewer and fewer sources of medical care.

As a nation, we have to be concerned about these trends and their impact on the poor, but we must also consider their potential impact on our whole community. Very few of us can afford to pay for care in a serious or even minor illness without a generous insurance plan. Those in well-paying jobs are usually protected as long as they are employed, but as millions in the "smokestack" industries can attest, that insurance protection vanishes after a layoff, at just the time when workers are least equipped to pay private premium rates and are most prone to illness from stress. Even full-time work is no guarantee of insurance protection. People who work for the lowest wages typically have no employee benefits such as health insurance even after eight years in their jobs. In addition, widows and divorced women and their children usually lose medical benefits they cannot afford to replace, and chronically ill and disabled workers often go uninsured for years before establishing eligibility for a public insurance program. Who can be secure that his or her insurance will still be in force when it is most needed?

Lack of health insurance does not mean just running up unpaid medical bills. All too often the uninsured go without care. They are regularly turned away from essential services that could prevent serious illness or disabling conditions that could ease shattering pain, improve functioning and lengthen life. Numerous studies show that the uninsured have significantly fewer doctors' visits, days in the hospital, and prescriptions filled, although their health status is considerably worse.

In their 1981 pastoral letter on health care, the American Catholic bishops strongly reminded us that health care is neither a commodity to be left to the free market nor an optional community service. Every person has a basic right to adequate health care which flows from the sanctity of life and the dignity of human persons. The bishops called on the federal government to be the guarantor of a basic level of health services for all, with special attention to the health needs of the poor, whose interests are usually most threatened.

What has traditionally been called the health care system is not described as the health care industry. Health care is not, after all, an industry in the same sense as automobile manufacturing, movie making, or banking. In our tradition, health care has focused on healing as a ministry, not only by providing care for the ill but by working to restore health and wholeness to each person and to the community. Other religious groups and local communities also developed hospitals dedicated to serving the needs of all those in need of care. Now those institutions as well as Catholic facilities face competition from a variety of medical enterprises specializing only in profitable care of the affluent and well-insured.

Our religious heritage and modern understanding convince us that works of mercy and works of justice are inseparable. Just as we minister directly to

372   the sick in our institutions, we also work to ensure that as a nation we guarantee that no one is denied adequate health care because of inability to pay or other kinds of discrimination. We cannot tolerate public policies or institutional arrangements that subordinate basic human rights to government cost savings or investors' profits.

54: Sacredness of Human Life

DOCUMENT 1:

SOURCE: Vatican Council II, "Pastoral Constitution on the Church in the Modern World" (Dec. 7, 1965), *Vatican Council II*, Vol. 1, pp. 913–15.

THE DIGNITY OF THE HUMAN PERSON
Man as the Image of God

12. Believers and unbelievers agree almost unanimously that all things on earth should be ordained to man as to their center and summit.

But what is man? He has put forward, and continues to put forward, many views about himself, views that are divergent and even contradictory. Often he either sets himself up as the absolute measure of all things, or debases himself to the point of despair. Hence his doubt and his anguish. The Church is keenly sensitive to these difficulties. Enlightened by divine revelation she can offer a solution to them by which the true state of man may be outlined, his weakness explained, in such a way that at the same time his dignity and his vocation may be perceived in their true light.

For Sacred Scripture teaches that man was created "to the image of God," as able to know and love his creator, and as set by him over all earthly creatures that he might rule them, and make use of them, while glorifying God. "What is man that thou are mindful of him, and the son of man that thou dost care for him? Yet thou hast made him little less than God, and dost crown him with glory and honor. Thou hast given him dominion over the works of thy hands; thou hast put all things under his feet" (Ps 8:5–8).

But God did not create man a solitary being. From the beginning "male and female he created them" (Gn 1:27). This partnership of man and woman constitutes the first form of communion between persons. For by his innermost nature man is a social being; and if he does not enter into relations with others he can neither live nor develop his gifts.

So God, as we read again in the Bible, saw "all the things that he had made, and they were very good" (Gn 1:31).

Sin

13. Although set by God in a state of rectitude, man, enticed by the evil one, abused his freedom at the very start of history. He lifted himself up against God, and sought to attain his goal apart from him. Although they had known God, they did not glorify him as God, but their senseless hearts were darkened, and they served the creature rather than the creator. What revelation makes known to us is confirmed by our own experience. For when man looks into

374   his own heart he finds that he is drawn towards what is wrong and sunk in many evils which cannot come from his good creator. Often refusing to acknowledge God as his source, man has also upset the relationship which should link him to his last end; and at the same time he has broken the right order that should reign within himself as well as between himself and other men and all creatures.

Man therefore is divided in himself. As a result, the whole life of men, both individual and social, shows itself to be a struggle, and a dramatic one, between good and evil, between light and darkness. Man finds that he is unable of himself to overcome the assaults of evil successfully, so that everyone feels as though bound by chains. But the Lord himself came to free and strengthen man, renewing him inwardly and casting out the "prince of this world" (Jn 12:31), who held him in the bondage of sin. For sin brought man to a lower state, forcing him away from the completeness that is his to attain.

Both the high calling and the deep misery which men experience find their final explanation in the light of this revelation.

The Essential Nature of Man

14. Man, though made of body and soul, is a unity. Through his very bodily condition he sums up in himself the elements of the material world. Through him they are thus brought to their highest perfection and can raise their voice in praise freely given to the creator. For this reason man may not despise his bodily life. Rather he is obliged to regard his body as good and to hold it in honor since God has created it and will raise it up on the last day. Nevertheless man has been wounded by sin. He finds by experience that his body is in revolt. His very dignity therefore requires that he should glorify God in his body, and not allow it to serve the evil inclinations of his heart.

Man is not deceived when he regards himself as superior to bodily things and as more than just a speck of nature of a nameless unit in the city of man. For by his power to know himself in the depths of his being he rises above the whole universe of mere objects. When he is drawn to think about his real self he turns to those deep recesses of his being where God who probes the heart awaits him, and where he himself decides his own destiny in the sight of God. So when he recognizes in himself a spiritual and immortal soul, he is not being led astray by false imaginings that are due to merely physical or social causes. On the contrary, he grasps what is profoundly true in this matter.

DOCUMENT 2 / Sacredness of Human Life

SOURCE: Pope John Paul II, "Celebrate Life" (Oct. 7, 1979), *The Pope Speaks* 24: no. 4, 1979, p. 372.

. . . I do not hesitate to proclaim before you and before the world that all human life—from the moment of conception and through all subsequent stages—is sacred, because human life is created in the image and likeness of God. Nothing surpasses the greatness or dignity of a human person.

Human life is not just an idea or an abstraction; human life is the concrete reality of a being that lives, that acts, that grows and develops; human life is the concrete reality of a being that is capable of love and of service to humanity.

WHOLE MORAL ORDER AFFECTED

Let me repeat what I told the people during my recent pilgrimage to my homeland: "If a person's right to life is violated at the moment in which he is first conceived in his mother's womb, an indirect blow is struck also at the whole of the moral order, which serves to ensure the inviolable good of man. Among those goods, life occupies the first place. The Church defends the right to life, not only in regard to the majesty of the Creator, who is the first giver of this life, but also in respect of the essential good of the human person" (June 8, 1979).

Human life is precious because it is the gift of God whose love is infinite. And when God gives life, it is forever.

Life is also precious because it is the expression and the fruit of love. This is why life should spring up within the setting of marriage, and why marriage and the parents' love for one another should be marked by generosity in self-giving. . . .

DOCUMENT 3 / Sacredness of Human Life

SOURCE: Joseph Cardinal Bernardin, "Call for a Consistent Ethic of Life" (Dec. 6, 1983), *Origins* 13: no. 29, Dec. 29, 1983, pp. 492–93.

II. A CONSISTENT ETHIC OF LIFE: A CATHOLIC PERSPECTIVE

... "The Challenge of Peace" provides a starting point for developing a consistent ethic of life, but it does not provide a fully articulated framework. The central idea in the letter is the sacredness of human life and the responsibility we have, personally and socially, to protect and preserve the sanctity of life.

Precisely because life is sacred, the taking of even one human life is a momentous event. Indeed, the sense that every human life has transcendent value has led a whole stream of the Christian tradition to argue that life may never be taken. That position is held by an increasing number of Catholics and is reflected in the pastoral letter, but it has not been the dominant view in Catholic teaching and it is not the principal moral position found in the pastoral letter. What is found in the letter is the traditional Catholic teaching that there should always be a presumption against taking human life, but in a limited world marked by the effects of sin there are some narrowly defined exceptions where life can be taken. This is the moral logic which produced the "just-war" ethic in Catholic theology. ...

Asking these questions along the spectrum of life from womb to tomb creates the need for a consistent ethic of life. For the spectrum of life cuts across the issues of genetics, abortion, capital punishment, modern warfare, and the care of the terminally ill. These are all distinct problems, enormously complicated and deserving individual treatment. No single answer and no simple responses will solve them. My purpose, however, is to highlight the way in which we face new technological challenges in each one of these areas; this combination of challenges is what cries out for a consistent ethic of life. ...

... It is therefore necessary to illustrate, at least by way of example, my proposition that an inner relationship does exist among several issues not only at the level of general attitude, but at the more specified level of moral principles. Two examples will serve to indicate the point.

The first is contained in "The Challenge of Peace" in the connection drawn between Catholic teaching on war and Catholic teaching on abortion. Both, of course, must be seen in light of an attitude of respect for life. The more explicit connection is based on the principle which prohibits the directly intended taking of innocent human life. The principle is at the heart of Catholic teaching on abortion; it is because the fetus is judged to be both human and not an aggressor that Catholic teaching concludes that direct attack on fetal life is always wrong. This is also why we insist that legal protection be given to the unborn.

The same principle yields the most stringent, binding, and radical conclusion of the pastoral letter: that directly intended attacks on civilian centers is always wrong. The bishops seek to highlight the power of this conclusion by specifying its implications in two ways: First, such attacks would be wrong even if our cities had been hit first; second, anyone asked to execute such attacks should refuse orders. These two extensions of the principle cut directly into the policy debate on nuclear strategy and the personal decisions of citizens. James Reston referred to them as "an astonishing challenge to the power of the state. . . ."

If one contends, as we do, that the right of every fetus to be born should be protected by civil law and supported by civil consensus, then our moral, political, and economic responsibilities do not stop at the moment of birth. Those who defend the right to life of the weakest among us must be equally visible in support of the quality of life of the powerless among us: the old and the young, the hungry and the homeless, the undocumented immigrant and the unemployed worker. Such a quality of life posture translates into specific political and economic positions on tax policy, employment generation, welfare policy, nutrition and feeding programs, and health care. Consistency means we cannot have it both ways: we cannot urge a compassionate society and vigorous public policy to protect the rights of the unborn and then argue that compassion and significant public programs on behalf of the needy undermine the moral fiber of the society or are beyond the proper scope of governmental responsibility. . . .

55: Scientific Knowledge

DOCUMENT 1:

SOURCE: Vatican Council II, "Pastoral Constitution on the Church in the Modern World" (Dec. 7, 1965), *Vatican Council II*, Vol. 1, pp. 915–16.

DIGNITY OF THE INTELLECT, OF TRUTH, AND OF WISDOM

15. Man, as sharing in the light of the divine mind, rightly affirms that by his intellect he surpasses the world of mere things. By diligent use of his talents through the ages he has indeed made progress in the empirical sciences, in technology, and in the liberal arts. In our time his attempts to search out the secrets of the material universe and to bring it under his control have been extremely successful. Yet he has always looked for, and found, truths of a higher order. For his intellect is not confined to the range of what can be observed by the senses. It can, with genuine certainty, reach to realities known only to the mind, even though, as a result of sin, its vision has been clouded and its powers weakened.

The intellectual nature of man finds at last its perfection, as it should, in wisdom, which gently draws the human mind to look for and to love what is true and good. Filled with wisdom man is led through visible realities to those which cannot be seen.

Our age, more than any of the past, needs such wisdom if all that man discovers is to be ennobled through human effort. Indeed, the future of the world is in danger unless provision is made for men of greater wisdom. It should also be pointed out that many nations, poorer as far as material goods are concerned yet richer as regards wisdom, can be of the greatest advantage to others.

It is by the gift of the Holy Spirit that man, through faith, comes to contemplate and savor the mystery of God's design.

DOCUMENT 2 / Scientific Knowledge

SOURCE: Pope Pius XII, "Moral Aspects of Genetics" (Sept. 7, 1953), *The Human Body: Papal Teachings,* pp. 252–56.

FUNDAMENTAL DEMANDS OF SCIENTIFIC KNOWLEDGE

... Truth is to be taken as an agreement between the judgment of man and the reality of being and of action of things; this is contrasted with the images and ideas fashioned by the mind. There was, and still is today, an opinion which holds that the message of objective reality penetrates the spirit as through a filter, being subject to modification quantitatively and qualitatively in the process. This is called dynamic thought, which gives its form to the object, unlike static thought which is the mere reflection of it, unless, on principle, it be asserted that the first is the only possible way of gaining human knowledge. Truth then would be reduced to personal thought agreeing with public or scientific opinion of the time. In every age, thought based on sound reason, and Christian thought particularly, is aware of the duty of upholding this essential principle: truth is the agreement of judgment with the very being of things. There is no need, however, to deny what was said above, about the concept of truth, which, though in the main erroneous, is yet justifiable in part. We touched on this question in Our Encyclical, *Humani Generis,* of Aug. 12, 1950, and stressed there a point which we think it well to repeat here: the necessity of preserving intact the great ontological laws, because without them it is impossible to understand reality. We mean, above all, the principles of contradiction, sufficient reason, causality, and finality.

From your writings, we understand that you are in agreement with our idea of truth. In your research you seek for truth, and it is on this that you base your conclusions and build your systems. You affirm that genes exist as a fact and not as a mere hypothesis. You admit then the existence of the objective facts and that science is both able to understand them and intends to do so, and not simply to work out fantasies that are purely subjective.

The distinction between sure facts and their interpretation or their orderly arrangement is as fundamental to the seeker as the definition of truth. A fact is always true because it can contain no ontological error; but it is not by any means the same in the matter of its scientific elaboration. Here, one runs the risk of coming to premature conclusions and committing errors of judgment.

All this makes it necessary to have respect for fact and for facts as a whole, to have prudence in declaring scientific propositions, to be sober in scientific judgment, to be possessed of that modesty so appreciated among the learned, inspired as it is by an awareness of the limits of human knowledge. This helps to broaden the mind and increase the docility of the real man of science, who will be loath to hold on to his own ideas when they are proved 379

380 to be not well-founded; and, finally, it enables one to examine the opinions of others, and judge them without prejudice.

When one possesses this disposition of soul, respect for truth will naturally be accompanied by truthfulness, that is to say, the agreement between one's personal convictions and the scientific position taken up in one's speech or writings.

The necessity for truth and truthfulness calls for another remark regarding scientific knowledge. Rarely is it that merely one science deals with a particular subject. Often there are many sciences dealing with a subject, each one treating it under a different aspect. If their research is correct, no contradiction is possible between their findings, because this would presuppose a contradiction in the ontological reality, and reality cannot contradict itself.

If, in spite of everything, contradictions arise, these can only be the result either of faulty observation, or of erroneous interpretation of a correct observation; or else they derive from the fact that the person engaged in the research has overstepped the limits of his special field, and advanced onto a terrain of which he had no knowledge. We feel that this remark, too, obviously, is necessary in all sciences.

If therefore, the theory of heredity, based on a knowledge of cellular structure—and, more recently, of the structure of the cytoplasm as well—and on knowledge of the immanent laws of hereditary transmission, is able to say why a man has certain characteristics, nevertheless it is not yet in a position to explain the whole life of that man. It must be completed by other sciences once the question arises regarding the existence and origin of the spiritual principle of his life, the human soul, which is essentially independent of matter. The conclusions of genetics regarding the primary cell and the development of the human body by normal divisions of cells under the influence of the genes, its statements about modifications, changes, and the partnership between inheritance and environment—all this is not enough to explain the unity of man's nature, his intellectual knowledge and his free will. Genetics, as such, has nothing to say to the fact that, in the unity of a human nature, a spiritual soul is joined to an organic substrate which enjoyed relative autonomy. It is here that psychology and metaphysics or ontology must enter in, not in opposition to genetics but in agreement, in order to further and substantially complete its findings. Neither, on the other hand, can philosophy neglect genetics if, in its analysis of psychic activities, it wants to remain in contact with reality. Insofar as the psychic is conditioned by the body, one cannot claim to make the entire psychic dependent on the *anima rationalis* as the *forma corporis,* and say that the amorphous *materia prima* receives all its determinations from the spiritual soul created directly by God, and none at all from the genes contained in the cells.

The many different sources of knowledge call attention to another fact of decisive importance: the distinction between the knowledge acquired by personal study, and that which one owes to the research and therefore to the witness of others. When one is sure that this witness is worthy of belief, then it constitutes a normal source of knowledge, which neither practical life nor science can overlook. Prescinding from the absolute necessity of having frequent

recourse to the witness of others, the truly learned man's disposition of soul, **381**
mentioned above, convinces him that in his field the proven specialist is always
in much closer touch with objective truth than anybody who is not versed in
the subject.

We cannot refrain from applying to the witness of God what we have
just said about the witness of man. Revelation, and therefore, the formal explicit
witness of the Creator, touches also certain fields of natural science and certain
theses of your specialized branch, such as the theory of hereditary transmission.
Now, the Creator fulfills, in the highest degree, the requirements of truth and
truthfulness. Judge, therefore, for yourselves whether it is compatible with
scientific objectivity to set aside that witness, since there is every guarantee
regarding its reality and its content.

As far as the theory of hereditary transmission is concerned, the essential
question is that of the origin of man's physical organism, (not of his spiritual
soul). Your science deals diligently with this problem, but theology, a science
which has revelation as its subject, also devotes very keen attention to it. On
two occasions—in our 1941 address to our Academy of Sciences, and, in 1950,
in the Encyclical referred to above—we ourselves called for more research in
the hope that some day, perhaps, results might be achieved of which one could
be sure, for, up to the present, nothing decisive has been obtained. We urged
that these questions be treated with the prudence and the maturity of judgment
which their great importance demands. From the writings on your special
subject, we took a quotation in which, after an outline of all the present-day
discoveries and of the opinions of specialists in their regard, the same sobriety
was recommended and definite judgment was reserved.

If you reflect on what we have said of research and of scientific knowledge,
it ought to be understood that, neither on the part of reason nor on the part
of thought inspired by Christian teaching, are any barriers placed in the way
of research for truth or of its attainment or its affirmation. Barriers there are,
but their purpose is not to imprison truth: their purpose is to prevent unproved
hypotheses from being accepted as established facts, to keep persons from
forgetting that it is necessary to complete one source of knowledge with another,
and to avoid wrong interpretations of the scale of values and of the degree of
certitude of a source of knowledge. It is to avoid those causes of error that
barriers exist, but there are no barriers to truth.

56: Sexuality

DOCUMENT 1:

Source: Pontifical Council for the Family, "The Truth and Meaning of Human Sexuality," *Origins* 25: no. 32 (Feb. 1, 1996), pp. 530–52.

Among the many difficulties parents encounter today despite different social contexts, one certainly stands out: giving children an adequate preparation for adult life, particularly with regard to education in the true meaning of sexuality. There are many reasons for this difficulty, and not all of them are new.

In the past, even when the family did not provide specific sexual education, the general culture was permeated by respect for fundamental values and hence served to protect and maintain them. In the greater part of society, both in developed and developing countries, the decline of traditional models has left children deprived of consistent and positive guidance, while parents find themselves unprepared to provide adequate answers.

This new context is made worse by what we observe: an eclipse of the truth about man which, among other things, exerts pressure to reduce sex to something commonplace. In this area society and the mass media most of the time provide depersonalized, recreational, and often pessimistic information. Moreover, this information does not take into account the different stages of formation and development of children and young people, and it is influenced by a distorted individualistic concept of freedom in an ambience lacking the basic values of life, human love, and the family.

. . . Aware of this family dimension of education for love and for living one's own sexuality properly, and conscious of the unique "experience of humanity" of the community of believers, our council wishes to put forward pastoral guidelines, drawing on the wisdom which comes from the word of the Lord and the values which illuminate the teaching of the Church.

. . . In this field the Church is strengthened by some unquestionable certainties that have also guided the preparation of this document.

Love is a gift of God, nourished by and expressed in the encounter of man and woman. Love is thus a positive force directed toward their growth in maturity as persons. In the plan of life which represents each person's vocation, love is also a precious source for the self-giving which all men and women are called to make for their own self-realization and happiness. In fact, man is called to love as an incarnate spirit, that is, soul and body in the unity of the person. Human love hence embraces the body, and the body also expresses spiritual love. Therefore, sexuality is not something purely biological, rather it concerns the intimate nucleus of the person. The use of sexuality as physical giving has its own truth and reaches its full meaning when it expresses the personal giving of man and woman even unto death.

As with the whole of the person's life, love is exposed to the frailty brought about by original sin, a frailty experienced today in many sociocultural contexts marked by strong negative influences, at times deviant and traumatic. Nevertheless, the Lord's redemption has made the positive practice of chastity into something that is really possible and a motive for joy, both for those who have the vocation to marriage (before in the time of preparation and afterward in the course of married life) as well as for those who have the gift of a special calling to the consecrated life.

In the light of the redemption and how adolescents and young people are formed, the virtue of chastity is found within temperance—a cardinal virtue elevated and enriched by grace in baptism. So chastity is not to be understood as a repressive attitude. On the contrary, chastity should be understood rather as the purity and temporary stewardship of a precious and rich gift of love, in view of the self-giving realized in each person's specific vocation. Chastity is thus that "spiritual energy capable of defending love from the perils of selfishness and aggressiveness, and able to advance it toward its full realization."

. . . Taking up the teaching of the Second Vatican Council, the Catechism of the Catholic Church says: "It is imperative to give suitable and timely instruction to young people, above all in the heart of their own families, about the dignity of married love, its role and its exercise."

. . . Parents in particular have the duty to let their children know about the mysteries of human life, because the family "is, in fact, the best environment to accomplish the obligation of securing a gradual education in sexual life. The family has an affective dignity which is suited to making acceptable without trauma the most delicate realities and to integrating them harmoniously in a balanced and rich personality." As we have recalled, this primary task of the family includes the parents' right that their children should not be obliged to attend courses in school on this subject which are not in harmony with their religious and moral convictions. The school's task is not to substitute for the family, rather it is "assisting and completing the work of parents, furnishing children and adolescents with an evaluation of sexuality as value and task of the whole person, created male and female in the image of God."

In this regard we recall what the Holy Father teaches in *Familiaris Consortio*: "The Church is firmly opposed to an often widespread form of imparting sex information dissociated from moral principles. That would merely be an introduction to the experience of pleasure and a stimulus leading to the loss of serenity while still in the years of innocence by opening the way to vice."

Therefore, four general principles will be proposed and afterward the various stages in a child's development will be examined.

Four Principles Regarding Information About Sexuality

Each child is a unique and unrepeatable person and must receive individualized formation. Since parents know, understand, and love each of their

384 children in their uniqueness, they are in the best position to decide what the appropriate time is for providing a variety of information, according to their children's physical and spiritual growth. No one can take this capacity for discernment away from conscientious parents.

Each child's process of maturation as a person is different. Therefore, the most intimate aspects, whether biological or emotional, should be communicated in a personalized dialogue. In their dialogue with each child, with love and trust, parents communicate something about their own self-giving which makes them capable of giving witness to aspects of the emotional dimension of sexuality that could not be transmitted in other ways. . . .

The moral dimension must always be part of their explanations. Parents should stress that Christians are called to live the gift of sexuality according to the plan of God, who is love, i.e., in the context of marriage or of consecrated virginity and also celibacy. They must insist on the positive value of chastity and its capacity to generate true love for other persons. This is the most radical and important moral aspect of chastity. Only a person who knows how to be chaste will know how to love in marriage or in virginity.

From the earliest age, parents may observe the beginning of instinctive genital activity in their child. It should not be considered repressive to correct such habits gently that could become sinful later and, when necessary, to teach modesty as the child grows. It is always important to justify the judgment of morally rejecting certain attitudes contrary to the dignity of the person and chastity on adequate, valid, and convincing grounds, both at the level of reason and faith, hence in a positive framework with a high concept of personal dignity. . . .

Formation in chastity and timely information regarding sexuality must be provided in the broadest context of education for love. It is not sufficient, therefore, to provide information about sex together with objective moral principles. Constant help is also required for the growth of children's spiritual life so that the biological development and impulses they begin to experience will always be accompanied by a growing love of God, the creator and redeemer, and an ever greater awareness of the dignity of each human person and his or her body. In the light of the mystery of Christ and the Church, parents can illustrate the positive values of human sexuality in the context of the person's original vocation of love and the universal call to holiness.

Parents should provide this information with great delicacy, but clearly and at the appropriate time. Parents are well aware that their children must be treated in a personalized way according to the personal conditions of their physiological and psychological development and taking into due consideration the cultural environment of life and the adolescent's daily experience. In order to evaluate properly what they should say to each child, it is very important that parents first of all seek light from the Lord in prayer and that they discuss this together so that their words will be neither too explicit nor too vague. Giving too many details to children is counterproductive. But delaying the first information for too long is imprudent, because every human person has natural curiosity in this regard, and sooner or later everyone begins to ask

themselves questions, especially in cultures where too much can be seen, even
in public. . . .

In light of these recommendations, education for love can take concrete form in four working principles.

Human sexuality is a sacred mystery and must be presented according to the doctrinal and moral teaching of the Church, always bearing in mind the effects of original sin. . . .

Only information proportionate to each phase of their individual development should be presented to children and young people. . . .

No material of an erotic nature should be presented to children or young people of any age, individually or in a group. . . .

No one should ever be invited, let alone obliged, to act in any way that could objectively offend against modesty or which could subjectively offend against his or her own delicacy or sense of privacy. . . .

DOCUMENT 2 / Sexuality

Source: Congregation for the Doctrine of the Faith, "Declaration on Certain Problems of Sexual Ethics" (Dec. 29, 1975), *Vatican Council II*, Vol. 2, 1982, pp. 486–96.

1. The human person, present-day scientists maintain, is so profoundly affected by sexuality that it must be considered one of the principal formative influences on the life of a man or woman. If fact, sex is the source of the biological, psychological, and spiritual characteristics which make a person male or female and which thus considerably influence each individual's progress towards maturity and membership of society. . . .

3. Nowadays people are increasingly convinced that man's dignity and destiny, and indeed his development, demand that they should apply their intelligence to the discovery and constant development of the values inherent in human nature and should give practical effect to them in their lives.

However, man may not make moral judgments arbitrarily: "Deep within his conscience man discovers a law which he has not laid upon himself, but which he must obey . . . . For man has in his heart a law inscribed by God. His dignity lies in observing this law and by it he will be judged. . . ."

Therefore, man's true dignity cannot be achieved unless the essential order of his nature be observed. It must, of course, be recognized that in the course of history civilization has taken many forms, that the requirements for human living have changed considerably, and that many changes are still to come. But limits must be set to the evolution of mores and lifestyles, limits set by the unchangeable principles based on the elements that go to make up the human person and on his essential relationships. Such things transcend historical circumstances.

These fundamental principles, which can be perceived by human reason, are contained in "the divine law itself—eternal, objective, and universal, by which God orders, directs, and governs the whole world and the ways of the human community according to a plan conceived in his wisdom and love. God has enabled man to participate in this law of his so that, under the gentle disposition of his divine providence, many may be able to arrive at a deeper and deeper knowledge of the unchanging truth." This divine law is accessible to our minds.

4. Consequently, it is wrong to assert as many do today that neither human nature nor revealed law provide any absolute and unchangeable norms as a guide for individual actions, that all they offer is the general law of charity and respect for the human person. Proponents of this view allege in its support that the norms of the natural law, as they are called, and the precepts of Sacred Scripture are to be seen rather as patterns of behavior found in particular
cultures at given moments of history. . . .

5. Since sexual ethics have to do with certain fundamental values of **387** human and Christian life, this general teaching applies equally to sexual ethics. There are principles and norms in sexual ethics which the Church has always proclaimed as part of her teaching and has never had any doubt about it, however much the opinions and mores of the world opposed them. These principles and norms in no way owe their origin to a particular culture, but rather to knowledge of the divine law and of human nature. They do not therefore cease to oblige or become doubtful because cultural changes take place.

These are the principles on which the Second Council of the Vatican based its suggestions and directives for the establishment and the organization of a social order in which due account would be taken of the equal dignity of men and women, while respecting the difference between them.

In speaking of "man's sexuality and the faculty of reproduction," the Council noted that they "wondrously surpassed the endowments of lower forms of life." It then dealt one by one with the principles and rules which relate to human sexuality in marriage and which are based on the specific purpose of sexuality.

With regard to the matter in hand, the Council declares that when assessing the propriety of conjugal acts, determining if they accord with true human dignity, "it is not enough to take only the good intention and the evaluation of motives into account. Objective criteria must be used, criteria based on the nature of the human person and of human action, criteria which respect the total meaning of mutual self-giving and human procreation in the context of true love."

This last quotation summarizes the Council's teaching on the finality of the sexual act and on the principal criterion of its morality: when the finality of the act is respected the moral goodness of the act is ensured. This teaching is explained in greater detail in the same Constitution.

This same principle, which the Church derives from divine revelation and from its authentic interpretation of the natural law, is at the core of its traditional teaching that only in legitimate marriage does the use of the sexual faculty find its true meaning and its probity.

6. It is not the intention of this Declaration to deal with all abuses of sex, nor with all that is involved in the cultivation of chastity. Its object is rather to re-state the Church's norms with regard to certain points of doctrine. It would seem that it has become a matter of urgent necessity to oppose the grave errors and depraved conduct which are now widespread.

7. Nowadays many claim the right to sexual intercourse before marriage, at least for those who have a firm intention of marrying and whose love for one another, already conjugal as it were, is deemed to demand this as its natural outcome. This argument is put with particular insistence when the celebration of marriage is impeded by external circumstances or when this intimate relationship is judged necessary for the preservation of love.

This opinion is contrary to Christian teaching, which asserts that sexual intercourse may take place only within marriage. No matter how definite the

388   intention of those who indulge in premarital sex, the fact is that such liaisons can scarcely ensure mutual sincerity and fidelity in a relationship between a man and a woman, nor, especially, can they protect it from inconstancy of desires or whim. Jesus willed that such a union be stable and he restored it to its original condition, based on the difference between the sexes: "Have you not read that the creator from the beginning made them male and female and that he said: 'This is why a man must leave father and mother, and cling to his wife, and the two become one body. They are no longer two, therefore, but one body. So then, what God has united, man must not divide.' St. Paul was more explicit, when he taught that if the unmarried or widows are unable to remain continent they have no alternative but to marry: "Better be married than burn with vain desire." In marriage the love of a couple for each other becomes part of Christ's unfailing love for the Church. An incontinent union of bodies defiles the temple of the Holy Spirit which the Christian himself has become. Sexual intercourse is not lawful, therefore, save between a man and a woman who have embarked upon a permanent, life-long partnership.

The Church has always understood this and taught it and has found the fullest confirmation of its teaching in natural philosophy and the testimony of history.

Experience teaches that love must be protected by the stability of marriage if sexual intercourse is really to meet the demands of its own finality and of human dignity. For this to be achieved there is need of a contract sanctioned and protected by society. The marriage contract inaugurates a state of life which is of the greatest importance. It makes possible a union between husband and wife that is exclusive and it promotes the good of their family and of the whole of human society. In fact, premarital liaisons very often exclude the expectation of a family. The love which, wrongly, is portrayed as conjugal will not be able to develop into paternal and maternal love, as it certainly should. Or, if children are born to partners in such a union it will be to their detriment. They will be deprived of a stable family life in which to grow up properly and through which to find their place in the community.

Those who wish to be united in matrimony should, therefore, manifest their consent externally and in a manner which the community accepts as valid. The faithful, for their part, should declare their consent to marry in the way prescribed by the laws of the Church. This makes their marriage one of Christ's sacraments. . . .

9. The traditional teaching of the Catholic Church that masturbation is gravely sinful is frequently doubted nowadays if not expressly denied. It is claimed that psychology and sociology show that, especially in adolescents, it is a normal concomitant of growth towards sexual maturity and that for this reason no grave fault is involved. The only exception is when a person deliberately indulges in solitary pleasure focused exclusively on self (*ipsatio*), since such an action would be totally opposed to that loving partnership between persons of opposite sexes which, indeed, they claim to be the principal object of sexual activity.

The opinion, however, is contrary to both the teaching and the pastoral practice of the Church. Whatever force there may be in certain biological and philosophical arguments put forward from time to time by theologians, the fact remains that both the Magisterium of the Church, in the course of a constant tradition, and the moral sense of the faithful have been in no doubt and have firmly maintained that masturbation is an intrinsically and gravely disordered action. The principal argument in support of this truth is that the deliberate use of the sexual faculty, for whatever reason, outside of marriage is essentially contrary to its purpose. For it lacks that sexual relationship demanded by the moral order and in which "the total meaning of mutual self-giving and human procreation in the context of true love" is achieved. All deliberate sexual activity must therefore be referred to the married state. Although it cannot be established that Sacred Scripture condemned masturbation by name, the tradition of the Church has rightly taken it to have been condemned by the New Testament when it speaks of "uncleanness" and "unchastity" and other vices contrary to chastity and continence.

Sociological investigations can disclose the incidence of masturbation in this or that region, among this or that people, in any circumstances of time or place that are chosen for investigation. That is how facts are collected. But facts do not furnish a rule for judging the morality of human acts. The incidence is linked, it is true, with the weakness implanted in man by original sin. But it is also linked with the loss of the sense of God, with the corruption of morals caused by the commercialization of vice, with the unrestrained license of so many public entertainments and publications, with the neglect of modesty, which is the guardian of chastity.

Modern psychology has much that is valid and useful to offer on the subject of masturbation. It is helpful for gauging moral responsibility more accurately and for directing pastoral activity along the right lines. It can enable one to understand how adolescent immaturity, which sometimes outlasts adolescence, the lack of psychological balance, and ingrained habit can influence a person's behavior, diminishing his responsibility for his actions, with the result that he is not always guilty of subjectively grave fault. But the absence of grave responsibility must not always be presumed. If it were it would scarcely be a recognition of men's ability to behave morally.

In the pastoral ministry itself, when there is a question of reaching a sound judgment on an individual case, the habitual general conduct of the person concerned should be taken into account, not only the practice of justice and charity but also the care given to the observance of the special precept of chastity. In particular, one should ascertain whether necessary natural and supernatural helps are being used which age-long Christian ascetical experience recommends for curbing passion and making progress in virtue.

10. There is nowadays a considerable threat to the observance of the moral law on sexual matters and to the practice of chastity, especially among less fervent Christians. The threat is posed by the current tendency to minimize the reality of grave sin as much as possible, at least in the concrete, and even

390 at times to deny its existence altogether. Some have gone on to assert that mortal sin, which separated man from God, is to be found only in the direct and formal refusal of God's call, or when a person deliberately chooses self-love, to the total exclusion of the neighbor. They say that only then is there question of a "fundamental option"—that is, a decision of the will which involves the person totally and without which there is no mortal sin. For it is by this option that from the depths of his personality a man adopts or ratifies a fundamental attitude towards God or people. On the contrary, they say, actions which are termed "peripheral" (in which, they say, the choice is often not definitive) do not succeed in changing a person's fundamental option. Indeed, since they are often done out of habit, there is then even less chance of their doing so. Therefore, while such actions can indeed weaken a person's fundamental option, they cannot change it completely. Now, according to these authors, it is more difficult to change a fundamental option for God in sexual matters, where normally it is not by fully deliberate and responsible actions that a person violates the moral order, but rather under the influence of passion or because of weakness or immaturity; sometimes it happens because a person wrongly thinks he can thus express love for his neighbor. Social pressures are often a further cause.

It is true that it is a person's fundamental option which ultimately defines adequately his moral stance. But it can be radically altered by individual actions, especially when, as often happens, they have already been prepared for by previous less deliberate actions. However that may be, it is scarcely correct to say that individual actions are not sufficient to constitute mortal sin (*mortale peccatum*).

According to the Church's teaching, mortal sin, which is opposed to God, is not found solely in the formal and direct refusal to obey the precept of charity. It is also found in that opposition to true love which is involved in every deliberate transgression of the moral law in a grave matter (*in re gravi*).

Christ designated the double law of charity as the foundation of moral life. "Everything in the law and the prophets hangs on these two commandments." They include therefore the other individual commandments. To the young man who asked him: 'What good must I do to gain eternal life?' Jesus replied: ". . . if you wish to enter into life, keep the commandments . . . . Do not murder; do not commit adultery; do not steal; do not give false evidence; honor your father and your mother; and love your neighbor as yourself."

A person commits mortal sin, therefore, not only when his actions stem from direct contempt for God and his neighbor, but also when knowingly and willingly, for whatever reason, he makes a choice which is gravely at variance with right order (*aliquid graviter inordinatum*). For in that choice, as has been said, contempt for the divine precept is already implied: it involves turning away from God and losing charity. According to Christian and the Church's teaching, and as right reason acknowledges, sexual morality encompasses such important human values that every violation of it is objectively grave (*objective . . . gravis*).

It must be acknowledged that, granted their nature and causes, totally **391** free consent may easily be lacking in sins of sex. Prudence and caution are needed therefore in passing any judgment on a person's responsibility. The words of Scripture are relevant here: "Man looks at appearances, but God looks at the heart." However, while prudence is recommended in judging the subjective gravity of an individual sinful action (*actus pravi*), it in no way follows that there are no mortal sins in matters of sex.

Pastors of souls must therefore be patient and kind. However, they may not set God's commandments at naught nor diminish men's obligations more than is right. "It is a great charity to souls to refuse to minimize any of the saving teaching of Christ, but this attitude must always go hand in hand with tolerance and charity. The Redeemer himself gave an example of it when talking to people and when dealing with them. He came not to judge but to save the world. He was unsparing in his condemnation of sin, but was patient and merciful towards sinners."

11. As has already been said, the purpose of this Declaration is to put the faithful on their guard against certain current errors and patterns of behavior. The virtue of chastity, however, does not at all consist solely in avoiding these faults. It demands something more as well: achievement of higher goals. It is a virtue which affects the whole person, both inwardly and in external behavior.

People should cultivate this virtue in a way that is suited to their state of life. Some profess virginity or consecrated celibacy which enables them to give themselves to God alone with undivided heart in a remarkable manner. Others live in the way prescribed for all by the moral law, whether they are married or single. However, in every state of life, chastity is not confined to an external bodily quality. It must purify the heart, as Christ said: "You have learned that they were told, 'Do not commit adultery.' But what I tell you is this: If a man looks on a woman with a lustful eye, he has already committed adultery with her in his heart."

Chastity is part of that continence which St. Paul numbers among the gifts of the Holy Spirit. Impurity, however, he condemns as a vice particularly unworthy of a Christian and as one which merits exclusion from the Kingdom. "This is the will of God, that you should be holy: you must abstain from fornication; each one of you must learn to gain mastery over his body, to hallow and honor it, not giving way to lust like the pagans who are ignorant of God; and no man must do his brother wrong in this matter . . . . For God called us to holiness, not to impurity. Anyone therefore who flouts these rules is flouting, not man, but God who bestows upon you his Holy Spirit." "Fornication and indecency of any kind, or ruthless greed, must not be as much as mentioned among you, as befits the people of God. No coarse, stupid, or flippant talk; these things are out of place; you should rather be thanking God. For be very sure of this: no one given to fornication or indecency, or the greed which makes an idol of gain, has any share in the Kingdom of Christ and of God. Do not let anyone deceive you with shallow arguments; it is for all these things that God's dreadful judgment is coming upon his rebel subjects. Have no part or

392   lot with them. For though you were once all darkness, now as Christians you are light. Live like men who are at home in daylight, for where light is, there all goodness springs up, all justice and truth."

Further, St. Paul indicates a specifically Christian motive for practicing chastity. He condemns the sin of fornication, but not merely because the action injures a person's neighbors or the social order. He condemns it because the fornicator offends Christ, by whose blood he was saved and whose member he is, and he offends the Holy Spirit, whose temple he is: "Do you know that your bodies are limbs and organs of Christ? .... Every other sin that a man can commit is outside his own body; but the fornicator sins against his own body. Do you know that your body is a shrine of the indwelling Holy Spirit, and the Spirit is God's gift to you? You do not belong to yourselves, you were bought at a price. Then honor God in your body."

The more the faithful appreciate the importance of chastity and its necessary role in their lives, the more clearly will they perceive, by a kind of spiritual instinct, its directives and counsels. It will also be easier for them, in obedience to the Magisterium of the Church, to accept and comply with the dictates of a right conscience in individual instances.

12. The apostle Paul has a vivid description of the bitter interior struggle, experienced by a man enslaved to sin, between "the law that . . . (his) reason approves" and another law, which is in his "bodily members' and which holds him captive. Man, however, can be liberated from "this body doomed to death" through the grace of Jesus Christ. This grace is given to men. They are justified through it and in Christ Jesus the life-giving law of the Spirit has set them free from the law of sin and death. St. Paul therefore implores them: "So sin must no longer reign in your mortal body, exacting obedience to the body's desires."

However, while it is true that this liberation fits us for the service of God in a new life, it does not remove the concupiscence which comes from original sin, nor does it remove the inducements to evil provided by this world which lies wholly "in the power of the evil one." Thus St. Paul encourages the faithful to overcome temptations by the power of God, to "stand firm against the devices of the devil," by faith, watchful prayer, and austerity of life, by which the body is brought into subjection to the Spirit.

The Christian life, which consists in following in the footsteps of Christ, requires of every one that "he must leave self behind; day after day must take up his cross," sustained by the hope of reward, for "if we died with him, we shall live with him; if we endure, we shall reign with him."

Granted the forcefulness of these admonitions, Christians of today—indeed, today more than ever before—should use the means which the Church has always recommended for living a chaste life. They are: discipline of the senses and of the mind, vigilance and prudence in avoiding occasions of sin, modesty, moderation in amusements, wholesome pursuits, constant prayer, frequent recourse to the Sacraments of Penance and the Eucharist. Young people especially should diligently develop devotion to the Immaculate Mother of God and should take as models the lives of the saints and of other Christians, especially young Christians, who excelled in the practice of chastity.

It is particularly important that everyone should hold the virtue of chastity **393** in high esteem, its beauty and its radiant splendor. This virtue emphasizes man's dignity and opens man to a love which is true, magnanimous, unselfish, and respectful of others.

DOCUMENT 3 / Sexuality

Source: Congregation for Catholic Education, "Educational Guidance in Human Love" (Nov. 1, 1983), *Origins,* 13: no. 27, Dec. 15, 1983, pp. 451–53.

Significance of Sexuality

4. Sexuality is a fundamental component of personality, one of its modes of being, of manifestation, of communicating with others, of feeling, of expressing, and of living human love. Therefore it is an integral part of the development of the personality and of its educative process: "It is, in fact, from sex that the human person receives the characteristics which, on the biological, psychological, and spiritual levels, make that person a man or a woman, and thereby largely condition his or her progress toward maturity and insertion into society."

5. Sexuality characterizes man and woman not only on the physical level, but also on the psychological and spiritual, making its mark on each of their expressions. Such diversity, linked to the complementarity of the two sexes, allows thorough response to the design of God according to the vocation to which each one is called.

Sexual intercourse, ordained toward procreation, is the maximum expression on the physical level of the communion of love of the married. Divorced from this context of reciprocal gift—a reality which the Christian enjoys, sustained and enriched in a particular way by the grace of God—it loses its significance, exposes the selfishness of the individual, and is a moral disorder.

6. Sexuality oriented, elevated, and integrated by love acquires truly human quality. Prepared by biological and psychological development, it grows harmoniously and is achieved in the full sense only with the realization of affective maturity, which manifests itself in unselfish love and in the total gift of self.

The Actual Situation

7. One can see—among Christians too—that there are notable differences with regard to sex education. In today's climate of moral disorientation a danger arises, whether of a harmful conformism or prejudice which falsifies the intimate nature of being human, ushered whole from the hands of the Creator. . . .

13. Also praiseworthy are the efforts of many who, with scientific seriousness, dedicate themselves to study the problem, moving from the human sciences and integrating the results of such research in a project which conforms with human dignity, a project by the light of the Gospel.

I. SOME FUNDAMENTAL PRINCIPLES
Christian Concept of Sexuality

22. In the Christian vision of man and woman, a particular function of the body is recognized, because it contributes to the revealing of the meaning

of life and of the human vocation. Corporeality is, in fact, a specific mode of existing and operating proper to the human spirit. This significance is first of all of an anthropological nature: the body reveals man, "expresses the person," and is therefore the first message of God to the same man and woman, almost a species of "primordial sacrament, understood as a sign which efficaciously transmits in the visible world the invisible mystery hidden in God from all eternity."

23. There is a second significance of a theological nature: the body contributes to revealing God and his creative love, inasmuch as it manifests the creatureliness of man and woman, whose dependence bestows a fundamental gift, which is the gift of love. "This is the body: a witness to creation as a fundamental gift and so a witness to love as the source from which this same giving springs. . . . "

25. The sexual distinction, which appears as a determination of human being, is diversity, but in equality of nature and dignity.

The human person, through his or her intimate nature, exists in relation to others, implying a reciprocity of love. The sexes are complementary: similar and dissimilar at the same time; not identical, the same, though, in dignity of person; they are peers so that they may mutually understand each other, diverse in their reciprocal completion.

26. Man and woman constitute two modes of realizing, on the part of the human creature, a determined participation in the divine being: they are created in the "image and likeness of God" and they fully accomplish such vocation not only as single persons, but also as couples, which are communities of love. Oriented to unity and fecundity, the married man and woman participate in the creative love of God, living in communion with him through the other. . . .

28. Since men and women in their time have been inclined to reduce sexuality to genital experience alone, there have been reactions tending to devalue sex, as though by its nature men and women were defiled by it. These present guidelines intend to oppose such devaluation. . . .

30. In the light of the mystery of Christ, sexuality appears to us as a vocation to realize that love which the Holy Spirit instills in the hearts of the redeemed. Jesus Christ has enriched such vocation with the Sacrament of Marriage.

31. Furthermore, Jesus has pointed out by word and example the vocation to virginity for the sake of the Kingdom of Heaven. Virginity is a vocation to love: it renders the heart more free to love God. Free of the duties of conjugal love, the virgin heart can feel, therefore, more disposed to the gratuitous love of one's brothers and sisters.

In consequence, virginity for the sake of the Kingdom of Heaven better expresses the gift of Christ to the Father on behalf of us and prefigures with greater precision the reality of eternal life, all substantiated in charity.

Virginity certainly is a renunciation of the form of love which typifies marriage, but committed to undertaking in greater profundity the dynamism, inherent in sexuality, of self-giving openness to others. It seeks to obtain its

396 strengthening and transfiguring by the presence of the Spirit, who teaches us to love the Father and the brethren, after the example of the Lord Jesus.

32. In synthesis, sexuality is called to express different values to which specific moral exigencies correspond. Oriented toward interpersonal dialogue, it contributes to the integral maturation of people, opening them to the gift of self in love; furthermore, tied to the order of creation, to fecundity, and to the transmission of life, it is called to be faithful to this inner purpose also. Love and fecundity are meanings and values of sexuality which include and summon each other in turn and cannot therefore be considered as either alternative or opposites.

33. The affective life, proper to each sex, expresses itself in a characteristic mode in the different states of life: conjugal union, consecrated celibacy chosen for the sake of the Kingdom, the condition of the Christian who has not yet reached marriage or who remains celibate or who has chosen to remain such. In all these cases the affective life must be gathered and integrated in the human person. . . .

Nature, Purpose, and Means of Sex Education

34. A fundamental objective of this education is an adequate knowledge of the nature and importance of sexuality and of the harmonious and integral development of the person toward psychological maturity, with full spiritual maturity in view, to which all believers are called.

To this end, the Christian educator will remember the principles of faith and the different methods of educational aid, taking account of the positive evaluation which actual pedagogy makes of sexuality.

35. In the Christian anthropological perspective, affective sex education must consider the totality of the person and insist therefore on the integration of the biological, psycho-affective, social, and spiritual elements. This integration has become more difficult because the believer also bears the consequences of sin from the beginning.

A true "formation" is not limited to the informing of the intellect, but must pay particular attention to the will, to feelings, and emotions. In fact, in order to move to maturation in affective-sexual life, self-control is necessary, which presupposes such virtues as modesty, temperance, respect for self and for others, openness to one's neighbor.

All this is not possible if not in the power of the salvation which comes from Jesus Christ. . . .

57: Sterilization

DOCUMENT 1:

SOURCE: Pope Pius XII, "Fundamental Laws Governing Conjugal Relations" (Oct. 29, 1951), *The Human Body: Papal Teachings*, pp. 161–62.

THE CONJUGAL ACT

It would be more than a mere want of readiness in the service of life if the attempt made by man were to concern not only an individual act but should affect the entire organism itself, with the intention of depriving it, by means of sterilization, of the faculty of procreating a new life. Here, too, you have a clearly established rule in the Church's teaching which governs your behavior both internally and externally. Direct sterilization—that is, the sterilization which aims, either as a means or as an end in itself, to render childbearing impossible—is a grave violation of the moral law, and therefore unlawful. Even public authority has no right, whatever "indication" it may use as an excuse, to permit it, and much less to prescribe it or to use it to the detriment of innocent human beings. This principle has already been enunciated in the above-mentioned Encyclical of Pius XI on marriage [*Casti Connubii*, Dec. 31, 1930]. So, therefore, ten years ago, when sterilization came to be more widely used, the Holy See was obliged to make an explicit and solemn declaration that direct sterilization, whether permanent or temporary, of the man or of the woman, is unlawful, and this by virtue of the natural law from which the Church herself, as you well know, has no power to dispense.

DOCUMENT 2 / Sterilization

Source: Congregation for the Doctrine of the Faith, "Sterilization in Catholic Hospitals" (Mar. 13, 1975), *Vatican Council II,* Vol. 2, 1982, pp. 454–55.

This sacred congregation has carefully examined the problem of therapeutic preventive sterilization and the various opinions put forward on how to solve it. It has also examined the problems posed by requests for collaboration in such sterilizations in Catholic hospitals. It offers the following replies to the questions asked of it:

1. Any sterilization whose sole, immediate effect, of itself, that is, of its own nature and condition, is to render the generative faculty incapable of procreation is to be regarded as direct sterilization, as this is understood in statements of the pontifical Magisterium, especially of Pius XII. It is absolutely forbidden, therefore, according to the teaching of the Church, even when it is motivated by a subjectively right intention of curing or preventing a physical or psychological ill-effect which is foreseen or feared as a result of pregnancy. The sterilization of the faculty itself is even more strongly prohibited than is the sterilization of individual acts, since it is nearly always irreversible. Nor can any public authority justify the imposition of sterilization as being necessary for the common good, since it damages the dignity and inviolability of the human person. Neither can one invoke the principle of totality in this case, the principle which would justify interference with organs for the greater good of the person. Sterility induced as such does not contribute to the person's integral good, properly understood, keeping things and values in proper perspective." Rather does it damage a person's ethical good, since it deprives subsequent freely chosen sexual acts of an essential element. Hence article 20 of the ethical code published by the conference held in 1971 faithfully reflects the correct teaching and its observance should be urged.

2. The congregation reaffirms this traditional Catholic teaching. It is aware that many theologians dissent from it, but it denies that this fact as such has any doctrinal significance, as though it were a theological source which the faithful might invoke, forsaking the authentic Magisterium for the private opinions of theologians who dissent from it.

3. With regard to the administration of Catholic hospitals:

   a. The following is absolutely forbidden: cooperation, officially approved or admitted, in actions which of themselves (that is of their own nature and condition) have a contraceptive purpose, the impeding of the natural effects of the deliberate sexual acts of the person sterilized. For the official approval of direct sterilization and, all the more so, its administration and execution according to hospital regulations is something of its nature—that is, intrinsically—objectively evil. Nothing can justify a Catholic hospital cooperating in it. Any such cooperation would accord ill with the mission confided to such an institution and would be contrary to the essential proclamation and defense of the moral order.

b. The traditional teaching on material cooperation, with its appropriate distinctions between necessary and freely given cooperation, proximate and remote cooperation, remains valid, to be applied very prudently when the case demands it.

c. When applying the principle of material cooperation, as the case warrants it, scandal and the danger of creating misunderstanding must be carefully avoided with the help of suitable explanation of what is going on.

This sacred congregation hopes that the criteria outlined in this document will meet the expectations of this episcopate, so that having removed the doubts of the faithful they may more easily perform their pastoral duty.

DOCUMENT 3 / Sterilization

SOURCE: National Conference of Catholic Bishops, "Commentary on: Reply of the Sacred Congregation for the Doctrine of the Faith on Sterilization in Catholic Hospitals" (Sept. 15, 1977), United States Catholic Conference, Washington, DC, 1978, pp. 6–8.

GUIDELINES FOR HOSPITAL POLICY

. . . Without repeating all the elements expressed in the Congregation's statement, we present the following guidelines for Catholic health facilities:

1. As it was stated in the Roman document, the Catholic hospital can in no way approve the performance of any sterilization procedure that is directly contraceptive. Such contraceptive procedures include sterilizations performed as a means of preventing future pregnancy that one fears might aggravate a serious cardiac, renal, circulatory, or other disorder. Freely approving direct sterilization constitutes formal cooperation in evil and would be "totally unbecoming the mission" of the hospital as well as "contrary to the necessary proclamation and defense of the moral order."

2. The Catholic health facility has the moral responsibility (and this is legally recognized) to decide what medical procedures it will provide services for. Ordinarily, then, there will be no need or reason to provide services for objectively immoral procedures. Material cooperation will be justified only in situations where the hospital because of some kind of duress or pressure cannot reasonably exercise the autonomy it has (i.e., when it will do more harm than good).

3. Because of the extraordinary nature of the decision concerning material cooperation, i.e., the exception to the ethical religious directives and the potential scandal, the bishop of the diocese or his representative must be involved in the decision.

4. In judging the morality of cooperation a clear distinction should be made between the reason for the sterilization and the reason for the cooperation. If the hospital cooperates because of the reason for the sterilization, e.g., because it is done for medical reasons, the cooperation can hardly be considered material. In other words the hospital can hardly maintain under these circumstances that it does not approve sterilizations done for medical reasons, and this would make cooperation formal. If the cooperation is to remain material, the reason for the cooperation must be something over and above the reason for the sterilization itself. Since, as mentioned above (¶2), the hospital has authority over its own decisions, this should not happen with any frequency.

5. In making judgments about the morality of cooperation each case must be decided on its own merits. Since hospital situations, and even individual cases, differ so much, it would not be prudent to apply automatically a decision made in one hospital, or even in one case, to another.

6. As was stated in the Roman document, the Catholic health facility must   **401**
take every precaution to avoid creating misunderstanding or causing scandal
to its staff, patients, or general public by offering a proper explanation when
necessary. It should be made clear that the hospital disapproves of direct sterilization and that material cooperation in no way implies approval.

Direct sterilization is a grave evil. The allowance of material cooperation
in extraordinary cases is based on the danger of an even more serious evil,
e.g., the closing of the hospital could be under certain circumstances a more
serious evil.

This is a commentary on the response of the Sacred Congregation for the
Doctrine of the Faith regarding the use of material cooperation on the part of
Catholic health care facilities in cases of sterilization. It is not meant to be a
general discussion of the application of material cooperation as such, and,
therefore, should not be extended to other areas. . . .

DOCUMENT 4 / Sterilization

SOURCE: National Conference of Catholic Bishops, "Statement on Tubal Ligation" (July 9, 1980), *Origins* 10: no. 11, Aug. 28, 1980, p. 175.

Since we note among Catholic health care facilities a certain confusion in the understanding and application of authentic Catholic teaching with regard to the morality of tubal ligation as a means of contraceptive sterilization (cf. nos. 18 and 20, Ethical and Religious Directives for Catholic Health Facilities), the National Conference of Catholic Bishops [NCCB] makes the following clarification:

1) The traditional teaching of the Church as reaffirmed by the Sacred Congregation for the Doctrine of the Faith [SCDF] March 13, 1975, clearly declares the objective immorality of contraceptive (direct) sterilization even if done for medical reasons.

2) The principle of totality does not apply to contraceptive sterilization and cannot be used to justify it.

3) Formal cooperation in the grave evil of contraceptive sterilization, either by approving or tolerating it for medical reasons, is forbidden and totally alien to the mission entrusted by the Church to Catholic health care facilities.

4) The reason for justifying material cooperation as described in the NCCB Commentary on the SCDF response refers not to medical reasons given for the sterilization but to grave reasons extrinsic to the case. Catholic health care facilities in the United States complying with the Ethical and Religious Directives are protected by the First Amendment from pressures intended to require material cooperation in contraceptive sterilization. In the unlikely and extraordinary situation in which the principle of material cooperation seems to be justified, consultation with the bishop or his delegate is required.

5) The local ordinary has responsibility for ensuring that the moral teachings of the Church be taught and followed in health care facilities which are to be recognized as Catholic. In this important matter there should be increased and continuing collaboration between the bishops, health care facilities, and their sponsoring religious communities. Local conditions will suggest the practical structures necessary to insure this collaboration.

6) The NCCB profoundly thanks the many physicians, administrators, and personnel of Catholic health care facilities who faithfully maintain the teaching and practice of the Church with regard to Catholic moral principles.

DOCUMENT 5 / Sterilization

SOURCE: Congregation for the Doctrine of the Faith, "Response on Uterine Isolation and Related Matters," *Origins* 24: no. 12 (Sept. 1, 1994), pp. 211–12.

The cardinal members of the Congregation for the Doctrine of the Faith in answer to the questions examined in ordinary session decreed the following replies:

Q.1. When the uterus becomes so seriously injured (e.g. during a delivery or a Caesarean section) so as to render medically indicated even its total removal (hysterectomy) in order to counter an immediate serious threat to the life or health of the mother, is it licit to perform such a procedure notwithstanding the permanent sterility which will result for the woman?

R. Affirmative.

Q.2. When the uterus (e.g. as a result of previous Caesarean sections) is in a state such that while not constituting in itself a present risk to the life or health of the woman, nevertheless is foreseeably incapable of carrying a future pregnancy to term without danger to the mother, danger which in some cases could be serious, is it licit to remove the uterus (hysterectomy) in order to prevent a possible future danger deriving from conception?

R. Negative.

Q.3. In the same situation as in No. 2, is it licit to substitute tubal ligation, also called uterine isolation, for the hysterectomy since the same end would be attained of averting the risks of a possible pregnancy by means of a procedure which is much simpler for the doctor and less serious for the woman and since, in addition, in some cases, the ensuing sterility might be reversible?

R. Negative.

Explanation

In the first case, the hysterectomy is licit because it has a directly therapeutic character, even though it may be foreseen that permanent sterility will result. In fact, it is the pathological condition of the uterus (e.g. a hemorrhage which cannot be stopped by other means), which makes its removal medically indicated. The removal of the organ has as its aim, therefore, the curtailing of a serious present danger to the woman independent of a possible future pregnancy.

From the moral point of view, the cases of hysterectomy and "uterine isolation" in the circumstances described in Nos. 2 and 3 are different. These fall into the moral category of direct sterilization which in the Congregation for the Doctrine of the Faith's document *Quaecumque Sterilizatio* (*Acta Apostolicae Sedis* LXVIII (1976), pp. 738–40, no. 1) is defined as an action "whose sole, immediate effect is to render the generative faculty incapable of procreation." And the same document continues: "It [direct sterilization] is absolutely

404 forbidden . . . according to the teaching of the Church, even when it is motivated by a subjectively right intention of curing or preventing a physical or psychological ill effect which is foreseen or feared as a result of pregnancy."

In point of fact, the uterus as described in No. 2 does not constitute in and of itself any present danger to the woman. Indeed the proposal to substitute "uterine isolation" for hysterectomy under the same conditions shows precisely that the uterus in and of itself does not pose a pathological problem for the woman. Therefore, the described procedures do not have a properly therapeutic character but are aimed in themselves at rendering sterile future sexual acts freely chosen. The end of avoiding risks to the mother, deriving from a possible pregnancy, is thus pursued by means of a direct sterilization, in itself always morally illicit, while other ways which are morally licit remain open to free choice.

The contrary opinion, which considers the interventions described in Nos. 2 and 3 as indirect sterilizations, licit under certain conditions, cannot be regarded as valid and may not be followed in Catholic hospitals.

During an audience granted to the undersigned prefect, the sovereign pontiff John Paul II approved these responses adopted in an ordinary session of the Congregation for the Doctrine of the Faith and ordered them to be published.

58: Suffering

DOCUMENT 1:

SOURCE: Pope John Paul II, "The Christian Meaning of Human Suffering" (Feb. 11, 1984), *Origins* 13: no. 37, Feb. 23, 1984, pp. 609, 611–12, 618–19.

I. INTRODUCTION

1. Declaring the power of salvific suffering, the apostle Paul says: "In my flesh I complete what is lacking in Christ's afflictions for the sake of his body, that is, the church. . . . "

4. . . . About the theme of suffering these two reasons seem to draw particularly close to each other and to become one. The need of the heart commands us to overcome fear, and the imperative of faith—formulated, for example, in the words of St. Paul quoted at the beginning—provides the content, in the name of which and by virtue of which we dare to touch what appears in every man so intangible; for man, in his suffering, remains an intangible mystery.

II. THE WORLD OF HUMAN SUFFERING

5. Even though in its subjective dimension, as a personal fact contained within man's concrete and unrepeatable interior, suffering seems almost inexpressible and not transferable, perhaps at the same time nothing else requires as much as does suffering, in its "objective reality," to be dealt with, meditated upon, and conceived as an explicit problem; and that therefore basic questions be asked about it and the answers sought. It is evident that it is not a question here merely of giving a description of suffering. There are other criteria which go beyond the sphere of description and which we must introduce when we wish to penetrate the world of human suffering.

Medicine, as the science and also the art of healing, discovers in the vast field of human suffering the best known area, the one identified with greater precision and relatively more counterbalanced by the methods of "reaction" (that is, the methods of therapy). Nonetheless, this is only one area. The field of human suffering is much wider, more varied, and multidimensional. Man suffers in different ways, ways not always considered by medicine, not even in its most advanced specializations. Suffering is something which is still wider than sickness, more complex, and at the same time still more deeply rooted in humanity itself. A certain idea of this problem comes to us from the distinction between physical suffering and moral suffering. This distinction is based upon the double dimension of the human being and indicates the bodily and spiritual element as the immediate or direct subject of suffering. Insofar as the words   **405**

406 "suffering" and "pain" can, up to a certain degree, be used as synonyms, physical suffering is present when "the body is hurting" in some way, whereas moral suffering is "pain of the soul." In fact, it is a question of pain of a spiritual nature and not only of the "psychological" dimension of pain which accompanies both moral and physical suffering. The vastness and the many forms of moral suffering are certainly no less in number than the forms of physical suffering. But at the same time, moral suffering seems as it were less identified and less reachable by therapy.

7. . . . It can be said that man suffers whenever he experiences any kind of evil. In the vocabulary of the Old Testament, suffering and evil are identified with each other. In fact, that vocabulary did not have a specific word to indicate "suffering." Thus it defined as "evil" everything that was suffering. Only the Greek language, and together with it the New Testament (and the Greek translation of the Old Testament), use the verb *pascho* ("I am affected by . . . ; I experience a feeling; I suffer"); and, thanks to this verb, suffering is no longer directly identifiable with (objective) evil, but expresses a situation in which man experiences evil and in doing so becomes the subject of suffering. Suffering has indeed both a subjective and a passive character (from *patior*). Even when man brings suffering on himself, when he is its cause, this suffering remains something passive in its metaphysical essence.

This does not, however, mean that suffering in the psychological sense is not marked by a specific "activity." This is in fact that multiple and subjectively differentiated "activity" of pain, sadness, disappointment, discouragement, or even despair, according to the intensity of the suffering subject and his or her specific sensitivity. In the midst of what constitutes the psychological form of suffering there is always an experience of evil, which causes the individual to suffer.

Thus the reality of suffering prompts the question about the essence of evil: What is evil?

This question seems in a certain sense inseparable from the theme of suffering. The Christian response to it is different, for example, from the one given by certain cultural and religious traditions which hold that existence is an evil from which one needs to be liberated. Christianity proclaims the essential good of existence and the good of that which exists, acknowledges the goodness of the Creator, and proclaims the good of creatures. Man suffers on account of evil, which is a certain lack, limitation, or distortion of good. We could say that man suffers because of a good in which he does not share, from which in a certain sense he is cut off or of which he has deprived himself. He particularly suffers when he "ought"—in the normal order of things—to have a share in this good and does not have it.

Thus, in the Christian view, the reality of suffering is explained through evil, which always in some way refers to a good.

8. In itself human suffering constitutes as it were a specific "world" which exists together with man, which appears in him and passes, and sometimes does not pass, but which consolidates itself and becomes deeply rooted in him.

This world of suffering, divided into many, very many subjects, exists as it were "in dispersion." Every individual, through personal suffering, constitutes not only a small part of that "world," but at the same time that "world" is present in him as a finite and unrepeatable entity. Parallel with this, however, is the interhuman and social dimension. The world of suffering possesses as it were its own solidarity. People who suffer become similar to one another through the analogy of their situation, the trial of their destiny, or through their need for understanding and care, and perhaps above all through the persistent question of the meaning of suffering. Thus, although the world of suffering exists "in dispersion," at the same time it contains within itself a singular challenge to communion and solidarity. We shall also try to follow this appeal in the present reflection.

Considering the world of suffering in its personal and at the same time collective meaning, one cannot fail to notice the fact that this world, at some periods of time and in some eras of human existence, as it were becomes particularly concentrated. This happens, for example, in cases of natural disasters, epidemics, catastrophes, upheavals, and various social scourges. One thinks, for example, of a bad harvest and connected with it—or with various other causes—the scourge of famine. . . .

V. SHARERS IN THE SUFFERING OF CHRIST

19. . . . One can say that with the passion of Christ all human suffering has found itself in a new situation. And it is as though Job had foreseen this when he said: "I know that my Redeemer lives," and as though he had directed toward it his own suffering, which without the redemption could not have revealed to him the fullness of its meaning. In the cross of Christ not only is the redemption accomplished through suffering, but also human suffering itself has been redeemed. Christ—without any fault of his own—took on himself "the total evil of sin." The experience of this evil determined the incomparable extent of Christ's suffering, which became the price of the redemption. The song of the suffering servant in Isaiah speaks of this. In later times the witnesses of the New Covenant, sealed in the blood of Christ, will speak of this. These are the words of the apostle Peter in his first letter: "You know that you were ransomed from the futile ways inherited from your fathers, not with perishable things such as silver or gold, but with the precious blood of Christ, like that of a lamb without blemish or spot." And the apostle Paul in the Letter to the Galatians will say: "He gave himself for our sins to deliver us from the present evil age," and in the First Letter to the Corinthians: "You were bought with a price. So glorify God in your body."

With these and similar words the witnesses of the New Covenant speak of the greatness of the redemption accomplished through the suffering of Christ. The Redeemer suffered in place of man and for man. Every man has his own share in the redemption. Each one is also called to share in that suffering through which the redemption was accomplished. He is called to share in that suffering through which all human suffering has also been redeemed. In

408 bringing about the redemption through suffering, Christ has also raised human suffering to the level of the redemption. Thus each man in his suffering can also become a sharer in the redemptive suffering of Christ.

23. . . . Suffering, in fact, is always a trial—at times a very hard one—to which humanity is subjected. The Gospel paradox of weakness and strength often speaks to us from the pages of the letters of St. Paul, a paradox particularly experienced by the apostle himself and together with him experienced by all who share Christ's sufferings. Paul writes in the second letter to the Corinthians: "I will all the more gladly boast of my weaknesses, that the power of Christ may rest upon me." In the second letter to Timothy we read: "And therefore I suffer as I do. But I am not ashamed, for I know whom I have believed." And in the letter to the Philippians he will even say: "I can do all things in him who strengthens me."

Those who share in Christ's sufferings have before their eyes the paschal mystery of the cross and resurrection, in which Christ descends, in a first phase, to the ultimate limits of human weakness and impotence. Indeed, he dies nailed to the cross. But if at the same time in this weakness there is accomplished his lifting up, confirmed by the power of the resurrection, then this means that the weaknesses of all human sufferings are capable of being infused with the same power of God manifested in Christ's cross. In such a concept, to suffer means to become particularly susceptible, particularly open, to the working of the salvific powers of God offered to humanity in Christ. In him, God has confirmed his desire to act especially through suffering, which is man's weakness and emptying of self, and he wishes to make his power known precisely in this weakness and emptying of self. . . .

DOCUMENT 2/ Suffering

SOURCE: John Paul II, "The Gospel of Life" (Mar. 25, 1995), *Origins* 24: no. 42, Apr. 6, 1995, pp. 701, 722.

31. ... More than anything else, it is the problem of suffering which challenges faith and puts it to the test. How can we fail to appreciate the universal anguish of man when we meditate on the Book of Job? The innocent man overwhelmed by suffering is understandably led to wonder: "Why is light given to him that is in misery, and life to the bitter in soul, who long for death, but it comes not, and dig for it more than for death, but it comes not, and dig for it more than for hid treasures?" (3:20–21). But even when the darkness is deepest, faith points to a trusting and adoring acknowledgment of the "mystery": "I know that you can do all things, and that no purpose of yours can be thwarted" (Jb 42:2).

32. ... The words and deeds of Jesus and those of his Church are not meant only for those who are sick or suffering or in some way neglected by society. On a deeper level they affect the very meaning of every person's life in its moral and spiritual dimensions. Only those who recognize that their life is marked by the evil of sin can discover in an encounter with Jesus the Savior the truth and the authenticity of their own existence. Jesus himself says as much: "those who are well have not need of a physician, but those who are sick; I have not come to call the righteous, but sinners to repentance" (Lk 12:20).

97. The work of education cannot avoid a consideration of suffering and death. These are a part of human existence, and it is futile, not to say misleading, to try to hide them or ignore them. On the contrary, people must be helped to understand their profound mystery in all its harsh reality. Even pain and suffering have meaning and value when they are experienced in close connection with love received and given. In this regard, I have called for the yearly celebration of the World Day of the Sick, emphasizing "the salvific nature of the offering up of suffering which, experienced in communion with Christ, belongs to the very essence of the redemption." Death itself is anything but an event without hope. It is the door which opens wide on eternity and, for those who live in Christ, an experience of participation in the mystery of his death and resurrection.

DOCUMENT 3 / Suffering

SOURCE: Pope Pius XII, "Christian Principles and the Medical Profession" (Nov. 12, 1944), *The Human Body: Papal Teachings*, pp. 56–58.

SUFFERING AND DEATH

The truths so far expounded can be known by the light of the reason alone. But there is another fundamental law which appears more to the eyes of the doctor than to others, whose complete meaning and purpose can be revealed and illustrated only by the light of revelation. We are thinking of the law of suffering and death.

Physical pain has no doubt a natural and salutary function as well: it is a danger signal which gives warning that some hidden sickness has been born and is developing, perhaps secretly; and thus it induces one to seek the remedy. But in the course of his scientific research, the doctor inevitably comes upon suffering and death like a locked door to which his mind does not hold the key. In the exercise of his profession, they loom inexorably and mysteriously, a law in the face of which his art often stands helpless and his compassion sterile. He can make his diagnosis according to the principles of the laboratory and clinic, plan the treatment in accordance with all the demands of science . . . , but in the depths of his being, as man and scientist, he feels that the explanation of that mystery continues to elude him. He suffers; a consuming anguish grips him until he asks of faith the answer which though now incomplete—it is complete in the mysterious designs of God and will be revealed as such in eternity—has yet the power of bringing him peace of soul.

And this is the answer faith gives. God, when he created man, had by a gift of grace made him exempt from that natural law which governs every living material being. God had not wished to include in man's destiny suffering and death. They were introduced by sin. But he, the Father of mercy, took them into his own hands, made them pass through the body, the veins, the heart of his beloved Son, God like himself, become man for the salvation of the world. And thus suffering and death became for every man who accepts Christ, a means of redemption and sanctification. And thus man's pilgrimage here below, continually shadowed by the sign of the cross and the law of suffering and death, develops and purifies the soul and leads it to happiness without end in eternal life.

To suffer . . . to die . . . . It is truly, to use the bold phrase of the Apostle of the Gentiles, the "folly of God"—a folly which is wiser than all the wisdom of men. (a) In the pale radiance of his weak faith, the poor poet sang: *L'homme est un apprenti, la douleur est son maître, Et nul ne se connait tant qu'il n'a pas souffert.* [Man is an apprentice, sadness is his master, and not one knows so much if he has not suffered.] (b) In the light of revelation, the holy author of the Imitation of Christ could pen the sublime twelfth chapter of his second book,

De regia via sanctae crucis, all aglow with the most wonderful understanding of   **411**
the noblest Christian conception of life.

In the face of the insistent problem of pain, what reply can the doctor
give? for his own satisfaction first? and to the unhappy person whom sickness
has reduced to a blind torpor, and in whom rises a vain sense of rebellion
against suffering and death? Only a heart impregnated with a deep and living
faith will find the words which carry the sincerity and deep conviction capable
of rendering acceptable the words of the divine Master: "It is necessary to
suffer and to die, and so enter into glory." The doctor will fight against sickness
and death with all the means and methods of his science and art, but not
with the desperate resignation of pessimism, nor yet with the "exasperated
resolution" which a certain modern philosophy has seen fit to exalt, but with
the calm peace of one who sees and knows what suffering and death mean in
the salvific designs of the omniscient and infinitely good and merciful Lord.

DOCUMENT 4 / Suffering

SOURCE: Congregation for the Doctrine of the Faith, "Declaration on Euthanasia" (May 5, 1980), *Vatican Council II*, Vol. 2, pp. 513–15.

THE MEANING OF SUFFERING FOR CHRISTIANS AND THE USE OF PAINKILLERS

Death does not always come in dramatic circumstances after barely tolerable sufferings. Nor do we have to think only of extreme cases. Numerous testimonies which confirm one another lead one to the conclusion that nature itself has made provision to render more bearable at the moment of death separations that would be terribly painful to a person in full health. Hence it is that a prolonged illness, advanced old age, or a state of loneliness or neglect can bring about psychological conditions that facilitate the acceptance of death.

Nevertheless the fact remains that death, often preceded or accompanied by severe and prolonged suffering, is something which naturally causes people anguish.

Physical suffering is certainly an unavoidable element of the human condition; on the biological level, it constitutes a warning of which no one denies the usefulness; but, since it affects the human psychological makeup, it often exceeds its own biological usefulness and so can become so severe as to cause the desire to remove it at any cost.

According to Christian teaching, however, suffering, especially suffering during the last moments of life, has a special place in God's saving plan; it is in fact a sharing in Christ's passion and a union with the redeeming sacrifice which he offered in obedience to the Father's will. Therefore one must not be surprised if some Christians prefer to moderate their use of painkillers, in order to accept voluntarily at least a part of their sufferings and thus associate themselves in a conscious way with the sufferings of Christ crucified (cf. Mt 27:34). Nevertheless it would be imprudent to impose a heroic way of acting as a general rule. On the contrary, human and Christian prudence suggest for the majority of sick people the use of medicines capable of alleviating or suppressing pain, even though these may cause as a secondary effect semiconsciousness and reduced lucidity. As for those who are not in a state to express themselves, one can reasonably presume that they wish to take these painkillers, and have them administered according to the doctor's advice.

59: Suicide

DOCUMENT 1:

Source: Pope John Paul II, "The Gospel of Life" (Mar. 25, 1995), *Origins* 24: no. 42, Apr. 6, 1995, p. 712.

66. Suicide is always as morally objectionable as murder. The Church's tradition has always rejected it as a gravely evil choice. Even though a certain psychological, cultural, and social conditioning may induce a person to carry out an action which so radically contradicts the innate inclination to life, thus lessening or removing subjective responsibility, suicide, when viewed objectively, is a gravely immoral act. In fact, it involves the rejection of love of self and the renunciation of the obligation of justice and charity toward one's neighbor, toward the communities to which one belongs, and toward society as a whole. In its deepest reality, suicide represents a rejection of God's absolute sovereignty over life and death as proclaimed in the prayer of the ancient sage of Israel: "You have power over life and death; you lead men down to the gates of Hades and back again" (Wis 16:13; cf. Tb 13:2). . . .

60: Surgery

DOCUMENT 1:

SOURCE: Pope Pius XII, "Surgery" (May 20, 1948), *The Human Body: Papal Teachings*, pp. 95–100.

... The decision to operate is a grave decision to make. Have all the resources of medicine been tried to see whether they alone can be efficacious? Is the operation still necessary? What dangers does it present? On the other hand, what would be the risks of its omission? Again, is this the most opportune moment for the operation? Would it be better postponed, or is it rather necessary to hurry and act at once? Which risk is to be taken? that of speeding up the process or that of waiting longer? What is to be the attitude towards the patient's doctor? For each physician has his own opinion, so that, especially in complex cases, there can be discord. Each one them, while defending his own opinion, can understand, too, the motives which prompt the other decisions.

But once the surgeon has well considered everything, including the moral aspect of the act, he should hesitate no longer. Even after this judgment has been conscientiously and duly formed, however, he still has a very delicate duty to carry out. He must explain the usefulness or the necessity of the operation—and the uncertainties, too—to the patient and his family. And he must determine to what extent he will counsel or suggest or insist with them. How can he enlighten them quite sincerely, leaving them at the same time the freedom to decide?

Other cases arise which we could not call embarrassing, for in these one's duty is clear, but cases which are very sad on account of the tragic consequences which can derive from the observance of that duty. These are the cases in which the moral law imposes its veto. If you alone were concerned, it would not perhaps be difficult to ignore the suggestion of a misguided pity, and to make reason prevail over emotion. But often you must react not only against the presumptions of base and wicked passions, but also against the well understandable anguish of conjugal and paternal love.

DOCUMENT 2 / Surgery

SOURCE: Pope Pius XII, "Removal of a Healthy Organ" (Oct. 8, 1953), *The Human Body: Papal Teachings*, pp. 277–79.

The first question you have posed is in the form of a particular case, typical of its kind: a healthy organ is amputated in order to eliminate or arrest the evil effects on another organ, with the sufferings and dangers they bring. And you ask whether this is permissible.

Three conditions govern the moral licitness of a surgical operation which causes anatomic or functional mutilation: first that the continued presence or functioning of a particular organ within the whole organism is causing serious damage or constitutes a menace to it; next, this damage must be remediable or at least can be measurably lessened by the mutilation in question, and the operation's efficacy in this regard should be well assured; finally, one must be reasonably certain that the negative effect, that is, the mutilation and its consequences, will be compensated for by the positive effect: elimination of danger to the whole organism, easing of pain, and so forth.

The decisive point rests not in the fact that the organ which is amputated or paralyzed be itself infected, but that its continued presence or functioning cause either directly or indirectly a serious menace for the whole body. It is quite possible that in functioning normally a healthy organ could cause harm to one which is unhealthy, in such a way as to aggravate the evil and the repercussions of this last on the organism as a whole. Or it can happen that the removal of a healthy organ and the paralyzing of its function remove from the evil—cancer, for example—the possibility of extending further, or else change the effect of this evil on the body. If there is no other alternative available, in both cases a surgical operation on the healthy organ is permissible.

Our conclusion is based on the right which man has received from the Creator over his body. This right is founded on the principle of totality, in virtue of which every particular organ is subordinated to the body as a whole, and, in case of conflict, must cede to the good of the whole. As a result, man, who has received the use of the whole organism, has the right to sacrifice a particular organ if its continued presence or functioning causes notable harm to the whole, a harm which cannot otherwise be avoided.

Since in the case proposed, you assure us that the removal of the seed-producing glands permits the evil to be combated, this removal meets with no objection from the moral point of view.

We would like, however, to draw your attention to an erroneous application of the principle of totality which we have enunciated.

It not rarely happens that, either when gynecological complications demand an operation, or quite independently of such complications, the healthy fallopian tubes are removed or put out of action to prevent any new conception

416 and the grave dangers which could arise therefrom either to the health or life of the mother; these dangers arise from other unhealthy organs—kidneys, heart, lungs—whose condition would be aggravated in case of childbearing. To justify the removal of the oviducts, appeal is made to the principle of totality, and it is asserted that the removal of healthy organs is permitted when the good of the whole organism demands it.

The appeal to this principle here is unjustified, for in this case, the danger which threatens the mother does not derive at all either directly or indirectly from the presence of normal functioning of the oviducts, nor from the influence they exercise over the diseased organs—kidneys, heart, or lungs. The danger comes only when free sexual intercourse causes a conception which can menace the organs mentioned, because these are too weak or diseased. But the conditions which permit a part to be disposed of in favor of the whole, in virtue of the principle of totality, do not exist. Therefore the operation on the healthy oviducts is morally illicit. . . .

61: Surrogate Mothers

DOCUMENT 1:

SOURCE: Congregation for the Doctrine of the Faith, "Instruction on Respect for Human Life in Its Origin and on the Dignity of Procreation" (Feb. 22, 1987), *Origins,* 16: no. 40, Mar. 19, 1987, p. 705.

II. INTERVENTIONS UPON HUMAN PROCREATION
3. Is "Surrogate" Motherhood* Morally Licit?

No, for the same reasons which lead one to reject heterologous artificial fertilization: For it is contrary to the unity of marriage and to the dignity of the procreation of the human person.

---

*By surrogate mother the instruction means:

a) The woman who carries in pregnancy an embryo implanted in her uterus and who is genetically a stranger to the embryo because it has been obtained through the union of the gametes of "donors." She carries the pregnancy with a pledge to surrender the baby once it is born to the party who commissioned or made the agreement for the pregnancy.

b) The woman who carries in pregnancy an embryo to whose procreation she has contributed the donation of her own ovum, fertilized through insemination with the sperm of a man other than her husband. She carries the pregnancy with a pledge to surrender the child once it is born to the party who commissioned or made the agreement for the pregnancy.

Surrogate motherhood represents an objective failure to meet the obligations of maternal love, of conjugal fidelity, and of responsible motherhood; it offends the dignity and the right of the child to be conceived, carried in the womb, brought into the world, and brought up by his own parents; it sets up, to the detriment of families, a division between the physical, psychological, and moral elements which constitute those families.   **417**

DOCUMENT 2 / Surrogate Mothers

Source: New Jersey Catholic Conference, "New Jersey Bishops' Statement 'On Surrogate Motherhood' " (Nov. 28, 1986), *Origins,* 16: no. 30, Jan. 8, 1987, p. 551.

. . . It is the position of the Catholic bishops of New Jersey that the concept of surrogate motherhood is legally wrong because it violates the public policy of this state (by making licit the sale of a child, albeit through the subterfuge of renting the womb of a woman) and is morally wrong because it violates the biological and spiritual unity of the husband and wife and the parental relationship of parents and child.

The concept of surrogate motherhood as a legal wrong is firmly grounded in the public policy of this state for a myriad of reasons but most significantly because it exploits a child as a commodity and exploits a woman as a "baby-maker." In the former situation it promotes injustice and, in the latter, it utterly disregards social responsibility.

Children are a gift of God. As such they can never be treated as chattels or commercial pawns or as commodities to be produced as service rendered in exchange for a service fee. The practice of surrogate motherhood is an affront to the human dignity of a child. This human dignity is not only recognized but is protected by the state under the doctrine of *parens patriae,* a doctrine that is traceable to our heritage at common law. In conformity with this doctrine, the New Jersey adoption laws not only prohibit the payment or the receiving of money or any valuable consideration in exchange for the placement of a child for adoption, but also makes the material assistance of an agent, finder, or intermediary a criminal act. The entire concept of surrogate motherhood reduces the creation of a child, a human being, to the level of a commercial transaction. The womb is leased to produce rather than to love a child into existence. When the natural mother surrenders her child for financial remuneration, she is exploiting the most precious thing she can bring into existence, her own child.

The rights of the child itself are also violated. Every child has a right to true parents. Surrogate mothering confuses the relationship by introducing a second mother. The natural attachment a woman has with the child in whose creation she has participated is denied. The process destroys the parent-child bond and is a grave injustice to the child.

The concept exploits women as a part of a "human machine." The surrogate mother uses her womb for commercial use. When her days are accomplished and her contract labor is finished, she is made to surrender an integral part of her life, her child, and with it to surrender any natural claim or bond to the child. She has allowed herself to be used for financial gain and all that remains is the money—and the broken bond and, perhaps, some broken dreams.

The probability cannot be ignored that this concept may also put undue pressure

upon poor women to use their bodies to support themselves or their families. **419**
It would not be unfair to say that the concept of surrogate motherhood would
not be the subject of discussion today if money was not involved; money for
the mother, money for the clinics that invented the concept, and money for the
legal community which has mapped out the particulars of its operation. . . .

62: Truthtelling

DOCUMENT 1:

SOURCE: Pope Pius XII, "Christian Principles and the Medical Profession" (Nov. 12, 1944), *The Human Body: Papal Teachings*, pp. 62–63.

THE INTANGIBILITY OF HUMAN LIFE

The eighth commandment likewise has its place in the morality of medicine. According to the moral law, no one may tell a lie. And yet there are cases when a doctor, even when asked, though he cannot give an answer which is positively untrue, at the same time cannot crudely tell the whole truth, especially when he knows that the patient has not the strength to stand such a revelation. But there are other cases when the doctor has most certainly the duty of speaking out clearly, a duty before which every other medical or humanitarian consideration must give way. It is not lawful to lull the sick person or his relations into a false sense of security when there is the risk of compromising the eternal salvation of the former, or his fulfillment of his duties in justice and charity. It would be wrong to try to justify or excuse such conduct under the pretext that the physician always says what, in his opinion, will best contribute to the patient's well-being, and that it is the fault of his hearers if they take his words too literally.

DOCUMENT 2 / Truthtelling

SOURCE: Pontifical Council Cor Unum, *Questions of Ethics Regarding the Fatally Ill and the Dying*, Vatican Press, 1981.

6. COMMUNICATING WITH DYING PEOPLE

6.1 The Right to Know the Truth

The communication with dying patients brings up the moral question of their right to know the truth. The clergy, pastorally, and doctors and nurses, professionally, must consider what sort of behavior a dying person has a right to expect from those around him. The dying, and, more generally, anyone with an incurable disease, have a right to be told the truth. Death is too essential an event for the envisioning of it to be avoided. In the case of a believer, its approach requires preparation and specific actions made in full consciousness. In the case of any human being, dying brings the responsibility of fulfilling certain duties towards one's family, of putting order to business affairs, bringing accounts up to date, settling debts, etc. In any case, preparation for dying should begin long before the approach of death and while a person is still in good health.

6.1.2 The Responsibility of Those Surrounding a Dying Person

Whoever is nearest the patient must inform him of the possibility of his dying. The family, the chaplain, and the group providing medical care, must assume their share in this duty. Each case is different, depending on the sensitivities and capabilities of all concerned, and on the condition of the patient and his ability to relate to others. How he will react to the truth—by rebellion, depression, resignation, and so on—is what those surrounding him must try to foresee, in order to be able to behave with tact and calm. A ray of hope may licitly be held out to the patient; death may even be presented as not 100 percent certain—but only provided that doing this does not totally conceal the possibility of dying, the serious probability.

63: Withholding Life Support

DOCUMENT 1:

Source: Pope John Paul II, "The Gospel of Life" (Mar. 25, 1995), *Origins* 24: no. 42, Apr. 6, 1995, p. 712.

65. . . . Euthanasia must be distinguished from the decision to forgo so-called "aggressive medical treatment," in other words, medical procedures which no longer correspond to the real situation of the patient either because they are by now disproportionate to any expected results or because they impose an excessive burden on the patient and his family. In such situations, when death is clearly imminent and inevitable, one can in conscience "refuse forms of treatment that would only secure a precarious and burdensome prolongation of life, so long as the normal obligation to care for oneself and to allow oneself to be cared for, but this duty must take account of concrete circumstances. It needs to be determined whether the means of treatment available are objectively proportionate to the prospects for improvement. To forgo extraordinary or disproportionate means is not the equivalent of suicide or euthanasia; it rather expresses acceptance of the human condition in the face of death. . . .

DOCUMENT 2 / Withholding Life Support

SOURCE: Pope Pius XII, "The Prolongation of Life" (Nov. 24, 1957), *The Pope Speaks* 4: no. 4, 1958, pp. 395–98.

THREE QUESTIONS

The problems that arise in the modern practice of resuscitation can therefore be formulated in three questions:

First, does one have the right, or is one even under the obligation, to use modern artificial respiration equipment in all cases, even those which, in the doctor's judgment, are completely hopeless?

Second, does one have the right, or is one under obligation, to remove the artificial respiration apparatus when, after several days, the state of deep unconsciousness does not improve if, when it is removed, blood circulation will stop within a few minutes? What must be done in this case if the family of the patient, who has already received the last sacraments, urges the doctor to remove the apparatus? Is Extreme Unction still valid at this time?

Third, must a patient plunged into unconsciousness through central paralysis, but whose life—that is to say, blood circulation—is maintained through artificial respiration, and in whom there is no improvement after several days, be considered *de facto* or even *de jure* dead? Must one not wait for blood circulation to stop, in spite of the artificial respiration, before considering him dead?

BASIC PRINCIPLES

We shall willingly answer these three questions. But before examining them we would like to set forth the principles that will allow formulation of the answer.

Natural reason and Christian morals say that man (and whoever is entrusted with the task of taking care of his fellowman) has the right and the duty in case of serious illness to take the necessary treatment for the preservation of life and health. This duty that one has toward himself, toward God, toward the human community, and in most cases toward certain determined persons derives from well ordered charity, from submission to the Creator, from social justice and even from strict justice, as well as from devotion toward one's family.

But normally one is held to use only ordinary means—according to circumstances of persons, places, times, and culture—that is to say, means that do not involve any grave burden for oneself or another. A more strict obligation would be too burdensome for most men and would render the attainment of the higher, more important good too difficult. Life, health, all temporal activities are in fact subordinated to spiritual ends. On the other hand, one is not forbidden to take more than the strictly necessary steps to preserve life and health, as long as he does not fail in some more serious duty. . . .

424 THE FACT OF DEATH

The question of the fact of death and that of verifying the fact itself (*de facto*) or its legal authenticity (*de jure*) have, because of their consequences, even in the field of morals and of religion, an even greater importance. What we have just said about the presupposed essential elements for the valid reception of a sacrament has shown this. But the importance of the question extends also to effects in matters of inheritance, marriage and matrimonial processes, benefices (vacancy of a benefice), and to many other questions of private and social life.

It remains for the doctor, and especially the anesthesiologist, to give a clear and precise definition of "death" and the "moment of death" of a patient who passes away in a state of unconsciousness. Here one can accept the usual concept of complete and final separation of the soul from the body; but in practice one must take into account the lack of precision of the terms "body" and "separation." One can put aside the possibility of a person being buried alive, for removal of the artificial respiration apparatus must necessarily bring about stoppage of blood circulation and therefore death within a few minutes.

In case of insoluble doubt, one can resort to presumptions of law and of fact. In general, it will be necessary to presume that life remains, because there is involved here a fundamental right received from the Creator, and it is necessary to prove with certainty that it has been lost.

We shall now pass to the solution of the particular questions.

A DOCTOR'S RIGHTS AND DUTIES

1. Does the anesthesiologist have the right, or is he bound, in all cases of deep unconsciousness, even in those that are considered to be completely hopeless in the opinion of the competent doctor, to use modern artificial respiration apparatus, even against the will of the family?

In ordinary cases one will grant that the anesthesiologist has the right to act in this manner, but he is not bound to do so, unless this becomes the only way of fulfilling another certain moral duty.

The rights and duties of the doctor are correlative to those of the patient. The doctor, in fact, has no separate or independent right where the patient is concerned. In general he can take action only if the patient explicitly or implicitly, directly or indirectly, gives him permission. The technique of resuscitation which concerns us here does not contain anything immoral in itself. Therefore the patient, if he were capable of making a personal decision, could lawfully use it and, consequently, give the doctor permission to use it. On the other hand, since these forms of treatment go beyond the ordinary means to which one is bound, it cannot be held that there is an obligation to use them nor, consequently, that one is bound to give the doctor permission to use them.

The rights and duties of the family depend in general upon the presumed will of the unconscious patient if he is of age and *sui juris*. Where the proper and independent duty of the family is concerned, they are usually bound only to the use of ordinary means.

Consequently, if it appears that the attempt at resuscitation constitutes in 425 reality such a burden for the family that one cannot in all conscience impose it upon them, they can lawfully insist that the doctor should discontinue these attempts, and the doctor can lawfully comply. There is not involved here a case of direct disposal of the life of the patient, nor of euthanasia in any way: this would never be licit. Even when it causes the arrest of circulation, the interruption of attempts at resuscitation is never more than an indirect cause of the cessation of life, and one must apply in this case the principle of double effect and of *voluntarium in causa*.

DOCUMENT 3 / Withholding Life Support

Source: Congregation for the Doctrine of the Faith, "Declaration on Euthanasia" (May 5, 1980), *Vatican Council II*, Vol. 2, pp. 514–16.

DUE PROPORTION IN THE USE OF REMEDIES

Today it is very important to protect, at the moment of death, both the dignity of the human person and the Christian concept of life against a technological attitude that threatens to become an abuse. Thus, some people speak of a "right to die," which is an expression that does not mean the right to procure death either by one's own hand or by means of someone else, as one pleases, but rather the right to die peacefully with human and Christian dignity. From this point of view, the use of therapeutic means can sometimes pose problems.

In numerous cases, the complexity of the situation can be such as to cause doubts about the way ethical principles should be applied. In the final analysis, it pertains to the conscience either of the sick person, or of those qualified to speak in the sick person's name, or of the doctors, to decide in the light of moral obligations and of the various aspects of the case.

Everyone has the duty to care for his or her own health or to seek such care from others. Those whose task it is to care for the sick must do so conscientiously and administer the remedies that seem necessary or useful.

However, is it necessary in all circumstances to have recourse to all possible remedies?

In the past, moralists replied that one is never obliged to use "extraordinary" means. This reply, which as a principle still holds good, is perhaps less clear today, by reason of the imprecision of the term and the rapid progress made in the treatment of sickness. Thus some people prefer to speak of "proportionate" and "disproportionate" means. In any case, it will be possible to make a correct judgment as to the means by studying the type of treatment to be used, its degree of complexity or risk, its cost, and the possibilities of using it, and comparing these elements with the result that can be expected, taking into account the state of the sick person and his or her physical and moral resources.

In order to facilitate the application of these general principles, the following clarifications can be added:

—If there are no other sufficient remedies, it is permitted, with the patient's consent, to have recourse to the means provided by the most advanced medical techniques, even if these means are still at the experimental stage and are not without a certain risk. By accepting them, the patient can even show generosity in the service of humanity.

—It is also permitted, with the patient's consent, to interrupt these means, where the results fall short of expectations. But for such a decision to be made, account will have to be taken of the reasonable wishes of the patient and the patient's family, as also of the advice of the doctors who are specially competent in the matter. The latter may in particular judge that the investment in instruments and personnel is disproportionate to the results foreseen; they may also judge that the techniques applied impose on the patient strain or suffering out of proportion with the benefits which he or she may gain from such techniques.

—It is also permissible to make do with the normal means that medicine can offer. Therefore one cannot impose on anyone the obligation to have recourse to a technique which is already in use but which carries a risk or is burdensome. Such a refusal is not the equivalent of suicide; on the contrary, it should be considered as an acceptance of the human condition, or a wish to avoid the application of a medical procedure disproportionate to the results that can be expected, or a desire not to impose excessive expense on the family or the community.

—When inevitable death is imminent in spite of the means used, it is permitted in conscience to take the decision to refuse forms of treatment that would only secure a precarious and burdensome prolongation of life, so long as the normal care due to the sick person in similar cases is not interrupted. In such circumstances the doctor has no reason to reproach himself with failing to help the person in danger.

CONCLUSION

The norms contained in the present Declaration are inspired by a profound desire to serve people in accordance with the plan of the Creator. Life is a gift of God, and on the other hand death is unavoidable; it is necessary therefore that we, without in any way hastening the hour of death, should be able to accept it with full responsibility and dignity. It is true that death marks the end of our earthly existence, but at the same time it opens the door to immortal life. Therefore all must prepare themselves for this event in the light of human values, and Christians even more so in the light of faith.

As for those who work in the medical profession, they ought to neglect no means of making all their skill available to the sick and the dying; but they should also remember how much more necessary it is to provide them with the comfort of boundless kindness and heartfelt charity. Such service to people is also service to Christ the Lord, who said, "As you did it to one of the least of these my brethren, you did it to me" (Mt 25:40).

DOCUMENT 4 / Withholding Life Support

SOURCE: National Conference of Catholic Bishops Committee for Pro-Life Activities, "Guidelines for Legislation on Life-Sustaining Treatment" (Nov. 10, 1984), *Origins* 14: no. 32, Jan. 24, 1985, pp. 526–28.

MORAL PRINCIPLES

Our Judeo-Christian heritage celebrates life as the gift of a loving God and respects the life of each human being because each is made in the image and likeness of God. As Christians we also celebrate the fact that we are redeemed by Christ and called to share eternal life with him. From these roots the Roman Catholic tradition has developed a distinctive approach to fostering and sustaining human life. Our tradition not only condemns direct attacks on innocent life, but also promotes a general view of life as a sacred trust over which we can claim stewardship but not absolute dominion. As conscientious stewards, we see a duty to preserve life while recognizing certain limits to that duty, as was reiterated most recently in the Vatican Declaration on Euthanasia. This and other documents have set forth the following moral principles defining a "stewardship of life" ethic:

1. The Second Vatican Council condemned crimes against life, including "euthanasia or willful suicide" (*Gaudium et Spes*, 27). Grounded as it is in respect for the dignity and fundamental rights of the human person, this teaching cannot be rejected on grounds of political pluralism or religious freedom.

2. As human life is the basis and necessary condition for all other human goods, it has a special value and significance; both murder and suicide are violations of human life.

3. "Euthanasia" is "an action or an omission which of itself or by intention causes death, in order that all suffering may in this way be eliminated" (*Declaration on Euthanasia*). It is an attack on human life which no one has a right to make or request. Although individual guilt may be reduced or absent because of suffering or emotional factors which cloud the conscience, this does not change the objective wrong of the act. It should also be recognized that an apparent plea for death may really be a plea for help and love.

4. Suffering is a fact of human life and has special significance for the Christian as an opportunity to share in Christ's redemptive suffering. Nevertheless there is nothing wrong in trying to relieve someone's suffering as long as this does not interfere with other moral and religious duties. For example, it is permissible in the case of terminal illness to use painkillers which carry the risk of shortening life, so long as the intent is to relieve pain effectively rather than to cause death.

5. Everyone has the duty to care for his or her own health and to seek necessary medical care from others, but this does not mean that all possible remedies must be used in all circumstances. One is not obliged to use "extraordinary" means—that is, means which offer no reasonable hope of benefit or which involve excessive hardship. Such decisions are complex and should be made by the patient in consultation with his or her family and physician whenever possible.

Although these principles have grown out of a specific religious tradition, they appeal to a common respect for the dignity of the human person rather than to any specific denominational stance. We offer them without hesitation to the consideration of men and women of goodwill, and commend them to the attention of legislators and other policy makers. We see them as especially appropriate to a society which, whatever its moral and political pluralism, was founded on the belief that all human beings are created equal as bearers of the inalienable right to life.

LEGISLATIVE GUIDELINES

Today the application of these principles to the legislative debate regarding treatment of the terminally ill is both difficult and necessary. The medical treatment of terminally ill patients, including the withdrawal of extraordinary means, has always been subject to legal constraints. Since 1975, however, an increasing number of court decisions and legislative enactments have interpreted and changed these constraints. Some decisions and enactments have been constructive, but others have not. Technological changes in medicine occur so rapidly that it is difficult to keep pace with them. These changes have had a drastic effect on the physician-patient relationship and make much more difficult the decision process by which a patient determines treatment with the counsel and support of physician and family.

As problems and confusions surrounding the treatment of terminally ill patients continue to multiply, new legislation dealing with this subject is being enacted in some states and proposed in many others. Yet the law relating to the treatment of terminally ill patients still differs from state to state and does not always adequately reflect the moral principles which we endorse. The Church therefore feels an obligation to provide its guidance through participation in the current debate.

In light of these considerations, we suggest the following as ways of respecting the moral principles listed above as well as related concerns of the Church whenever there is a debate on whether existing or proposed legislation adequately addresses this subject. Such legislation should:

(a) Presuppose the fundamental right to life of every human being, including the disabled, the elderly, and the terminally ill. In general, phrases which seem to romanticize death, such as "right to die" or "death with dignity," should be avoided.

(b) Recognize that the right to refuse medical treatment is not an independent right, but is a corollary to the patient's right and moral responsibility to request reasonable treatment. The law should demonstrate no preference for protecting *only* the right to *refuse* treatment, particularly when *life-sustaining* treatment is under consideration.

(c) Place the patient's right to determine medical care within the context of other factors which limit the exercise of that right—e.g., the state's interest

430 in protecting innocent third parties, preventing homicide and suicide, and maintaining good ethical standards in the health care profession. Policy statements which define the right to refuse treatment in terms of the patient's constitutional rights (e.g., a "right of privacy") tend to inhibit the careful balancing of all the interests that should be considered in such cases.

(d) Promote communication among patient, family, and physician. Current "living will" laws tend to have the opposite effect—that of excluding family members and other loved ones from the decision-making process. As a general rule, documents and legal proceedings are no substitute for a physician's personal consultation with the patient and/or family at the time a decision must be made on a particular course of treatment.

(e) Avoid granting unlimited power to a document or proxy decision maker to make health care decisions on a patient's behalf. The right to make such decisions on one's own behalf is itself not absolute and in any event cannot be fully exercised when a patient has had no opportunity to assess the burdens and benefits of treatment in a specific situation. Laws which allow a decision to be made on behalf of a mentally incompetent patient must include safeguards to ensure that the decision adequately represents the patient's wishes or best interests and is in accord with responsible medical practice.

(f) Clarify the rights and responsibilities of physicians without granting blanket immunity from all legal liability. No physician should be protected from liability for acting homicidally or negligently. Nor should new legal penalties be imposed on a physician for failing to obey a patient's or proxy's wishes when such obedience would violate the physician's ethical convictions or professional standards.

(g) Reaffirm public policies against homicide and assisted suicide. Medical treatment legislation may clarify procedures for discontinuing treatment which only secures a precarious and burdensome prolongation of life for the terminally ill patient, but should not condone or authorize any deliberate act or omission designed to cause a patient's death.

(h) Recognize the presumption that certain basic measures such as nursing care, hydration, nourishment, and the like must be maintained out of respect for the human dignity of every patient.

(i) Protect the interests of innocent parties who are not competent to make treatment decisions on their own behalf. Life-sustaining treatment should not be discriminatorily withheld or withdrawn from mentally incompetent or retarded patients.

(j) Provide that life-sustaining treatment should not be withdrawn from a pregnant woman if continued treatment may benefit her unborn child.

These guidelines are not intended to provide an exhaustive description of good legislation or to endorse the viewpoint that every state requires new legislation on treatment of the terminally ill. They outline a general approach which, we believe, will help clarify rights and responsibilities with regard to such treatment without sacrificing a firm commitment to the sacredness of human life.

DOCUMENT 5 / Withholding Life Support

SOURCE: Pontifical Council Cor Unum, *Question of Ethics Regarding the Fatally Ill and the Dying,* Vatican Press, 1981, pp. 3–7; 21–22.

2. FUNDAMENTAL CONCEPTS

2.1 Life

2.1.1. *The Christian meaning of life.* Life is given to mankind by our Creator. It is a gift bestowed in order for man to accomplish a mission. Thus, a person's "right to live" is not what is of foremost importance, since this right is not man's but, rather, belongs to God, who does not give life to human beings as something of which they may dispose as they see fit. Life is directed towards an end towards which it is the responsibility of human beings to direct themselves; towards the perfecting of themselves according to God's plan.

The first corollary of this fundamental concept, is that to give up life of one's own choice is to give up striving towards an end which not we but God has established. Man has been called upon to make his life useful; he may not destroy it at will. His duty is to care for his body, its functions, its organs; to do everything he can to render himself capable of attaining to God. This duty implies giving up things which in themselves may be good. This duty sometimes requires that we sacrifice health and life; our concern for them cannot allow us to deny the claim of superior values. All the same, in the matter of cares to be taken for maintaining good health and preserving life, a correct proportion must be arrived at, regarding both the superior goods perhaps at stake and also the concrete conditions in which man lives out his existence on earth.

2.1.2. *We cannot freely dispose of the life of someone else.* If one may not destroy one's own life at will, this is also true, a fortiori, of someone else's life. A sick person cannot simply be made the object of decisions which he himself does not make—or of which, if he is unable to make them, he would not morally approve. Each human individual, as the person principally responsible for this life, must be at the center of all assistance. Others are present in order to help him, *not* substitute *for* him. This does not mean, however, that doctors or members of the family may not at times find themselves in the position of having to take decisions for a sick person, who for various reasons cannot do so himself, concerning therapeutic measures and treatments to be applied to him. But to the doctors and others in this position, more than to anyone else, it is absolutely forbidden to make an attempt on the life of the patient, even out of compassion and pity. . . .

2.2 Death

2.2.1. *The meaning which death has for Christians.* The death of a human being is the end of his corporeal existence. It brings to an end that phase of   **431**

432   his divine vocation which is his striving, within the compass of time, toward his total perfection. For a Christian, the moment of death is the moment of his finally being united forever to Christ. Today more than ever, it is pertinent to recall this religious and Christological conception of death. It must go hand in hand with a very real perception of the contingency of our living in our body and of the connection between death and our human condition of being sinners. "For . . . whether we live or whether we die, we are the Lord's" (Rom 14:8). Our attitude toward the dying must be inspired by this conviction, and must not merely be reduced to an effort made by science to put off death as long as possible. . . .

2.4 Therapeutic measures

2.4.1. *Ordinary measures and extraordinary measures.* The Working Group considered at some length the distinction between these two kinds of therapies. It is true that the terms are becoming somewhat outmoded in scientific terminology and medical practice, but in theology they are indispensable to the consideration of the validity or invalidity of points of great moral importance. For the theologian applies the term "extraordinary" to measures to which there never exists any obligation to have recourse.

The distinction permits us to draw certain complex realities more closely together. It acts as the "middle term." Life within the compass of time is a basic value but is not an absolute; and we find, consequently, that we must demarcate the limits of the obligation to keep oneself alive. The distinction between "ordinary" and "extraordinary" measures expresses this truth and applied these limits to concrete cases. The use of equivalent terms, particularly the words "care suited to the real needs," perhaps expresses the concept more satisfactorily.

2.4.2. *Criteria for distinguishing.* The criteria whereby we can distinguish *extraordinary* measures from *ordinary* measures are very many. Some of them are *objective*: such as the nature of the measures proposed, how expensive they are, whether it is just to use them, and what the options of justice are in the matter of using them. Other criteria are *subjective*: such as not giving certain patients psychological shocks, anxiety, uneasiness, and so on. It will always be a question, when deciding upon measures to be taken, of establishing to what extent the means to be used and the end being sought are proportionate.

2.4.3. *The criterion of the quality of life: its importance.* Among all the criteria for decision, particular importance must be given to the quality of the life to be saved or kept living by the therapy. The Letter of Cardinal Villot to the Congress of the International Federation of Catholic Medical Associations is very clear on this subject: "It must be emphasized that it is the sacred character of life which forbids a physician to kill and makes it a duty for him at the same time to use every resource of his art to fight against death. This does not, however, mean that a physician is under obligation to use all and every one of the life-maintaining techniques offered him by the indefatigable creativity of science. Would it not be a useless torture, in many cases, to impose vegetative reanimation during the last phase of an incurable disease?" (*Documentation* **433** *Catholique,* 1979, p. 963).

But the criterion of the quality of life is not the only one to be taken into account since, as we have said above, subjective considerations must enter into a properly cautious judgment as to what therapy to undertake and what therapy not. The fundamental point is that the decision should be made according to rational arguments that have taken well into account the many and various aspects of the situation, including what effect will be had upon the family. The principle to follow is, therefore, that no moral obligation to have recourse to extraordinary measures exists; and that, incidentally, a doctor must follow the wishes of a sick person who refuses such measures.

2.4.4. *Obligatory minimal measures.* On the contrary, there remains the strict obligation to apply under all circumstances those therapeutic measures which are called "minimal," that is, those which are normally and customarily used for the maintenance of life (alimentation, blood transfusions, injections, etc.). To interrupt these minimal measures would, in practice, be equivalent to wishing to put an end to the patient's life. . . .

7.2 The Choice of One Therapy or Another

As a general rule, and despite what the press leads people to believe, a doctor does not ask himself whether to allow or not allow a patient to die. He decides upon a certain medical treatment: what are its indications, what are its contraindications? These all require him to consider various factors. He does so in the light of moral principles as well as of scientific knowledge; this is how it becomes of great value to a doctor to consider them while he reflects: what must or must not be undertaken? when should extraordinary measures be recurred to and when not? and, if so, for what reasons and for how long? Too often, a doctor may come to question himself as to the advisability of continuing a certain treatment, and the question he may put to himself is: "Was it wise to have begun the treatment in the first place?" For, if there exist moral reasons for prolonging life, there also exist moral reasons for not opposing death with what is known as "therapeutic obstinacy."

7.3 Massive Therapy and Choosing the Persons to Receive It

Among the ethical questions brought up by "massive therapies" requiring very highly evolved and expensive equipment and techniques is to be considered the selection of patients to whom to apply a therapy that cannot be applied to everyone with the same malady. Is it legitimate to use the resources of refined medical techniques for the benefit of only one patient, while others are still not receiving the most elementary treatment? One has a right to ask. If certain persons believe that such a question is "going against progress," Christians, at least, should bear it in mind in their valuation.

Index